The Benevolent Heart of Practitioner:
Chinese Traditional Medical Ethics Culture

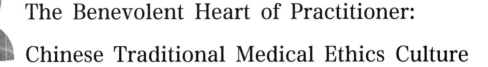

医者仁心
中国传统医德文化

黄　平　陈毅君 ◎ 顾问

付明明　李禄峰 ◎ 编著

西南交通大学出版社
·成都·

图书在版编目（CIP）数据

医者仁心：中国传统医德文化 = The Benevolent
Heart of Practitioner: Chinese Traditional Medical
Ethics Culture：英文 / 付明明，李禄峰编著. --成
都：西南交通大学出版社，2023.11
　ISBN 978-7-5643-9622-0

　Ⅰ. ①医… Ⅱ. ①付… ②李… Ⅲ. ①医务道德 – 文
化史 – 中国 – 古代 – 英文 Ⅳ. ①R192-092

中国国家版本馆 CIP 数据核字（2023）第 227029 号

The Benevolent Heart of Practitioner:
Chinese Traditional Medical Ethics Culture

Yizhe Renxin：Zhongguo Chuantong Yide Wenhua
医者仁心：中国传统医德文化

付明明　李禄峰　编著

责任编辑	孟　媛
封面设计	GT 工作室

出版发行　西南交通大学出版社
　　　　　（四川省成都市金牛区二环路北一段 111 号
　　　　　西南交通大学创新大厦 21 楼）
邮政编码　610031
营销部电话　028-87600564　　　028-87600533
网址　　　http://www.xnjdcbs.com
印刷　　　成都市新都华兴印务有限公司

成品尺寸	170 mm × 230 mm
印张	19.5
字数	457 千
版次	2023 年 11 月第 1 版
印次	2023 年 11 月第 1 次
书号	ISBN 978-7-5643-9622-0
定价	68.00 元

PREFACE

China, with a rich history spanning over 5,000 years, is the only country that has preserved its ancient civilization's legacy without cultural interruption among the four ancient civilizations. This glorious history has given us great cultural confidence, which represents the full recognition of a nation, a country and a political party of its own cultural value. Cultural confidence is the deepest spiritual pursuit and the unique spiritual symbol of the Chinese nation. The ethics of traditional Chinese medicine (TCM) practice is a typical aspect of China's excellent traditional culture, and embodies the Chinese people's expectation and value recognition of TCM practitioners for thousands of years. Over the TCM history, household names include Qibo, Hua Tuo, Bianque, Zhang Zhongjing, Sun Simiao, Song Ci, Qian Yi, Liu Wansu, Li Shizhen, Chen Shigong, and Xu Dachun, who exhibited not only noble medical ethics, but also exquisite medical skills. Their stories featuring medical ethics have become timeless anecdotes, passed down from generation to generation. They also set a model for us to cultivate medical ethics for medical students today.

In 2018, the Ministry of Education issued the *Opinions on Strengthening the Collaborative Implementation of Excellent Doctor Education and Training Program 2.0*, which clearly points out that moral education should be the priority of medical talent training. In 2020, the Ministry of Education issued the *Outline for the Ideological and Political Development of Curriculum in Institutions of Higher Learning*, which further emphasizes the leading roles of medical ethics education, the spirit of "respecting and protecting life, caring for the wounded and dying, and being dedicated to the medical and healthcare services" and the education of a doctor's benevolence in the training of medical students. This is a testament to our original purpose to write this textbook: to enhance medical ethics of current medical students with the strong appeal from the TCM ethics culture.

This book divides the TCM ethics culture into chapters according to historical periods, such as Pre-Qin, Qin and Han, Wei, Jin, Southern and Northern dynasties, Sui and Tang dynasties, Song dynasty, Jin and Yuan dynasties, Ming and Qing dynasties. Each chapter summarizes and discusses TCM ethics culture in different periods, medical ethics thoughts of famous TCM practitioners, and comments on their practice and medical ethics. In addition, as a reference material for modern medical education, each chapter also outlines medical education in the corresponding period. This book, featuring a clear structure, concise and easy-to-understand language, can serve as a reference book for medical students and workers as well as enthusiasts of traditional Chinese culture, to improve their knowledge about medical history and their level of medical ethics.

We would like to express our gratitude to the colleagues who have offered valuable suggestions and generous assistance during the compilation of this book. It is inevitable that this book might have certain deficiencies due to the limitations of our expertise. We warmly welcome constructive criticism and feedback from our readers to help us improve the quality of our work.

June, 2023

CONTENTS

1

Medical Ethics Culture
in the Pre-Qin Period

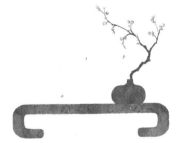

1.1 Overview of Medical Ethics

1.1.1 Social Background of Medical Ethics

1. Economic background

Nearly two million years ago, human beings have lived in ancient China, marking the beginning of the Chinese history. After more than one million years of evolution, human beings entered the stage of early Homo Sapiens 200,000 to 300,000 years ago. About 50,000 years ago, the early Homo Sapiens evolved into the late Homo Sapiens, who have acquired richer labor experience and skills. In the Xia, Shang and Zhou dynasties, our ancestors established the country with agriculture. After the emergence of Jingtian System (ancient farmland subdivision system), a lot of barren land was cultivated into fertile fields, and fallow and rotation in agriculture appeared. Grain yield increased, followed by the development of wine brewing, silkworm and mulberry breeding and animal husbandry. The famous Houmuwu Dafangding (Chinese ritual bronze) was cast in this period. During this period, there were pottery, bone ware, jade ware and other labor tools and ritual vessels. As Baigong (craftsmen) appeared, the development of handicraft industry also promoted the development of commerce and the emergence of currency.

2. Political background

As the primitive society disintegrated, the tribes gradually became united, and the Fang Guo (ancient united city-state system) appeared. By the time Qi inherited the throne from his father, Yu, the hereditary system of royal power was basically settled. The Xia dynasty was the first slave-owner's state in the history of China, marking the birth of state in the early stage. In the Shang dynasty, the military and criminal legal systems developed significantly. On the basis of the patriarchal system, the Zhou dynasty implemented the enfeoffment system and granted the title of feudal princes to maintain social stability and consolidate the hierarchical system of the patriarchal society.

3. Cultural background

According to *The Analects of Confucius: Wei Zheng*, "The House of Yin adopted the civilization of the Xia dynasty; what modifications they made are known. The present Zhou dynasty adopted the civilization of the House of Yin; what modifications this last dynasty made are also known." The etiquette system in the Xia dynasty set an example for later generations. In the Pre-Qin period, the astronomical calendar was well developed, and the earliest observation records of stars such as Nova, Mars, Jupiter and Daxing (the sun) in the world, confirming the "twenty-eight lunar mansions" as the star observation marks. There were mature inscriptions on bones, tortoise shells or bronze objects, which promoted the communication of people's ideas; the concept of five elements (water, fire, wood, gold and earth) represents the early simple materialist thought in China; in addition, there are also the Zhou Yi (The Book of Changes) and The Shi King (The Book of Songs) that are still praised by the world today.

Medical science was developed by human beings in their struggle against nature. In ancient times, with the development of economy, politics and culture, witchcraft gradually emerged. In the late Shang dynasty, some witches became healers with certain medical knowledge. Around the late Western Zhou dynasty, medical practice further differentiated, and the role of "medical practitioner" came into being. The destruction of rite system in the Spring and Autumn Period and the Warring States Period and the contention of a hundred schools of thought accelerated the liberation of people's "law of nature" thought. Confucianism, which stood out among hundred schools of thought, has always regarded the attention to the real society and people as the theoretical basis and the goal of endeavor, resulting in the emergence of simple medical ethics that values personnel and promotes humanity. In addition, Mohism, Taoism and Legalism also played their roles in promoting the development of medical ethics.

1.1.2　Main Contents of Medical Ethics Culture

1. Pray for the heaven to bless the people

During this period, due to low productivity and extremely limited medical technology, when someone had incurable diseases, our ancestors associated health and survival with ghosts and heavenly will. In this period, the boundary between witchcraft and medical skills was vague. People communicated with heaven, earth and ghosts through prayer, sacrificial ceremony, curse and other rite styles to express their awe to gods and pray for blessing. At the same time, the ritual of communicating with gods brought psychological hints and comfort to patients and stimulated their courage and perseverance to overcome diseases. This mythical approach fully demonstrated the piety of witch healers to gods and their care about the well-being of people, but it also reflected the lack of effective medical skills.

2. Treat diseases and save lives with full use of medical technologies

At that time, witch healers could take the life and health of patients as the starting point, master some simple medical knowledge and skills through years of experience in production and life, and apply them to the treatment of patients. The new means were more effective than witchcraft in the past. The patient recovered faster and better, and the recovery of the patient's health stimulated more witch healers to improve their skills and gradually develop beyond witchcraft. At the same time, the use of medicines and medical technologies had also made patients aware of the backwardness of witchcraft, which had led to the gradual shift of witchcraft to medical skills that could really cure diseases. With the joint attention of both healers and patients, medical skills were further promoted.

3. Attaching importance to the improvement of medical skills

With the recognition of medical skills and the improvement of productivity, more and more patients had turned to medical skills. They expressed their respect for medicine, and medical skills were promoted. The progress was a result of countless medical practitioners' studying efforts, and sometimes they even risked their lives. For example, the well-known story of "Shennong tasted hundreds of herbs" reflected the fact that the ancient TCM practitioners tasted herbs at the expense of their own health and even lives to understand the effect of herbs, which requires them to overcome timidity with the firm belief in treating diseases and saving people, and even put the threats of death aside. It is this spirit of keeping patients in mind and taking patient health as its own responsibility that promotes the improvement of medical technology.

1.1.3 Characteristics of Medical Ethics Culture

1. Affected significantly by the view of ghosts and gods

Due to the backward productivity, the treating of patients by wizards, witch healers and medical practitioners in early days were obviously affected by ghost theory. Therefore, they often used witchcraft and medical skills in the name of ghosts and gods to treat patients. This also fully demonstrated the awe and worship of ghosts and gods in this period.

2. The human-centered thought gradually appeared

With the improvement of productivity and medical skills, people were increasingly seeing the advantages of medical skills over witchcraft, realizing that mankind can compete with ghosts and gods and even heavenly will. At the same time, medical practitioners' sense of responsibility towards patients and proficiency in medical skills also enhanced the effect of treatment. The patients gradually realized that people's illness is not closely related to the will of ghosts and gods, and people increasingly felt that they were not restricted by ghosts and gods, that is, the human-centered thought was strengthened.

3. Mutual respect and trust between medical practitioners and patients

In the process of treating patients, medical practitioners and patients respect and trust each other, and the treatment plan, treatment attitude and personal conduct of medical practitioners are recognized by patients. At the same time, patients' expectation, respect and trust in medical practitioners also promote the development of treatment, and TCM practitioners and patients can reach a consensus on jointly curing diseases, which is not only beneficial to the treatment, but also beneficial to the recovery of patients.

1.2 Representative Medical Practitioners and Their Medical Ethics

This period was the origin period of TCM ethics culture, during which many famous stories about medical ethics passed down to this day were born. The stories demonstrated good examples of medical ethics and facilitated the inheritance of medical ethics culture in later generations.

1. Fuxi

Fuxi, also known as Mixi, was an ancient mythological figure. According to the records in *Taiping Yulan* (*Imperial Readings of the Taiping Era*), Fuxi was born in today's Tianshui, Gansu Province, and archaeological excavations show that the Dadiwan site is located in Tianshui, so Fuxi should be the leader of his primitive tribes in Dadiwan area. *Diwang Shiji* (*Emperor's Time in China*) called Fuxi one of the "Sanhuang (three primordial sovereigns)", and the other two are Xuanyuan and Shennong. *Diwang Shiji* also records that "Fuxi draws the eight trigrams to know the virtues of the heaven to compare with things in the nature. So, six qi, six fu-organs, five zang-organs, five elements, Yin and Yang, four seasons, ascending and descending of water and fire, can have manifestations; The reason of all kinds of diseases can be classified. So, he tastes hundreds of medicines and makes nine classical needles to save the people." *Lushi: Houji* (an unofficial history of China written by Luo Mi) records, "Fuxi tasted herbs and made it to cure diseases." According to these records, Fuxi made nine classical needles to treat diseases for the people. Although this is still different from the acupuncture mentioned in our later generations, it can be said that Fuxi is the originator of acupuncture. The origin, efficacy and application of Fuxi's stone needle acupuncture are also summarized and affirmed in *Huangdi Neijing: Suwen* (*Yellow Emperor's Canon of Medicine: Plain Conversation*) and *Shan Hai Jing: Dong Shan Jing* (*Classic of Eastern Mountains and Rivers*). According to legend, Fuxi had also invented new means of production and explored new ways of life, which has freed mankind from the ignorance of the prehistoric era and laid the foundation for the prosperity and development of Chinese civilization. He also devoted himself to studying the eight trigrams, demonstrating the changes between heaven and earth and creating a philosophical system of life with the laws and regulations of Yin-Yang fish, and named it "the regulation of the eight trigrams".

The legend of Fuxi drawing the eight trigrams reflects that TCM practitioners in the early stage put forward specific treatment plans for the treatment of patients after comprehensively mastering and analyzing the occurrence, development, cure process and laws of diseases, which is the specific manifestation of studying professional skills and the embodiment of being responsible for patients. However, he tasted all kinds of herbs regardless of personal safety, recorded the efficacy of various herbs in detail, and explored the treatment and efficacy of stone needle acupuncture with himself as the test object, which showed the high professional dedication of TCM practitioners and the professional ethics of being fully responsible for patients, and laid a medical practice standard thought of revering life and being responsible for patients for later generations of medical practitioners.

2. Shennong

According to legend, Shennong was the leader of the tribal alliance of primitive society in China, the god of agriculture and the ancestor of medicine of the Chinese nation, and later generations respected him as one of the "Sanhuang (three primordial sovereigns)". The legend of "Shennong tasting hundreds of herbs" has been spread for thousands of years, which was first seen in *Huai Nan Zi: Necessity of Training* (a guide to the theory and practice of government in early Han China): "In immemorial times, ordinary people ate wild grass, drank raw water, plucked fruit from wild trees and ate clams' flesh. At that time, people often suffered from diseases and harm from poisonous things, therefore, Shennong taught them how to grow crops... Shennong tasted all kinds of plants himself as well as the water of various rivers and springs by himself in order to inform people know what they should choose and what they should avoid. At that time, Shennong suffered from toxicosis seventy times in a day." Later, it was found in the *Shiji: Sanhuang Benji* (*Records of the Historian: History of the Three Primordial Sovereigns*) that "Shennong tasted hundreds of herbs and was the originator of Chinese herbal medicine". Later generations praised him as the "ancestor of medicine". In order to save lives and prolong the longevity of the people, Shennong made an arduous journey. He traveled all over the land of Xiang (today's Hunan) and tasted herbs to know their effects such as calm, toxicity, cold and warm, and found medicine to diseases and antidotes to poisons. In the process of tasting herbs, he identified the types of herbs and found medicine that can cure diseases and maintain people's health. The legend of Shennong tasting herbs is a reflection of pragmatic medical practice, which has experienced a long period in the Chinese history. With the passage of time, the knowledge of medicine accumulated by our ancestors became more and more abundant and was continuously verified, and finally was gradually recorded in a book, *Shennong's Herbal Classic*. *Shennong's Herbal*

Classic has become the first classic work of Chinese herbal medicine in ancient China, and the medical works about herbs in later generations gradually developed and enriched base on it, so it has a positive effect on the development of TCM.

In the process of collecting and identifying herbs, Shennong ignored personal safety, trekked through mountains, rivers, and jungles. In order to comprehensively and carefully understand the growing environment, picking place, and efficacy of different herbs, he tasted all kinds of herbs around, which is the embodiment of being responsible for the herb picking and use of medicine.

3. Huangdi

According to legend, Yellow Emperor was the son of Shaodian. His original surname was Gongsun and he lived in Ji Shui for a long time, so his surname was changed to Ji. He was called Yellow Emperor because of the merits and virtues of earth (earth is one of five elements and corresponds to yellow). Yellow Emperor was recorded in the history books for unifying the Chinese nation, and became the ancestor of Chinese civilization because of spreading crops, grass and trees, vigorously developing production, creating characters, starting to make clothes, building boats, determining numbers, making rhythms, and creating medicine. The famous *Huangdi Neijing* (*Yellow Emperor's Canon of Medicine*) was named after Yellow Emperor. According to the *Gujin Yishi* (*History of Ancient and Modern Medicine*), "Heaven and earth are boundless. Yellow Emperor observes the five qi, knows the Wuyun (five-motions), and understands the laws of life and follows the number of Yin and Yang. Then he consults Qibo and writes the *Neijing* (*Canon of Medicine*), and invites Yufu, Qibo, Leigong to the Mingtang (Brightness Palace) for studying the breath and pulse of people. Wupeng and Tongjun are required to make prescriptions. For these reasons, people can live to their full age". It can be inferred that if the medical knowledge in the era of Shennong is still relatively primitive, then the medical knowledge in the Yellow Emperor era should be closer to rational knowledge.

Yellow Emperor's Canon of Medicine is a comprehensive medical book, which is divided into two parts: Lingshu (Spiritual Pivot) and Suwen (Plain Conversation). It is the earliest medical classic in China and one of the four classic works of traditional medicine, and the other three are *Nan Jing* (*Classic of Difficult Issues*), *Shanghan Zabing Lun* (*Treatise on Cold Pathogenic and Miscellaneous Diseases*) and *Shennong*

Bencao Jing (*Shennong's Herbal Classic*). *Shu Wu Guo Lun* (*Discussion on the Five Frequently Made Diagnostic Errors*) and *Zheng Si Shi Lun* (*Discourse on Evidence of the Four Failures*) are special articles on medical ethics. On the basis of the Huang-Lao school (the Yellow Emperor-Lao Zi school), the book established "theories of Yin-Yang and the five elements", "theory of pulse manifestation", "theory of the meridian and collateral", "theory of causes of disease", "theory of mechanism of disease", "diseases and symptoms", "diagnostic method" and "theory of health maintenance" and "theory of five phases and six climatic factors" in TCM practice. Its basic materials come from the long-term observation of life phenomena by ancient Chinese, a large number of clinical practices and simple anatomical knowledge. This book has laid the foundation for understanding human physiology, pathology, diagnosis and treatment, and is a medical masterpiece with great influence.

Yellow Emperor clearly pointed out the morality and knowledge that medical practitioners must have in treating and saving patients. He stressed that medical practitioners should be serious and responsible, cautious in words and actions, make no mistakes in the treatment of patients, and have specialized and sophisticated skills, extensive knowledge of astronomy, geography, humanity, etc. In terms of teaching, he also clearly pointed out that people who do not meet the standards of being a medical practitioner should not be admitted to study medicine. In addition, what is not the true meaning of medicine should not be taught to students. Yellow Emperor has clear requirements for the morality and quality of TCM practitioners and students that would be practitioners some day, which fully reflects Yellow Emperor's respect for medicine and life, and sets a model for later generations of medical practitioners and educators to practice and teach medicine.

4. Qibo

Qibo was the most prestigious "ancestor of Chinese traditional medicine" and "medical sage" in ancient China. He was born in Qishan (now Qishan County, Shaanxi Province), who was versatile and intelligent. After seeing many people died of diseases, he determined to study medicine, traveled around to look for good teachers to study. Later, he gradually became proficient in medical skills and a famous TCM practitioner. According to legend, Qibo, as an official served for Yellow Emperor, tasted various herbs at the order of Yellow Emperor, and also discussed meridians with Leigong (a mythological medical practitioner). *Yellow Emperor's Canon of Medicine* was written by Yellow Emperor and Qibo based on their discussions about medical theories, which is the cornerstone of "Qi Huang" or "Medical skills of Qi & Huang" in TCM practice.

Qibo could not bear to see people suffering from disease. Therefore, he was determined to study medicine and succeed in his studies. This is a vivid portrayal of the common people's sympathy and love for people, and is the original aspiration and motivation of Qibo to practice medicine. Qibo expressed his love for people with his actions, setting an example for the motivation, purpose and significance of studying medicine for later generations.

5. Yufu

Yufu was an ancient medical practitioner and was said to be one of the three famous TCM practitioners in the period of Yellow Emperor (the other two are Leigong and Qibo). He was good at surgery. In his medical practice, he not only gave the right prescription for an illness, but also knew how to use the surgical therapy of skin resection and muscle decomposition, cleansing the five zang-organs, which was named as the "surgical pioneer" by later generations. Three literary historians in the Western Han dynasty, Han Ying, Sima Qian, and Liu Xiang, all recorded Qin Yueren's (Bianque) discussions about Yufu's deeds, which showed his influence in the medical field in the ancient times.

Yufu pioneered surgical therapy, expanded medical treatment methods, and improved the efficacy, which was a manifestation of deep sympathy for the patient's suffering. Yufu could do skin resection and muscle decomposition, cleansing the five zang-organs, because he can accurately locate the internal structure of the human body below the epidermis and fully understand the lesions. The deeds of Yufu reflected that, if surgery is carried out, it is not only to see the surface of the body, but also to have an insight into the inside of the body through the surface, which puts forward higher requirements for the medical knowledge of surgeons, as well as the medical literacy and medical ability of surgeons.

6. Bianque

Bianque was a famous medical practitioner in the Spring and Autumn Period and the Warring States Period. His surname was Ji, clan name, Qin, and given name, Yueren. He was also known as Lu Yi (a medical practitioner from Lu), and Bianque was his nickname. The origin of this nickname may be related to the saying of "spiritual magpie indicates happiness" in the *Qin Jing* (*Book of Birds*). Medical practitioners treat and save patients. Wherever they go, they bring good news and health, just like flying magpies. Therefore, ancient people used to call those skilled TCM practitioners "Bianque". Bianque traveled around and relieved people of the pain of disease with his best efforts, so he had earned people's respect. Bianque studied hard and summarized the experience of his predecessors, and made bold innovations to become a knowledgeable and skilled TCM practitioner. Combined with its own medical practice, he made outstanding contributions to TCM on the aspects of diagnosis, pathology and treatment. Bianque's medical experience plays an important role in the medical history of China and has a great impact on the medical development of China. Therefore, the medical community has always regarded Bianque as the ancestor of ancient Chinese medicine, calling him "the medical sage of China" and "the founder of ancient medicine". Sima Qian praised Bianque by calling him the ancestor of TCM practitioners. His medical skill was exquisite and brilliant. The later generations should follow the law and not change it. "Historian Fan Wenlan called him the first person to summarize experience" in the *Zhongguo Tongshi Jianbian* (*Compendium of General History of China*). For thousands of years, Bianque has been deeply loved and respected by people. Tombs, stone tablets, and temples were built to commemorate him generation after generation.

The most widely known story of Bianque is Bianque Jian Duke Huan of Qi (Bianque's Meetings with Duke Huan of Qi). When Bianque passed by Linzi, the capital of the State of Qi, he saw Duke Huan of Qi, the monarch of the State of Qi. Seeing that Duke Huan of Qi looked ill, he concluded that he was ill, so he bluntly said to him, "You have a disease on the skin, which will be aggravated if you don't treat it as soon as possible." Duke Huan of Qi didn't take it seriously and said, "I'm not sick." Bianque left seeing his advice was not taken. At this time, Duke Huan of Qi said to the people around him, "All medical practitioners long for fame and benefit. They have no real skills but treat healthy people as if they are sick to show their skills and get the fame and benefit." Five days later, Bianque came to see Duke Huan of Qi again. After observation, he said to Duke Huan of Qi, "Your disease is in your blood and vessels now and it will be aggravated if you are not cured." Duke Huan of Qi was very unhappy after hearing this and did not take Bianque's words seriously. Another five days later, Bianque came to see Duke Huan of Qi again. After careful observation, he seriously said to him, "Your disease has entered the middle of your stomach and intestines. If you don't treat it, it will be incurable!" Duke Huan of Qi was very angry, and he ignored Bianque's advice again. When Bianque came to see Huanhou for the fourth time, he glanced at him and hurried away. Seeing that Bianque ignored himself, Duke Huan of Qi sent someone to ask. Bianque said, "The disease on the surface can be cured by cleansing with warm medicinal decoction; the disease in the blood and vessels and can be cured by acupuncture; the disease reaches the intestines and stomach can be cured by medicinal liquor. Now that Duke Huan of Qi's disease has gone deep into the bone marrow and there is no cure, I had to avoid it." Five days later, Duke Huan of Qi was seriously ill and sent someone to invite Bianque to treat him. Bianque had already escaped from the State of Qi, and Duke Huan of Qi died soon because he missed the opportunity for curing. Bianque could observe the development of disease from the complexion of Duke Huan of Qi, which was remarkable. Therefore, Zhang Zhongjing, a famous medical practitioner in the Han dynasty, praised Bianque by saying, "Each time I read about Yueren entering the Kingdom of Guo to examine patients and inspect the complexion of Duke Huan of Qi, I am always awed by his superb talents."

Bianque broke through the restriction of medical schools, and not limited to one style. He earnestly summarized predecessors' practice, folk experience and personal accumulation, and spent his lifetime summarizing the experience and lessons that were useful to patients and promote medical progress. This is a high degree of responsibility for medical undertakings and a true portrayal of high professional dedication, enriching the ways for later generations of medical practitioners to inherit and develop medicine. It also sets an example of patient-centered, disease-centered and comprehensive treatment with multiple treatment experiences.

7. Wen Zhi

Wen Zhi, a good official in the State of Song during the Warring States Period, was proficient in medical science and skills. Wen Zhi's treatment technique was very excellent. He properly treated the disease according to the patient's condition. Sometimes, he did not even use medicines or acupuncture, but used the principle of "the generation and restriction of Yin-Yang and five elements" to treat the disease by changing patients' emotions.

The treatment of patients not only started from the clinical manifestation of the disease, but also further explored the causes of the disease and the surrounding influencing factors from the source of the lesion, which broke through bio-medicine and applied the treatment methods of social medicine. Wen Zhi's innovation has provided practical exploration for later generations of medical treatment methods and promoted the development of medical treatment methods in multiple fields and channels.

1.3 Evaluation of Medical Practitioners and Their Medical Ethics

1.3.1 Official Evaluation of Medical Ethics Represented by the *Zhouli* (*Rites of Zhou*)

According to the *Zhouli-Tianguan: Yishi* (*Rites of Zhou—The Ministry of Official Personnel Affairs in Feudal China: Medical Practitioners*), "Medical practitioners are in charge of the order to gather medicines for medical treatment. Those with diseases and scars should be treated by the medical practitioners. At the end of the year, evaluate the treatment effect of medical practitioners and determine their grades. All diseases that can be diagnosed accurately are of the first class, one tenth of which cannot be diagnosed accurately are of the second class, two tenths are of the second class, three tenths are of the second class, and four tenths are of the second class." This is the earliest record of medical practitioner assessment. At the end of each year, medical practitioners are assessed according to the quantity and quality of treatment, and the assessment results are used as the basis for determining their salaries. From the perspective of assessment quality, it has high standards for physicians, reflecting the consideration of putting patients' safety in the first place, that is, including the assessment of physicians' medical ethics.

1.3.2 Evaluation of Medical Ethics in *Yellow Emperor's Canon of Medicine*

Yellow Emperor's Canon of Medicine has a special article on medical ethics in Suwen (Plain Conversation), which marked the initial formation of TCM ethics theory, and also indicated the importance of medical ethics in the society at that time, and it was an important content concerned by medical practitioners and patients.

1. Emphasize the vitality and priority of people's lives

Suwen: Baoming Quanxing Lun (*Plain Conversation: Discussion on Preserving Health and Protecting Life*) points out, "The covering of the heavens (in the upper) and the support of the earth (in the lower) have paved the way for the creation of all things (in nature), among which the noblest one is the man who exists." This emphasizes that man is the most precious of all things. Medical practitioners must realize the importance of human life and treat patients wholeheartedly. *Lingshu: Yuban* (*Spiritual Pivot: Jade Plate*) emphasizes that between the heaven and the earth, the most precious one is the man. And it emphasizes that man is the master of heaven and earth and highlights the important position of human life.

2. Emphasize a sense of responsibility towards patients

In *Suwen: Zhengsishi Lun* (*Plain Conversation: Discussion on the Four Therapeutic Errors*), it is said, "The reason that TCM practitioners cannot achieve perfect result in treating diseases lies in the fact that they cannot concentrate their mind, make logical analysis and take both the external manifestations and the internal disorders into consideration. That is why they are frequently confused and fail in treating diseases." If the medical practitioner is not focused, and cannot comprehensively analyze the patient's pulse and internal condition, there will be diagnostic errors, delays in treatment and even life-threatening situations. According to *Suwen: Shuwuguo Lun* (*Plain Conversation: Discussion on Five Errors Frequently Made in Diagnosis*), "Careless diagnosis of diseases is called violation of normal practice. If one can strictly follow these rules, his treatment of diseases will certainly conform to the principles suggested in the canons, he will be able to thoroughly understand the ideas expressed in the canons entitled Shangjing (Upper Canon) and Xiajing (Lower Canon)." If the medical practitioner fails to review carefully, it means that the patient is not diagnosed and treated according to the common practice of medicine. If the patient can be diagnosed and treated according to the diagnosis and treatment method, the medical practitioner will naturally know the patient's condition and take treatment according to the symptoms.

3. Propose standards for medical ethics

According to *Lingshu: Xieqi Zangfu Bingxing* (*Spiritual Pivot: Symptoms of*

Zangfu—Organs due to Attack of Pathogenic Factors), "Those who understand a disease by observing the complexion is known as excellent practitioners, those who understand a disease by taking pulse is known as magic practitioners and those who understand the location of a disease by inquiring the patient is known as ordinary practitioners.", "Those who can make a synthetic analysis of the complexion, pulse and skin over the cubit region are excellent practitioners. Excellent practitioners can cure nine patients out of ten. Those who can make good use of two of the three methods mentioned above are ordinary practitioners who cure seven patients out of ten. Those who can just make use of one of the three methods mentioned above are poor practitioners who can just cure six patients out of ten." This means that the person who knows the condition by observing the change of the patient's look is called an excellent practitioner, the person who knows the condition by taking pulse is called a magic practitioner, and the person who knows the part of the disease by asking the patient is called an ordinary practitioner. Those who are good at diagnosing the skin over the cubit region can know the condition without waiting to observe the pulse condition of the mouth; those who are good at diagnosing the pulse condition can know the condition without waiting to observe the five colors in TCM theory. If one makes a synthetic analysis of the complexion, pulse and skin over the cubit region, one can make the diagnosis more correct, which is excellent, and the cure rate can reach 9/10. If two diagnostic methods can be used, it is ordinary, and the cure rate can reach 7/10. If only one diagnostic method can be used, it is bad and the cure rate can reach 6/10.

4. Put forward requirements for the knowledge categories that TCM practitioners need to master

According to *Suwen: Zhuzhijiao Lun* (*Plain Conversation: Discussion on the Abstruse and Profound Theory of Medicine*), "As far as medicine is concerned, only when the practitioner has explored the knowledge of astronomy, geography and mankind, can the practitioner teach people medical knowledge without any doubt. In fact, only such medical theory can be handed down to the latter generations and taken as treasure." This emphasizes that medical practitioners should have extensive and rich knowledge, and understand the code of conduct in the world, so that they can become good medical practitioners, not only cure diseases, but also teach the general public, and his accumulated treatment experience and personal morality can be passed down.

1.3.3 Evaluation of Medical Ethics in *The Classic of Difficult Issues*

1. Put forward corresponding requirements for the medical skills and ethics of TCM practitioners

According to *Nan Jing: Shi'er Nan* (*The Classic of Difficult Issues: The Twelfth Difficult Issue*), "To fill the Yin (depots) when the Yang (depots) are cut off, or to fill the Yang (depots) when the Yin (depots) are cut off, means to replenish what is replete already, and to deplete what is depleted already, to diminish what is not enough, and to add where a surplus exists already. If anybody dies due to such therapies, the physician has killed the respective patient". The heart and lung qi belonging to Yang is deprived of, to tonify the kidney and liver belonging to Yin; the kidney and liver qi belonging to Yin is deprived of, to tonify the heart and lung belonging to Yang. This is to use Yang to replenish deficiency and use deficiency to replenish Yang, which is a fundamental mistake in treatment. Such death is caused by the mistake of medical practitioners.

2. Put forward corresponding requirements for medical practitioners to master medical skills systematically and holistically

According to *The Classic of Difficult Issues: The Seventy-Seventh Difficult Issue*: the superior practitioner treats what is not yet ill; the mediocre practitioner treats what is ill already.

When one sees an illness in the liver, one should know that the liver will transmit it to the spleen. Hence one prevents this transmission by filling the influences of the spleen, with the effect that it will not accept the evil influences from the liver. When a mediocre practitioner sees an illness in the liver, he does not know about mutual transmission, and he will focus all his efforts on treating the liver. According to *Yellow Emperor's Canon of Medicine*, a good TCM practitioner can stop the transform of disease and control the course of disease in advance. The aforementioned treating of what is not yet ill is to stop the deterioration of disease and control the disease in advance. For example, if the liver is diagnosed with disease, it may harm the spleen in the future. Therefore, it is necessary to tonify the function of the spleen first, and strengthen the spleen qi, and protect it from the evil qi of the liver, which is called preventive treatment. Ordinary TCM practitioners can also diagnose liver diseases, but they may not know the mutual transmission between diseases and only focus on treating the liver. This is a treatment for the disease that has already occurred.

1.3.4 Folk Evaluation of Medical Practitioners Represented by People's Evaluation of Bianque

Bianque was an outstanding representative of folk medical practitioner in this period. He was proficient in inspection, listening and smelling examination, inquiry and palpation, especially famous for inspection and palpation. Because of his medical skills, patients can often "return to life", and he was praised as "miracle-working practitioner" by the people, while Bianque said humbly: "I can't bring the dead back to life. This is all because he should live. All I can do is to help him recover." It can be seen that Bianque has excellent medical skills and is modest and simple.

Another reason why Bianque was welcomed by people was that he had comprehensive medical skills and could treat patients according to different diseases. *According to Shiji: Bianque Cang Gong Liezhuan (Records of the Historian: Biography of Bianque and Cang Gong)*, "When Bianque goes to Handan, he hears that people in Handan respect women, so he becomes a gynecologist; When in Luoyang, he hears that people in the Luoyang respect and love the elderly, so he becomes a TCM practitioner for the treatment of ear diseases, eye diseases and polio; When in Xianyang, he hear that people in the State of Qin loved children, so he becomes a pediatrician." Bianque can rescue local patients according to their needs. In addition, Bianque can also establish a very harmonious and mutually trustful treatment relationship with patients. It can be seen that the ways and means of diagnosis and treatment, personal morality and conduct, and the way of getting along with the people of Bianque are very worth learning from today.

1.3.5 Evaluation of Medical Ethics in *The Analects of Confucius*

In *The Analects of Confucius*, Confucius remarked, "The southern people have a saying, 'A man without perseverance cannot be a medical practitioner or a witch healer.'" Regardless of witchcraft, as for TCM practitioners, it is a recognition of the perseverance, and diligence required for TCM practitioners to learn medical skills, and also a praise for the quality of TCM practitioners.

1.4　Medical Education

From the perspective of medical education development, this period became the initial development period of TCM. Although medical education, management and assessment are not institutionalized, they play a good demonstration role in future medical education.

1.4.1　Medical Inheritance Mode

1. Inheritance of survival experience

The so-called inheritance of survival experience mainly occurs in the early days of human society, when human beings gathered and hunted everywhere for survival. A child follows an adult to collect what an adult picks. An adult teaches children what to eat and what not to eat in the collection practice; as well as which can be eaten raw, and which is needed to cook; which is poisonous, which is not poisonous, etc. Therefore, medicine is an inheritance generated solely for the need of survival and multiply. Sometimes due to extreme ignorance of nature and hunger, people might suffer from vomiting and diarrhea after mistakenly eating some toxic plants, and of course, sometimes people also accidentally eat something happen to relieve or eliminate the pain. It is through generations of attempts to survive that experience in identifying food, poisons, and medicine materials is accumulated. The legendary Shennong's taste of hundreds of herbs is actually a portrayal of people's accumulation of survival experience. By the end of the primitive society, people had mastered the treatment of snakebites, sword injuries, bleeding, sprains, swelling and pain, knife wounds, burns, dysentery, etc. The accumulation of these medical knowledge is actually the accumulation of experience in the struggle with nature for survival.

2. Pass from master to apprentice

The master-apprentice model in medical education was once the main model of medical training, which played an important role in the continuation, development and innovation of TCM. The master-apprentice education model represented by

Yellow Emperor and Qibo is a model for later generations. According to legend, Qi Daiji was a teacher of Qibo, who was proficient in medical knowledge. Qibo was a minister in the period of Yellow Emperor, and at the same time taught Yellow Emperor medical knowledge. He was a teacher of Yellow Emperor. Leigong was also a minister in the period of Yellow Emperor and a disciple of Yellow Emperor. According to the *Lushi* (an unofficial history of China written by Luo Mi), "Yellow Emperor consulted Qibo and Leigong and completed *Neijing* (*Canon of Medicine*)". It also illustrates the relationships among Yellow Emperor, Qibo and Leigong. In history, there is a clear record of the relationship between master and apprentice, which is the relationship between Chang Sangjun and Bianque. It is recorded in the *Records of the Historian: Biography of Bianque and Cang Gong* that "When Bianque was young, he was the director of a guest house. A guest named Chang Sangjun came to the guest house. Only Bianque thought he was unique and treated him respectfully. Chang Sangjun also knew that Bianque was not an ordinary person. He has been coming and going for more than ten years. One day, he asked Bianque to sit with him and said quietly: 'I have a secret prescription. I am old and want to pass it on to you. Don't let it out.' Bianque said, 'I promise with respect.' Then he took a medicine in his arms and gave it to Bianque. He said, 'Take this medicine with dew on the plants, and you will know a lot in 30 days.' Then he took out all the secret prescriptions and gave them to Bianque. All of a sudden, he disappeared. Maybe he was not a mortal. Bianque could see the people on the other side of the wall after taking the medicine for 30 days as he said. Therefore, when diagnosing other people's diseases, he can see all the diseases in the five zang-organs, but on the surface, he still does a palpation for the patient." Although the story between Chang Sangjun and Bianque is mythical, it still reflects the inheritance mode of medical education in this period. The disciples of Bianque include Zi Yang, Zi Ming, Zi You, Zi Yi, Zi Yue, Zi Rong, etc. The expansion of the inheritance scale of masters and apprentices is also a manifestation of the development of folk medical education.

It is worth emphasizing that in the process of apprentice selection before the establishment of the master-apprentice relationship, the talent and character of the apprentice need to be observed and tested for a long time. For example, Chang Sangjun's test of Bianque has gone through a long investigation period, and Bianque's years of respect for Chang Sangjun also shows Bianque's high moral cultivation. After the test of the master, it is determined that a serious and cautious apprenticeship ceremony is required. *Huangdi Neijing-Suwen: Sanbu Jiuhou Lun* (*Yellow Emperor's Canon of Medicine-Plain Conversation: Discussion on the Three Regions and Nine Divisions*) records that Yellow Emperor asked Qibo for advice, "I'd like to know the main idea, hoping to pass it on to my descendants and to hand it down to the later generations who should always memorize it and engrave it on their mind. When receiving it, they must take oath and never reveal it rashly." "Take oath" is the etiquette taught by the master and apprentice.

3. Family inheritance

In the *Zhou Li: Kao Gong Ji* (*Rites of Zhou: The Artificers' Record*), "Zhushi", "Yeshi" and "Guishi" are used to call baigong (craftsmen), indicating that individual occupations had developed into family business in the Spring and Autumn Period and the Warring States Period. Although the widely existing model of medical family inheritance was clearly recorded in the Western Han dynasty, the inheritance of medical family should have existed in the Zhou dynasty. Family inheritance is actually one of the special forms of master-apprentice inheritance, which is special in that the teacher integrates father and master.

1.4.2 Teaching Content

In the Zhou dynasty, medicine not only had an obvious boundary with "witchcraft", but also had detailed divisions within itself, including preventive medicine and clinical medicine. *Zhou Li: Qiu Guan* (*Rites of Zhou: Record of the Officials*) recorded "Shushi", "Jianshi", "Chifashi", "Huishi" and "Huzhuoshi" are set to record the health and epidemic prevention work in different seasons and fields across the country. In clinical medicine, there were physicians in the Zhou dynasty, who both treated officials of the dynasty and implemented medical affairs management. Official medical practitioners are divided into four departments: Shi Yi (nutritionist), Ji Yi (internist), Yang Yi (surgeon) and Shou Yi (veterinarian). In the Spring and Autumn Period and the Warring States Period, with the war and the needs of people's production and life, "Jun Yi (military medical practitioner)" and "Ru Yi (scholar medical practitioner)" appeared.

From the classification of medical practitioners, it can be inferred that medical education in the Pre-Qin period was also very rich in content, covering the talents needed by medical officers. The classic of medical education in the Pre-Qin period,

Yellow Emperor's Canon of Medicine is now taken as an example.

1. Learning of medical knowledge

As recorded in *Suwen: Jiejingwei Lun (Plain Conversation: Discussion on the Elucidation of Abstruse Theory)*, "Yellow Emperor sat in the Mingtang (Brightness Palace). Leigong asked, I have studied medicine from (Your Majesty) and taught others the theory (described in the medical) canons (such as the principles of) Congrong (diagnostics), Xingfa (anatomy), Yin and Yang, acupuncture, moxibustion and decoction'." *Suwen: Shuwuguo Lunpian (Plain Conversation: Discussion on Five Errors Frequently Made in Diagnosis)* also writes, "That is why it is said (that when) treating diseases sages (excellent TCM practitioners) must know Yin and Yang in the heavens and the earth, order of the four seasons, the five zang-organs and the six fu-organs, male and female, external and internal, acupuncture and moxibustion, stone-needle and indication of toxic drugs. (So that they can) consider human affairs carefully and decide the right ways (to diagnose diseases). (By inquiring about the) noble, humble, poor or rich (states of the patient), (they are able to) differentiate the constitution and characteristics (of the patient)" Theory canons means ancient classics. Yin and Yang means the four seasons of heaven and earth. Xingfa means the five zang-organs and the six fu-organs, male and female, external and internal, are roughly equivalent to today's biological anatomy. These three courses are basic courses. Congrong is equivalent to diagnostics. *Suwen: Shicongrong Lun (Plain Conversation: Discussion on How to Diagnose Diseases)* talks about how to make a differential diagnosis by comparing similar symptoms. Congrong in other discussions also refers to syndrome differentiation according to the patient's condition and social status.

In addition, the *Lingshu: Jingbie Pian (Spiritual Pivot: Separate Channels)* also lists the twelve Channels as "what the beginners (in medicine) have to study first and the excellent TCM practitioners are working hard to explore", that is, meridians are not only the content of basic courses, but also the topic of in-depth discussion by senior TCM practitioners. It can be seen that medical education at that time was quite extensive and included most courses of modern TCM teaching. Relatively speaking, basic courses, internal medicine and acupuncture account for a large proportion, while surgery, traumatology, gynecology, pediatrics and ENT have not yet formed independent disciplines.

2. Improvement of medical ethics

The cultivation of TCM practitioners' medical ethics is always an important part of medical education. In terms of the purpose of studying medicine, *Suwen* (*Plain Conversation*) emphasizes that "abstruse and profound theory can be practiced efficiently", and *Lingshu* (*Spiritual Pivots*) emphasizes that "treat (diseases for) the people and protect oneself". Put "treating (diseases for) the people" above "protecting oneself." *Suwen: Sanbu Jiuhou Lun* (*Plain Conversation: Discussion on the Three Regions and Nine Divisions*) also requires that medical knowledge "should pass on to descendants and to hand down to the later generations"; According to *Lingshu: Jiuzhen Shi'er Yuan* (*Spiritual Pivot: Nine Needles and Twelve Yuan -Primary Acupoints*), "it can be kept forever and will never be lost", and *Suwen: Wuchangzheng Dalunpian* (*Plain Conversation: Major Discussion on the Administration of Five-Motions*) repeatedly warned TCM practitioners not to "bring the patient calamities" and "lest the life of the patient be threatened". For behaviors that violate medical ethics and use medical skills to achieve selfish purposes, Lingshu: Shizhong (Spiritual Pivot: Beginning and Ending) uses a severe curse to express indignation, "If one does not follow this theory and is self-opinionated, he will surely suffer from disasters".

3. Put forward the teaching methods of read, aware, distinguish, understand and promote

Read, aware, distinguish, understand and promote are the five stages required by ancient medical education for students and are also classic learning methods. *Suwen: Zhuzhijiao Lun* (*Plain Conversation: Discussion on the Abstruse and Profound Theory of Medicine*) recorded: "Yellow Emperor sat in the Mingtang (Brightness Palace). He called in Leigong and asked, 'Do you know the theory of medicine?' Leigong answered, 'I have read medical books, but I cannot understand completely; sometimes I have understood, but I cannot analyze; sometimes I'm able to analyze, but I cannot grasp the gist; sometimes I have grasped the gist, but I cannot expound and use it'." Song is to read loudly. Through familiar reading, one can memorize and understand the content. This is the first step of learning. The second step is Jie, that means to understand what you don't understand. Bie means compare, distinguish, this is the third step. The fourth step Ming is to grasp knowledge from the perspective of the whole and internal contacts. Zhang means expound and use the knowledge, which makes medical knowledge learned reach a higher level. This is the fifth step. The five-step learning method is simple and clear, and is also an important method for medical learning today.

In addition, another important aspect of medicine is practice, and the theoretical knowledge of medicine need to be fully applied and improved. *Yellow Emperor's Canon of Medicine* repeatedly emphasizes the integration of theoretical study and practice. In *Suwen: Qijiaobian Dalun (Plain Conversation: Major Discussion on the Changes of Qi-Convergence)*, it is said that "Those who are good at explaining Tiandao (law of the heavens) always apply it to human affairs. Those who are good at discussing things in ancient times certainly apply them to the present. Those who are good at expounding qi are undoubtedly related it to the activities of all things. Those who are good at interpreting interaction are able to integrate it with the transformation of the heavens and the earth. Those who are good at elucidating transformation and change certainly understand Shenming (rules of nature)." According to *Suwen: Jutong Lun (Plain Conversation: Discussion on Pains)*, "Those who are good at explaining the heavens must be able to prove it with human affairs, those who are good at discussing history must be able to relate it to the present situation and those who are good at talking about others must be able to delineate themselves." These discussions emphasize the importance of testing theory and experience.

Chapter Summary

1. Life first, improving medical skills is the essential requirement of medical practitioners

No matter Fuxi, Shennong or Bianque, they always respect life first in their practice of medicine and practice medicine with a pious heart of revering and respecting life. In order to obtain better treatment effect and relieve the pain of patients, it is necessary to actively improve medical skills to treat patients and save lives.

2. Patient-centered, respect for patients is the mission and requirement for medical practitioners

In the process of treating and saving people, TCM practitioners always focus on patients, fully respect patients, empathize with patients' pain, and formulate treatment plans based on the dual needs of patients' condition and psychology. They should not only see patients' physiological diseases, but also carry out physiological treatment and psychological comfort for patients at the same time, so as to shorten the treatment time. It is also the mission of TCM practitioners to improve the curative effect.

3. Improving medical ethics is the lifelong practice of medical practitioners

Medical ethics cultivation is an important part of medical education and an important indicator for the assessment of TCM practitioners. The level of medical ethics of a medical practitioner even determines the growth level of medical skills of a medical practitioner. Only when medical ethics and skills go hand in hand can the cause of a medical practitioner be promoted.

Application in Contemporary Times

1. Medical ethics embodies the comprehensive requirements of social foundation in the spiritual field

The medical ethics described in this chapter is formed on the basis of the political, economic, cultural and other social backgrounds in the Pre-Qin period. Its content and characteristics reflect the expectations of the people in the Pre-Qin period for the code of conduct shown by witch healers and medical practitioners engaged in the treatment of diseases and pains. Today, socialist medical ethics is the specific requirement of Xi Jinping Thought on Socialism with Chinese Characteristics for a New Era for the professional ethics of medical practitioners, reflecting the people's earnest expectation for the dedication and fulfillment of medical practitioners in the diagnosis and treatment of patients.

Medical students and practitioners should keep in mind the oath of medical students that "health related, life entrusted", stay true to the original aspiration and mission of medical practice, cultivate the medical spirit of "respecting and protecting life, healing the wounded and rescuing the dying, and being dedicated to the cause", and practice the noble medical ethics of benevolence in the front-line clinical work.

2. Medical practitioners should have the spirit of bravely exploring to solve difficult medical problems

The TCM practitioners introduced in this chapter witnessed patients suffering from diseases. Without exception, they actively explored new medicines and treatment while proposing treatment plans. They walked through mountains and rivers to find herbs and folk prescriptions, and even tried new medicines and tested treatment methods personally regardless of their own safety. After obtaining stable efficacy, they applied the herbs to patients and continuously adjusted the combination, in order to improve the effect or apply to more kinds of diseases.

In the daily work and study, medical students and practitioners should carry forward the spirit of hard work with courage and perseverance of the ancients in the face of clinical pain points or medical difficulties, hold a high sense of responsibility for patients, fear no difficulties and obstacles, and move forward bravely until difficulties are overcome.

2

Medical Ethics Culture in the Qin and Han Dynasties

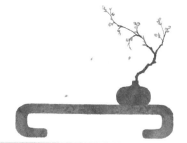

2.1　Overview of Medical Ethics

2.1.1　Background of Medical Ethics

1. Social background

The Qin and Han dynasties were the periods when the feudal system was established, consolidated and developed in ancient China. After the unification of the six states by Qin Shihuang (the first emperor of Qin), a series of measures were taken to consolidate the centralization system and reform the feudal system. The reform of feudal system has brought opportunities for medicine to completely get rid of witchcraft and establish an independent medical system.

The establishment of a unified state has strengthened medical management, and the medical system from the state to the local is more rigorous, with more distinct levels and clearer division of labor. In the Qin and Han dynasties, the medical organization was improved. There were official posts for medical practitioners such as the minister of imperial medical affairs, assistant officer of imperial medical affairs, and emperor's physician in the Qin dynasty. From 213—212 BC, Qin Shihuang burned books and buried scholars. The atrocity caused great losses to the preservation of ancient documents and reserve of cultural knowledge. However, medical books were not burned, which reflected the importance Qin dynasty attached to medicine. In the Han dynasty, a more complex medical management organization was established than in the Qin dynasty, with imperial medical affairs, assistant officer of imperial medical affairs, and various emperor's TCM practitioners under their jurisdiction serving the imperial court. There were also emperor's physician with different positions in the baron palaces. Temporary hospitals were set up during the pandemic. Medical institutions were also set up in the army.

In general, the Qin and Han dynasties were the first period of great unification in China's history. The initial economic development, the strengthening of economic and cultural exchanges between the inland and the border areas, and new breakthroughs in science and technology laid the foundation for the development and improvement of medicine and medical ethics.

2. Ideological and cultural background

In the early Western Han dynasty, Huang-Lao thought prevailed, which greatly affected the development of medicine. These influences are reflected in classics such as the *Lüshi Chunqiu* (*Master Lü's Spring and Autumn Annals*) and *Huai Nan Zi*. *Yellow Emperor's Internal Canon of Medicine* is one of the earliest medical classics in China and the earliest monograph on independent discussion of medical ethics in China. It is said to be a book on medicine by Yellow Emperor and his ministers Qibo and Leigong, which is actually a supplement to the inheritance, creation and development of Huang-Lao TCM practitioners in China in all ages, and its idea is widely accepted by later TCM practitioners.

In the middle of the Western Han dynasty, Emperor Wu adopted Dong Zhongshu's suggestion of "venerate Confucianism", which made Confucianism achieve a high status, and Confucianism had a deeper and wider impact on medicine and medical ethics. Dong Zhongshu proposed to "ban from hundred philosophers, venerate Confucianism", and combined Yin, Yang and five elements with Confucianism to establish the doctrines of "interactions between Heaven and Mankind" and "unification". Confucianism has gradually become an orthodox thought in Chinese society, and the thought of "a man of benevolence loves others" has replaced Huang-Lao thought as the leading thought in the medical field.

3. Medical background

In Qin and Han dynasties, both Qin Shihuang and Emperor Wu pursued immortality. They respected alchemists and encouraged the development of immortality medicine. Qin Shihuang sent alchemists many times to seek immortality medicine, which objectively promoted medical research. Since the Qin dynasty, the government has strengthened the management of medicine. Medical knowledge has been widely spread in more diverse ways, and there have been more and more folk TCM practitioners. Most of these folk TCM practitioners practice medicine individually, forming the main body of the traditional medical team.

At the end of the Eastern Han dynasty, eunuchs and consorts took turns to exercise power, deepening the social contradiction. Due to the brutality and squeezing of the ruling class, the Yellow Turban Uprising (a large popular rebellion) broke out at the end of the Eastern Han dynasty. The war caused a large number of deaths and severe damage to production. Diseases and hunger also made the plague epidemic rapidly. Many TCM practitioners wrote books while healing the wounded and rescuing the dying. Zhang Zhongjing studied medicine because of the epidemic disease in his hometown and most of his family died of cold diseases. So, he extensively collected medical prescriptions and wrote the great book *Treatise on Febrile and Miscellaneous Diseases*. All these have promoted the development of medicine.

During Qin and Han dynasties, great progress was made in the prevention of diseases and the improvement of sanitation facilities. In terms of disease prevention, attention was paid to water hygiene. In the treatment of infectious patients, attention was paid to isolation treatment; in terms of sanitation facilities, attention was paid to dredging ditches and building sewers and other facilities during the Qin dynasty. During the reign of Emperor Wu of the Han dynasty, pots (spittoons) were used. In November 1972, in the Han dynasty tomb excavated in Hantanpo, Wuwei, Gansu, there were a total of 92 handwritten medical slips, which were originally named "Wuwei Handai Yijian (Wuwei Medical Bamboo Slips of the Han dynasty)", and later renamed "Prescriptions for the Treatment of All Diseases" due to the words in the slips. The contents of the slips are quite extensive, including diseases of various departments such as internal medicine, surgery, gynecology, pediatrics and ENT, and nearly 100 kinds of medicines are contained. There are also acupuncture, medicinal contraindications and medicine prices, which are a summary of TCM practitioners' experience in medical practice and medication at that time, and also reflect the medical level in the Qin and Han dynasties.

2.1.2 Formation of Medical Ethics

The unity of the state and the increasingly richness of thoughts and cultural life accelerated the development of medicine and the formation of a medical ethics system. In this period, on the one hand, medical thoughts and ethics penetrated into each other, that is, medical thoughts contained medical ethics, and vice versa. On the other hand, there were also two types of medical ethics, namely, official medical ethics tendency and practice and folk medical ethics consciousness and practice, which were mainly manifested in medical ethics stories, medical theories and medical ethics speeches and myths and legends.

The purpose of medicine is to solve the primary problem in medical ethics. The purpose of medical science is to heal the wounded and rescue the dying, cure diseases and save people. Zhang Zhongjing clearly pointed out in *Treatise on Febrile and Miscellaneous Diseases* that: "the purpose of proficiently versed in the remedial art is to treat the illnesses of the sovereign and of their elders above, to relieve the suffering of the poor and destitute below and to safeguard their own body and sustain health at center, all in order to cultivate life", that is, the purpose of medical science is to cure diseases and save people. Moreover, Zhang Zhongjing called for focusing on medicine and proficiently versing in the remedial arts with the spirit of "loving and knowing others". Rigorous and extensive knowledge is also an important part of medical ethics. Rigor refers to the morality of TCM practitioners to treat medicine and medical skills seriously and prudently, and at the same time, only the knowledgeable can cope with the ever-changing development of diseases. An incompetent TCM practitioner who treats a disease against medical principles will cause a mild disease into a serious one and also put a patient who may survive to death.

Taoism had a certain impact on the development of medicine and medical ethics in the Qin and Han dynasties. The medical principles in *Master Lü's Spring and Autumn Annals* and *Huai Nan Zi* actually follow Taoism, mainly discussing the ways of health preservation while eliminating desires. Taoist doctrines in the Warring States Period developed to the direction of religious superstition in the Qin and Han dynasties. For example, in the last years of the Eastern Han dynasty, Zhang Daoling (a Chinese religious leader) honored Laozi as the religious ancestor and worshiped *Laozi Wuqian Wen* (*Dao De Jing*) as the highest classic. He created the "The Five Pecks of Rice Movement "(the founder and first patriarch of Taoism in China) and used the water mantra to cure people's diseases, with many followers. Taoist scholars attach more importance to their own lives than Confucian scholars do. They regard human life as the primary significance of life, and this thought of attaching great importance to life has a positive impact on the formation of medical ethics. It is the sacred duty of medical practitioners to heal the wounded and rescue the dying. *Yellow Emperor's Canon of Medicine*, which is deeply influenced by Taoist culture, clearly puts forward that "the covering of the heavens in the upper and the support of the earth in the lower have paved the way for the creation of all things in nature, among which the noblest one is man", that is, the most basic moral requirement of medical practitioners is to attach importance to human life, and medical practitioners should be skilled and noble in medical ethics.

Confucianism's thought of "benevolence" has a great impact on the medical science of the Qin and Han dynasties. For more than 2,000 years, ancient medical practitioners have always called medicine "benevolent act". Confucianism believes that the essence of human nature is "benevolent heart" and is a moral life. TCM practitioners pursue the value of life with the benevolence of society and integrate Confucian knowledge and understanding of people and human nature, which has a deeper effect on the shaping of traditional medical ethics. This is mainly reflected in TCM practitioner's understanding of people through the theory of "the heart of the sage". In *Gujin Yitong Daquan (Complete Compendium of Medical Tradition)*, it is recorded that "medicine takes living people as the heart, so it is called the benevolence act". In *Yixue Qiushi (Seeking Truth in Medicine)*, it is recorded that "medicine is a kind of benevolent act, and man can have a sense of compassion". It can be seen that "medicine is a kind of benevolence act" is the most fundamental understanding of medicine by TCM practitioners. Medical ethics and TCM practitioners are inseparable. The idea of "loving and knowing others, loving and knowing themselves" advocated by Zhang Zhongjing in Han dynasty also reflects the purpose of "benevolence" in medical practice and the moral characteristics of Confucianism in practice. It can be seen that medical ethics is the soul of a medical practitioners. Medical ethics not only exists in medical books, but also is reflected in medical practice. There are many TCM practitioners in the Han dynasty, including Hua Tuo, Zhang Zhongjing, Chunyu Yi, Dong Feng, Guo Yu, Su Dan, Hu Gong, Han Kang, etc. Their moral performance in medical practice reflects the level and characteristics of medicine and medical ethics in this period.

2.1.3　Medical Practitioner's Sentiment

The research on traditional Chinese medical ethics is mainly based on the words and deeds of famous TCM practitioners, who have profound knowledge. Therefore, we call them "Yi Jia" (esteemed medical practitioner). The medical practitioners are those who conduct medical activities, and their lofty sentiment is the main content of medical moral thoughts. The medical motivation reflects the life value of TCM practitioners. Medical motivation is the original intention of TCM practitioners to engage in medical activities, which reflects their value pursuit. We can have a deeper understanding of the values and the moral world of TCM practitioners through medical motivation.

TCM practitioners influenced by Taoist thoughts have the pursuit of "practice Taoism and attain immortality, reach longevity and accumulate virtue" in the process of medical practice. Among them, the practice of Taoism and attainment of immortality represents their ultimate value pursuit, while reaching longevity and accumulating virtue are the direct value pursuit in the process of medical practice for the practice of Taoism and attainment of immortality. In addition to the pursuit of immortality, accumulating virtue is also an important factor that prompts TCM practitioners to study medicine and improve their medical skills. *Laozi Xianger Zhu* is regarded as a Taoist classic, in which it is clearly stated that "Taoists prefer giving to others than being given by others". Practicing medicine and treating diseases have the function of "giving to others". Therefore, the significance of studying medical prescriptions is highly valued in Taoism. Mastering medical skills can not only protect life by self-healing, but also "give to others" by virtue of this ability in diagnosing diseases and accumulating virtue.

"Medicine is a benevolent skill", in which medicine refers to medical affairs, including medical skills of TCM practitioners, reflecting the socialization and professionalization of TCM practitioners' medical behavior. The sentence "medicine is a benevolent skill" represents the understanding of medical affairs, that is, the essence of medical affairs is the practice of benevolence. The concept of "medicine is a benevolent skill" reflects the characteristic that TCM practitioners associate medical affairs with benevolence, which cannot be equated with the professional ethics of TCM practitioners in the modern sense. In the TCM practitioners' concept, benevolence and humanity are the internal basis of medical activities, while medical activities are the external manifestation of benevolence and humanity, and the concrete practice and implementation of benevolence and humanity. At the same time, this is also reflected in the relationship between medical ethics and human nature. TCM practitioners believe that only by engaging in medical activities with benevolence can they feel "at ease". Therefore, ancient TCM practitioners believed that practicing medicine was practicing benevolence, and then put forward the statement that hanging a pot to help the world and knowing medicine to practice filial piety. They believed that medical practitioners should have rigorous academic spirit, modest and prudent style and noble morality; they should treat patients with courtesy and care. Medical practice should follow the principles of life first, equal treatment, justice first and benefits second, and should be prudent and appropriate in the process of diagnosis and treatment of diseases.

TCM practitioners associate medical affairs with a wide range of moral practices, which fully reflects the value pursuit of practicing medicine and accumulating morality. Zhang Zhongjing inherited the academic thoughts of *Yellow Emperor's Canon of Medicine* and *The Classic of Difficult Issues*, summarized rich clinical experience, and wrote *Treatise on Cold Diseases and Miscellaneous Diseases*. It is precisely the achievement of Zhang Zhongjing who saw the serious harm of cold diseases to people's health and studied medicine with a lofty sense of social responsibility. *Treatise on Cold Diseases and Miscellaneous Diseases* lays the theoretical foundation of principle, rule, prescription and medicine, and has a profound impact on the development of TCM. Due to the rigorous academic treatment of Zhang Zhongjing, his theory has experienced more than 1,000 years of testment and clinical verification, and still maintains strong vitality, effectively guiding the research and practice of TCM clinical practice and integration TCM and Western medicine.

Medical ethics cultivation is the moral qualities that TCM practitioners must possess, and it is also the concentrated embodiment of TCM practitioners' morality. TCM practitioners believe that moral cultivation plays a very important role, which is directly related to whether they can learn medicine and master medical knowledge. In history, when many famous TCM practitioners admit apprentices, the first thing was to examine their morality. According to the concept of "medicine is a benevolent skill", the traditional Chinese medical ethics is based on benevolence, and requires medical ethics. Therefore, TCM practitioners are usually considered to have moral cultivation of benevolence, wisdom, integrity and non-deception. "Benevolence" is the most important medical ethics. As a TCM practitioner, whether he has "benevolence" will directly affect the medical practice. The cultivation of "wisdom" is also very important. *Yellow Emperor's Canon of Medicine* pointed out that medical learning needs to "know astronomy, geography and people", which are the knowledge and skills that must be mastered for medical science, and need to be mastered with "wisdom". Medical theories are extensive and profound. Medical learners need not only natural wisdom, but also acquired continuous efforts, even hardships and extraordinary efforts. If they want to learn something, they must diligently seek ancient precepts and learn from others. Both innate qualifications and acquired efforts mean the qualities of "wisdom". In order to avoid TCM practitioners taking medical practice as a way to make profits, ancient TCM practitioners emphasized the quality of "integrity". Many TCM practitioners in the Qin and Han dynasties showed the noble quality of "integrity". The diseases of both the ruling class and the ruled class should be treated. At that time, the laboring people had poor living conditions and harsh environment, and were too poor to afford disease treatment. Therefore, sometimes medical practitioners could not get paid, and they may even help the patients financially. Without the moral quality of "integrity", they could not be like this.

The moral qualities of "not deceiving yourself" and "not deceiving others" embody the moral qualities of "not deceiving", making it an absolute intellectual authority in the Qin and Han dynasties when medical knowledge was not yet popularized. Patients are completely passive and fully trust TCM practitioners to some extent. Physicians must be practical and realistic in all aspects of pulse diagnosis, disease differentiation and medication, and allow no deception in any form. This is because patients can only accept the treatment as they completely rely on the inner heart of the TCM practitioner to identify whether the condition is really clear and whether the prescription is suitable for the disease. Therefore, TCM practitioners oppose any form of deception and drug abuse, and maintain a spirit of modesty and caution, without publicity or pride. Chunyu Yi is a TCM practitioner who followed such principles. Although he has excellent medical skills and can determine life and death when diagnosing diseases, he is not arrogant. Emperor Wen of Han once asked Chunyu Yi, "Can you diagnose disease and determine life and death without any error?" Chunyu earnestly replied: "There could be errors, and I can't be that perfect." In addition, Chunyu Yi also truthfully recorded cases that he did not cure in the process of medical practice, which reflected his moral qualities of being modest, cautious and non-deceptive.

2.1.4　Medical Ethics

Medical skill is a philosophical thought spread in ancient China. There is a description of Chinese medical skills in *Plain Conversation—Ancient Ideas on How to Preserve Natural Healthy Energy*: "Zhenqi in the body will be in harmony,

Jingshen (Essence-Spirit) will remain inside, and diseases will have no way to occur... inhaling fresh air, cultivating their spirit and keeping their muscles integrated". The term "harmony" here refers to nature, and "integrated" refers to the integration of nature and man. Medical ethics is an important part of traditional Chinese medical ethics, which reflects the overall characteristics of traditional Chinese medical ethics from one perspective.

The most important manifestation of TCM practitioners' understanding of medical skills is the saying "medicine is a benevolent skill". As mentioned earlier, "medicine" refers to medical activities, "benevolence" refers to benevolent heart, and "skill" refers to the method of medical practice. Medical skills are the means and skills of medical activities. They serve medical affairs and are guided by medical affairs, while medical affairs are guided by benevolence. Therefore, medical skills must be developed from benevolence, and the morality of medical skills plays a role. *The Book of Han: Records of Arts and Literature* pointed out, "Skilled people in medicine are born with tools, and one of the posts set by the emperor." Mastering medicine skill can master the law of life. Those who mastered medicine skills could hold relevant official positions in the imperial court. For example, Qibo mastered such skills and could handle everything from minor illnesses to the governance of the country. TCM practitioners always give full play to medical ethics, which is reflected in their participation in medicine and medical practice. It is because TCM practitioners attach importance to medical ethics that the social status of TCM practitioners has been improved.

Emperor Wu of Han adopted Dong Zhongshu's idea of "deposing all schools of thought and respecting Confucianism", and established the humanitarian concept of "the benevolent loves others" to lead the development of medicine. In addition to "loving others", TCM practitioners also emphasize safeguarding personal life in the understanding of medical skills. Zhang Zhongjing advocated the combination of loving others with medical skills and the maintenance of life. In his *Treatise on Cold Diseases and Miscellaneous Diseases*, he emphasized that TCM practitioners should have the spirit of exquisite prescriptions and loving people and knowing people, and should diligently seek ancient precepts and learn from others. He emphasized a serious attitude to cure the illness of the lord and his parents, save the poor, and protect his own health. He claimed that in treating patients TCM practitioners should not only diagnose part of the body such as the Cun pulse and hands and ignore the

Chi pulse and the feet. He opposed those who only pursue fame and fortune and emphasized the knowledge of broad spirit. Without medical skills, medical ethics cannot be realized. Without medical ethics, medical skills become evil talents. If a TCM practitioner has medical ethics but no medical skills, then the state of no medical skills is only temporary, and if he can make up for it with all his strength, and be careful in the practice, he would at least not kill people. However, if he has a problem in medical ethics, even with excellent medical skills, he may deceive patients, and cause endless harms. Therefore, medical ethics is more important than medical skills.

The value of medical science is embodied in helping people with medical skills, and good medical ethics requires exquisite medical skills as the carrier. Therefore, TCM practitioners of all dynasties have attached great importance to taking "exquisite skills" as the basis of "moral practice". During the Qin and Han dynasties, Chunyu Yi, Zhang Zhongjing and Hua Tuo made great achievements in medicine. Chunyu Yi is the pioneer of China's medical records. He loved medicine since childhood, and had been studying hard from his master Gongcheng Yangqing. After three years of study, he can "determine life and death" by treating people's diseases. Zhang Zhongjing's *Treatise on Febrile and Miscellaneous Diseases* not only contributed to the development of China's medicine at that time, but also made great contributions to later generations, which also influenced Japan, Democratic People's Republic of Korea, Vietnam and other countries. Zhang Zhongjing was also respected as the "sage of medicine", which is inseparable from his saying of "diligently seeking ancient precepts and learning from others". Hua Tuo invented Anesthesia Powder. It is said that he also successfully performed abdominal surgery, known as the originator of surgery. Medical ethics and medical skills are integrate and complementary to each other. Ethics is the prerequisite and skills are embodied in practice. Ancient TCM practitioners who pursued moral self-worth must devote themselves to medicine and improve their medical skills.

With the emergence of medical activities, related medical evaluations have also emerged. *Yellow Emperor's Canon of Medicine* points out that "disease is the root, medical skills are the leaves". This evaluation also reveals that in medical activities, when facing patients, TCM practitioners should not regard patients as experimental objects in their consciousness and conception to pursue the growth of medical knowledge and the accumulation of medical experience, but should serve patients as the purpose of medical practice, and regard service for patients as the purpose of pursuit to guide the application of medical skills. This opinion deeply reflects the spiritual essence of life-oriented TCM in ancient medical ethics.

The norms of medical skills are also very important. *Yellow Emperor's Canon of Medicine* is a very authoritative work in TCM, which puts forward many medical norms. The norms have been continued and developed in the history of medicine and become the most important medical norms. *Plain Conversations: Major Discussion on the Theory of Yin and Yang and the Corresponding Relationships Among All the Things in Nature* mentions that "the treatment of diseases must be based on the nature of changes in Yin and Yang", which means that the treatment of diseases is to restore the original balance of life by using medical methods according to the way of Yin and Yang, so as to achieve the purpose of mental and physical health. From the perspective of medical norms, the ultimate goal of TCM practitioners to treat patients is to restore the original state of their life. Therefore, in the process of use of medical skills, TCM practitioners do not pursue the proficiency and exquisiteness of medical skills, but to better serve the life. Therefore, patients are the main part of the medical practice process, and serving patients is the purpose of medical skills. *Yellow Emperor's Canon of Medicine* also makes specific regulations on the psychological state of TCM practitioners in the diagnosis and treatment of diseases, and puts forward detailed requirements for TCM practitioners to take the pulse of patients. *Plain Conversations: Discussion on the Essentials of Pulse* has the saying that "the best time for taking pulse is dawn". That is to say, when diagnosing and treating patients, we should maintain a calm and peaceful mind, so as to truly diagnose the patient's pulse condition and identify the condition. Floating heart and impetuousness would lead to bad diagnosis. Only a good mental and psychological state can ensure the correct diagnosis and formulate appropriate treatment plans to achieve effective treatment.

As the saying goes, "It is necessary to have effective tools to do good work". The fundamental task of medicine lies in saving people, which must be based on exquisite medical skills, and good medical ethics must also be based on exquisite medical skills. Therefore, TCM practitioners attach great importance to taking "exquisite skills" as the foundation and basis of "moral establishment" and medicine as the "skill of saving people", which is "subtle" and "life-critical". To realize the career ideal of "benevolence, saving people and benefiting the world", they must rely on excellent medical skills.

2.1.5 Connotation of Medical Ethics

In Chinese history, TCM practitioner was one of the earliest independent professions, which appeared in the Zhou dynasty. By the Qin and Han dynasties, the medical organization was quite complete. Influenced by Confucianism, Taoism and Buddhism, traditional medical ethics has distinctive features and rich connotations.

1. Benevolence in medical practice, sincerity to benefit the world

Influenced by the Confucian thought of "benevolence", TCM practitioners formed the medical ethics concept of "benevolence in medical practice". The essence of "benevolence" is love, which is a universal care for life. Physicians should take good care of people's lives, pay attention to their health, respect their personality, and treat diseases by giving benevolence to others. "Benevolence in medical practice" is the basic principle and core of traditional Chinese medical ethics, the cognition and practice of ancient TCM practitioners on medical undertakings and personal social responsibilities, and the embodiment of the highest realm of medical ethics.

2. Treat all people equally

In the diagnosis and treatment of patients, it is a key content of medical ethics to treat patients with right attitude and concept. "Treating all people equally" requires treating them regardless of their status, property, and affinity without discrimination. TCM practitioners practiced the medical norms of treating people equally in their own practice, which had a profound impact on the formation of medical ethics in later generations. In the Han dynasty, Chunyu Yi, Zhang Zhongjing, and Hua Tuo treated patients equally.

3. Medicine is subtle and needs wide medical sources

It is a consensus of TCM practitioners that exquisite medical skills are needed as the premise and foundation to treat and save people. Zhang Zhongjing has excellent medical skills, but he believes that he is not a genius, but masters prescriptions through acquired efforts, that is, "diligently seeking ancient precepts and learning from others". As he said, "if you are not a talent, how can you find out the truth?" All famous TCM practitioners in the past dynasties have studied medical books, assiduously studied medical skills, and continuously improved their medical level and medical skills in medical practice. It can be seen that TCM practitioners in the Qin and Han dynasties have high technical requirements for themselves and they are proficient in medical science. Learning from others and studying medical skills have also become the medical ethics adhered to by TCM practitioners throughout their lives.

4. Emphasizing righteousness over profit, being indifferent to fame and fortune

Emphasizing righteousness over profit is a kind of value advocated by Mencius' theories of good nature, and it is also one of Confucian classical ethics. TCM practitioners are deeply influenced by Confucian values of valuing righteousness over profit, and advocate that "TCM practitioners save people and do not rely on it to earn a living", that is, TCM practitioners should, with the ideal of saving people from suffering, put away the gains and losses of money and fame and wealth, and emphasize righteousness as the first. Zhang Zhongjing stressed that TCM practitioners must always be patient-oriented. In the preface of *Treatise on Febrile and Miscellaneous Diseases*, he criticized the TCM practitioners who were enthusiastic about fame and fortune at that time, and opposed "competing for prosperity, chasing the powerful, and diligently fishing fame and fortune". He also practiced in person and took the lead.

5. Respect the peers and value harmony

In medical activities, the interpersonal relationship in medical practice activities is not only the doctor-patient relationship, but also the peer relationship. How to deal with the peer relationship will not only affect the interests of patients, but also reflect the personal morality of TCM practitioners. Therefore, ancient TCM practitioners attached great importance to it. Ancient TCM practitioners absorbed the Confucian idea of "what you do not want to be done to yourself, do not do to others". Physicians believed that they should respect and love peers, help each other, learn from each other's strengths and make up for each other's weaknesses, and improve together. They should be modest and prudent in doing things, and not flaunt themselves or demean others. Therefore, the medical ethics concept of respecting peers and valuing harmony was formed.

6. Practice medicine with courtesy, be pure and upright

In the process of medical practice, courtesy also reflects the medical ethics of TCM practitioners. *Yellow Emperor's Canon of Medicine: Spiritual Pivot* emphasizes that TCM practitioners should "ask about customs when entering a country, ask about taboos when entering a home, ask about courtesy when going to the hall, and ask about likes and dislikes when facing patients", and advocates that patients should be treated "gently without arrogance", requiring TCM practitioners to maintain a conscious respectful attitude when communicating with patients. Respect for the patient also involves the privacy of the patient's family. Because some diseases have special causes, patients have special physical conditions or bad living habits, these information needs to be obtained by the TCM practitioner from the patient or his family for the needs of diagnosis and treatment. The patient could be unwilling to let others know such information. Therefore, TCM practitioners need to keep the privacy of patients confidential, which is also an important aspect for TCM practitioners to respect patients. Ancient TCM practitioners attached great importance to this, demonstrating the pure and upright medical ethics of TCM practitioners.

2.1.6　Doctor-patient Ethics

Ancient TCM practitioners followed the principle of value righteousness over benefits. In terms of charging patients for remuneration, TCM practitioners held an attitude of "receiving whatever they are paid". In practicing medicine, the relationship between TCM practitioners and patients was not based on economy, but relied on moral standards for guidance. The saying "medicine is a benevolent skill" is the moral concept of ancient TCM practitioners in medical practice. Physicians should have "benevolence in saving people", focus on saving people, sympathize with and care for patients, and do their best to save patients. In the traditional medical ethics, the doctor-patient ethics should follow the relationship between the rescuer and the rescued. The TCM practitioner has the nature of "goodness" in medical practice, as people's lives are the most important and as precious as gold, so the TCM practitioners who help others have the virtue valued beyond gold. It can be seen that the ethical thought of benevolence runs through the traditional Chinese medical ethics.

The dominance of Confucianism in feudal society determines that TCM practitioners of all dynasties must advocate Confucianism before they can become

TCM practitioners. Many Confucian physicians regard medical practice as a way to realize their self-worth and social value. Confucianism's idea that "pay attention to self-improvement when unappreciated, and spare no efforts in helping people when appreciated" was believed by scholars in ancient times. When Confucian intellectuals were unfairly treated politically and could not serve the country, some would hide in the forest of medicine, and save the world and realize their self-worth by practicing medicine. The doctor-patient relationship model is also deeply influenced by Confucianism. Doctors pursue the realization of moral personality based on their inner consciousness of benevolence, and integrate the realization of this ideal of life into the process of medical practice. They regard the ability to cure diseases and recover patients from dying as the merits of the benevolent, and believe that this is accomplish themselves, that is, realizing the inner morality. At the same time, recover patients from dying is undoubtedly also saving others in the interests of patients. In this way, accomplishment of oneself is achieved with the help of saving others. In the treatment of diseases, the two have reached an agreement. Therefore, there is a high degree of unity between accomplishment of oneself and saving others, which is the spiritual essence of ethics between medical practitioners and patient in ancient China.

During the Qin and Han dynasty, the medical ethics of *Yellow Emperor's Canon of Medicine* was widely accepted by TCM practitioners. The ideal personality of "benevolence" and the value of emphasizing righteousness over benefits had a profound impact on ancient TCM practitioners. The famous TCM practitioner Chunyu Yi of the Western Han dynasty had excellent medical skills, and liked to travel to the local areas and treat diseases for the people, so he often offended the government. Likewise, Hua Tuo was reluctant to only treat Cao Cao and was willing to live among the people as a TCM practitioner. After that, the people respected the beloved TCM practitioner as "the rebirth of Hua Tuo". Dong Feng, a TCM practitioner of the Three Kingdoms period, lived in the mountains and treated diseases, but he did not take money and other benefits. If patients with serious disease were cured, he would ask them to plant five apricot trees, and if the disease is mild, he would ask one apricot tree be planted. After so many years, more than 100,000 apricot trees have been planted to form a forest. Every year, he sell apricots for grains and give the grains to the poor and travelers who had no food, with over 20,000 hu (a dry measure used in former times) of grains distributed each year. Since then, "apricot forest in the warm spring" has become a praise for TCM practitioners' virtues.

In addition, in the process of diagnosis and treatment of diseases, Chinese traditional medical ethics attaches great importance to doctor-patient communication, as the communication is very important and runs through the meetings between TCM practitioners and patients. Communication is not only a way to obtain information in all aspects and understand patients, but also a way for TCM practitioners to effectively guide and regulate the spirit and psychology of patients. Good communication can reflect TCM practitioners' knowledge and ethical literacy. It will also enable harmonious interaction between TCM practitioners and patients and effective diagnosis and treatment of diseases.

2.2 Representative Medical Practitioners and Their Medical Ethics

2.2.1 Hua Tuo

1. Brief biography

Hua Tuo, a famous TCM practitioner in the late Eastern Han dynasty, with a courtesy name Yuanhua and an alternative name of Zhuan, was born in Qiao of Pei area (now Bozhou, Anhui Province). Hua Tuo, Dong Feng and Zhang Zhongjing were collectively called "three divine TCM practitioners in Jian'an Period". He is one of the four famous TCM practitioners in ancient China, known as the "Surgical Master" and the "Originator of Surgery", and is said to be the first medical practitioner in China to start general anesthesia surgery. When he was young, he once studied outside of hometown, focused on medical skills without seeking an official career, and had comprehensive medical skills. He was especially good and proficient at surgery, and proficient in internal medicine, gynecology, pediatrics, acupuncture and moxibustion. He tended to use less medicine, generally only a few, and took them out accurately without weighing. He had practiced medicine in Anhui, Henan, Shandong, Jiangsu and other places. According to the *Biography of Hua Tuo*, he used "anesthesia powder" to anesthetize patients and then perform laparotomy, which is the earliest record of general anesthesia in the world medical history. He also imitated the dynamics of tigers, deer, bears, apes, birds and other animals to create gymnastics called "Five-Animal Gymnastics", teaching people to strengthen their body. Later, he was killed because he refused to accept Cao Cao's conscription. He wrote many works such as *The Book of Blue Sacks (Qing Nang Shu)* and *The Pillow Moxibustion Sutra (Zhen Zhong Jiu Ci Jing)*, but unfortunately, they have all been lost.

2. Medical ethics

Hua Tuo lived in the late Eastern Han dynasty and the early Three Kingdoms period. At that time, warlords were fighting, floods and drought disasters were frequent, epidemics were spreading, and people were in an abyss of suffering. Seeing the suffering of the people, Hua Tuo hated the evil-doing feudal powers and sympathized with the oppressed and exploited laboring people. For this reason, he was not willing to be an official, and would rather travel around and treat diseases for people. Hua Tuo could see through the symptoms. He used simple medicine and was well aware of the physical and mental interaction. He attached great importance to prevention and health care, observed the natural ecology, taught people to regulate breath and feel harmonious with nature. However, for patients who were seriously ill, he would not proceed meaningless treatment and just told the truth.

Hua Tuo did not seek fame and fortune and did not admire wealth, which enabled him to concentrate on the research of medicine. According to *The Book of the Later Han Dynasty: Biography of Hua Tuo*, he "knows well about several cannons" and "understands how to nourish the nature", especially "is good at prescriptions and medicines". People call him "a divine TCM practitioner". He compiled his rich medical experience into a medical book called *The Book of Blue Sacks (Qing Nang Shu)*, but it was not passed down to today. Hua Tuo critically inherited the academic achievements of his predecessors and created new theories on the basis of summarizing the experience of his predecessors. At the same time, Hua Tuo also had in-depth research on the theory of Zhang Zhongjing in his contemporary times. When he read Volume 10 of *Treatise on Febrile and Miscellaneous Diseases* written by Zhang Zhongjing, he said with joy, "This is a book that can really save people". It can be seen that Zhang Zhongjing's theory has a great impact on Hua Tuo. Hua Tuo followed the paths pioneered by his predecessors to firmly create a new world. For example, he invented the external chest compression and mouth-to-mouth artificial respiration at that time. His most outstanding achievements should be the anesthesia, the invention of anesthesia powder taken with alcoholic drinks and the creation of sports therapy "Five-Animal Gymnastics". Some drugs with anesthesia properties were used as anesthesia before Hua Tuo, but they were used for war, assassination, execution, not for surgery. Hua Tuo summed up the experience in this field, observed the sleeping state of people when intoxicated, and invented the anesthesia powder taken with alcohol, which was officially used in medicine, thus greatly improving the technology and efficacy of surgery and expanding the scope of surgical treatment.

3. Medical allusions

In Luo Guanzhong's *Romance of the Three Kingdoms*, there is a story about Hua Tuo treating Guan Yu by bone scraping. The plot is that Guan Yu's right arm was injured by Wei army poison arrow during the Battle of Xiangyang. Later, the wound gradually enlarged and was very painful, causing Guan Yu unable to move. Hua Tuo scraped the bones of Guan Yu's arms to remove the toxicity on the bones, while Guan Yu remained his face unchanged while playing chess. This story not only celebrates the courage, perseverance and patience of Guan Yu, but also reflects the excellent medical skills of Hua Tuo, who has won praise and admiration from people. This is a fictional story widely spread among the people. It is partly based on the *Romance of the Three Kingdoms* and *Xiangyang Prefecture Annals in Hubei*.

In addition, Hua Tuo was good at applying psychotherapy to treat diseases. One governor was seriously ill and Hua Tuo went to see him. The governor asked Hua Tuo to treat him. Hua Tuo said to the governor's son, "Your father's disease is different from the general disease. There is congestion in his abdomen, so he should be irritated to vomit the congestion, so that he can be cured, otherwise he will die. Can you tell me everything wrong your father did? I would send a letter to rebuke him." The son said, "If it can cure my father's disease, I would tell you everything." So he told Hua Tuo all the unreasonable things his father had done for a long time. Hua Tuo wrote a letter scolding the governor. After the governor got the letter, he was angry and sent someone to arrest Hua Tuo. However, he didn't catch Hua Tuo. The governor spat out a lot of black blood due to the anger, and his illness was cured.

There is also a story about Cao Cao's intermittent headache. Hua Tuo was well-known for his rapid improvement in medical skills due to his effective learning. While Hua Tuo was enthusiastic about contributing his own exquisite medical skills to the common people, Cao Cao, a warlord rose in the turmoil of the Central Plains, heard and summoned him. It turned out that Cao Cao had been bothered by intermittent headache since his early years. The syndrome became more serious after he entered middle age. From time to time, he felt dizzy and unbearable headache, and the treatment of various TCM practitioners was of very little effect. After Hua Tuo came, he inserted a needle into the Geshu acupuncture point on Cao Cao's chest. After a while, Cao Cao started to feel eased, and the pain stopped immediately. Cao Cao was very happy, but Hua Tuo told the truth, "Your disease is a chronic brain disease, which is difficult to eradicate in a short time. It must be treated for a long time and gradually relieved to prolong life." Cao Cao listened, thought that Hua Tuo was using intrigues and tricks, so he was unhappy, but did not show it on his face. Later, Cao Cao suffered from headache several times and sent people to invite Hua Tuo. Hua Tuo always found an excuse to refuse, and Cao Cao killed him out of anger. Before Hua Tuo's death, he handed over a volume of medical books to a jail guard, hoping to pass on his lifelong experience of diagnosing diseases to later generations. Unfortunately, the jail guard burned the books for fear that he was involved into troubles.

4. Evaluation of later generations

According to the *Records of the Three Kingdoms*, "The medical diagnosis of Hua Tuo, the music of Du Kui, the physiognomy of Zhu Jianping, the dream explanation of Zhou Xuan, and the fortune telling skill of Guan Lu are all mysterious and ingenious skills. In the past, the legends of Bianque, Cang Gong and the fortune telling talents written by Sima Qian were to spread the strange news and things. Therefore, it is recorded here."

Hua Tuo is one of the few outstanding surgeons in the history of Chinese medicine. He takes it as his duty to rescue the people. His sense of social responsibility makes him practice medicine and save people without hesitation, fearless of power and ashamed to be an official. His excellent medical skills and noble medical ethics have made him popular among the people, and he is known as a "divine medical practitioner". He is good at using anesthesia, acupuncture and other methods, thinking in the shoes of patients, and has the medical ethics of respecting patients' opinions. In terms of health care, Hua Tuo invented the "Five-Animal Gymnastics" to raise people's awareness of disease prevention and control. Hua Tuo's qualities of fearlessness of power and dignity, valuing justice over interests, indifference to fame and fortune, sophistication and professionalism, and bold innovation, as well as the spirit of passing on lifelong medical experience to later generations and benefiting later generations before death, are all manifestations of good medical ethics.

2.2.2 Chunyu Yi

1. Brief biography

Chunyu Yi, born in Linzi (now Zibo, Shandong Province) in the early Western Han dynasty, is also known as Cang Gong because he once served as the head of capital warehouse. Chunyu Yi was skilled in medical doctrines, syndrome differentiation and pulse examination, and treatment of diseases. He once learned medicine from Gongsun Guang, *Yellow Emperor's Canon of Medicine* from Gongcheng Yangqing and pulse examination from Bianque. Later, he was sentenced for a crime, and his daughter Chunyu Tiying wrote to Emperor Wen of the Han dynasty that she was willing to be punished for his father, so he was exempted. In order to make himself professional in medicine, he resigned from the official position, did not operate businesses, and practiced medicine for a long time. Chunyu Yi paid attention to detailed records of medical cases when he diagnosed diseases, and sorted out typical cases, resulting in the first medical case book in the history of Chinese medicine—*Medical Cases (Zhen Ji)*. Due to his exquisite medical skills, noble medical ethics and pioneering contributions in medical history, Sima Qian established a biography for him in the *Records of the Historian*, and also recorded his 25 medical cases, which is the earliest existing medical history record in China.

Chunyu Yi was not only a famous medical scientist, but also an educator who was enthusiastic about spreading medical knowledge. He recruited many students and taught them meticulously. According to the *Records of the Historian: Biographies of Bianque and Cang Gong*, his students include Song Yi, Feng Xin, Tang An, Gao Qi, Wang Yu, Du Xin, etc. The first three were from Linzi. Bianque was the TCM practitioner with the largest number of students in the Qin and Han dynasties in the literature.

2. Medical allusions

Chunyu Yi was born in a poor family, and he liked reading medical books when he was young, but he had no curative effect at the beginning of treatment. Afterwards, he learned from Gongsun Guang, a famous TCM practitioner in Zichuan. Gongsun

Guang liked his modest character and willing to learn, so he taught him all his good prescriptions. Before long, Gongsun Guang found that he had nothing more to teach Chunyu Yi. He believed that Chunyu Yi would be a TCM practitioner with nationwide fame in the future. In order to allow Chunyu Yi to continue his further study, Gongsun Guang recommended him to learn from Gongcheng Yangqing. Gongcheng Yangqing, more than 70 years old, also appreciated the simplicity and progress of Chunyu Yi, so he explained all the secret and ancient prescriptions he collected to him. In the second year after Chunyu Yi graduated, he began to practice medicine. Three years later, he became a famous TCM practitioner. Chunyu Yi read classic medical books hard and could recite all the content. However, when diagnosing a patient, he would observe the actual condition of the patient, and not apply his knowledge rigidly. There was a health care TCM practitioner called Sui by the King of Qi state. He took the self-refined Wushi (Five Stones) Powder after getting sick, which aggravated his condition, so he invited Chunyu Yi. Chunyu Yi carefully examined his pulse and said, "You have internal heat, and the stone is the strongest medicine. Taking it will cause obstruction of urination and aggravate the condition. Do not take it again." He did not take it seriously, and retorted with examples: "Bianque once said, 'Yin stone can cure Yin disease, and Yang stone can cure Yang disease.'"Chunyu Yi smiled, "What you said is reasonable. Although Bianque said so, the patient's condition must be examined in detail, taking into consideration of the patient's general physical health, hobbies and condition of disease, so as to cure the disease." And Chunyu Yi predicted, if he fails to make a change, he will have carbuncle soon. Sure enough, more than a hundred days later, Sui had incurable carbuncle on his upper chest and died. This was a good reflection that Chunyu Yi studied flexibly and know how to vary treatment according to the syndrome.

According to the patient's condition, Chunyu Yi not only used medicine, but also adopted various physical therapies and acupuncture. When King Zichuan was ill, Chunyu Yi went to diagnose and felt his pulse. His illness was caused by falling asleep before drying the washed hair. The King got headache, fever, limb pain and upset, just like catching a cold in today's people's eyes. Chunyu Yi immediately applied ice water to the forehead of the King to help cool down, and applied needles on the three acupuncture points, namely Lidui, Xiangu and Fenglong on the Yangming Meridian to dissipate the heat on the muscle surface, and the disease was immediately cured. Putting ice bag or cold towel on the forehead of patient or wiping with alcohol is a commonly used physical cooling method for patients with high fever in modern times, but more than 2,000 years ago in the Han dynasty, it was an invention.

After being sentenced and pardoned, Chunyu Yi focused on medical treatment and used acupuncture and medicine, with remarkable efficacy. However, in the long-term medical practice, he also deeply felt that if the patient's condition and characteristics are not recorded, the medical practitioner can only rely on memory. If the medical practitioner's memory is inaccurate, it will affect the treatment effect and bring trouble to the patients. After long-term exploration and practice, Chunyu Yi came up with a good method. In the medical treatment, he recorded the patient's name, age, gender, occupation, place of origin, symptoms, name of disease, diagnosis, etiology, date of treatment, efficacy and outcome in detail, as well as the cured and dead cases in detail. Chunyu Yi called this record "medical cases". "Medical cases" not only greatly improves the curative effect, but also unintentionally preserves some of his medical academic thoughts, which is very beneficial to the inheritance and promotion of TCM theory in China. *The Records of the Historian: Biography of Bianque and Cang Gong* recorded 25 complete medical cases. Later, many TCM practitioners followed his example, and the "medical cases" gradually evolved into the "medical records" in modern times, and Chunyu Yi naturally became the founder of the medical records of TCM.

According to the records of "medical cases", it can be seen that Chunyu Yi practiced medicine all over Shandong, and cured diseases of King Jibei, King of Qi state and his grandson, the mansion chief of the imperial censor in the State of Qi, palace guards, talent recruiter, censor-in-chief, medium level minister, and the court physician of King of Qi state. When Liu Jianglu, King of Qi state, was the Marquis of Yangxu, Chunyu Yi cured a type of arthritis and diagnosed and treated hernia disease for Xiang Chu in Banli, Anling (now northeast Xianyang). It can be seen that Chunyu Yi treated many patients. In the eyes of Chunyu Yi, patients only have different diseases, and there is no difference in their status.

3. Medical ethics

In years of medical practice in different places, Chunyu Yi, like Bianque, has widely imparted his medical thoughts, experience and skills to others, without limiting the teaching of medical skills to an exclusive and narrow range according to the requirements of "no teaching others" put forward by his two teachers Gongsun Guang and Gongcheng Yangqing. He had many students and taught them in accordance with their aptitude. He cultivated Song Yi, Gao Qi, Wang Yu, Feng Xin, Du Xin, Tang An, and eunuchs and other people in the prime minister of Qi state. He was a TCM practitioner with the largest number of students in the Qin and Han dynasties according to historical records and an educator who was enthusiastic about spreading medicine.

What is valuable is that as a medical master, Chunyu Yi did not exaggerate his role as a TCM practitioner, but admit that he still has shortcomings and limitations. In response to the imperial court's edict that "can the treatment be always successful as it determines life and death", he frankly said, "The patients with defeated pulse cannot be cured, and those with obedient pulse can be cured... I cannot say that I make no mistakes." For some diseases, TCM practitioners cannot cure them.

Zhang Zhongjing, the medical sage, spoke highly of Chunyu Yi, and wrote in the preface to *Treatise on Febrile and Miscellaneous Diseases*: "In ancient times, there were great medical practitioners such as Shennong, Yellow Emperor, Qibo, Leigong, Shaoyu, Shaoshi and Zhongwen; in middle ages, there were Changsang and Bianque; in the Han dynasty, there were Gongcheng Yangqing and Cang Gong. After that, I have not heard such good medical practitioners." He compared Chunyu Yi with Yellow Emperor, Bianque and other famous TCM practitioners.

2.2.3　Zhang Zhongjing

1. Brief biography

Zhang Zhongjing, whose name is Ji and courtesy name is Zhongjing, was born in Nieyang County, Nanyang in the Eastern Han dynasty (now Zhangzhai Village, Rangdong Town, Dengzhou City, Henan Province). He was a famous medical scientist in the late Eastern Han dynasty, and was honored as the "medical sage" by later generations. He was one of the most outstanding medical scientists in China's history. His masterpiece, *Treatise on Febrile and Miscellaneous Diseases*, established the principles of syndrome differentiation and treatment of the Six Meridians, which is the basic principle of TCM clinical practice, the soul of TCM, and a must-read classic for later generations to study TCM.

The Eastern Han dynasty when Zhang Zhongjing lived was in great turmoil. The ruling class suffered from "the Disaster of Partisan Prohibitions" when relatives of the emperor, scholar-officials and eunuchs fought against each other. Warlords and the powerful also fought to take power in the Central Plains, and the peasant uprisings rose one after another. Countless people died on their way when escaping from the war. Zhang Zhongjing once had a large family with more than 200 members. Less than ten years since the beginning of Jian'an Period, two-thirds of them died of epidemics, of which seven out of ten died of cold pathogenic diseases. In the face of the plague and the corruption of the rulers, Zhang Zhongjing made up his mind to study the diagnosis and treatment of cold pathogenic diseases and subdue the plague. After traveling all over the country, he saw the serious consequences of various epidemic diseases on the people. He also took this opportunity to put his years of research on cold pathogenic diseases into practice, further enriched his own experience and improved his rational understanding. After decades of efforts, he finally wrote the *Treatise on Febrile and Miscellaneous Diseases*.

Cold pathogenic diseases are the general term for exogenous acute fever. *Plain Conversation: Discussion on Heat* records, "The fever today is a cold pathogenic disease." Based on this theory, Zhang Zhongjing analyzed the pathogenesis, places and features of cold pathogenic diseases at various stages, and established the syndrome differentiation system of cold pathogenic diseases. For various miscellaneous diseases, Zhang Zhongjing took the viscera meridians as the pivot for differentiation, and pioneered the viscera syndrome differentiation for later generations. There are 269 prescriptions and 214 kinds of medicines in the two books of *Treatise on Febrile and Miscellaneous Diseases* and the *Synopsis of the Golden Chamber*, which elaborate the processing and use of drugs, the compatibility and changes of prescriptions. Zhang Zhongjing's understanding of external fever and miscellaneous diseases and the guiding thoughts and methods of clinical syndrome treatment were summarized as syndrome differentiation and treatment systems by later generations. His achievements in pharmacy had a great impact on the development of later generations of medicine. *Treatise on Febrile and Miscellaneous Diseases* is a special book that collects the achievements of medical theories since the Qin and Han dynasties and is widely used in medical practice. It is one of the most influential classical medical works in the history of Chinese medicine and the first great work in clinical therapeutics in China.

According to historical records, Zhang Zhongjing's works include ten volumes of *Differentiation of Cold Pathogenic Diseases*, one volume of *Comments on Diseases, Medicines and Prescriptions*, two volumes of *Prescriptions for Women*, one volume of *On Five Internal Organs* and one volume of *On Mouth and Tooth*, but they have all been lost.

2. Medical allusions

The following is a story of suiting the remedy to the disease. Zhang Zhongjing was famous for his medical skills. He was also modest and learned from other TCM practitioners when possible. In the past, some TCM practitioners only passed on their medical skills to their descendants, and generally did not spread them to others. At that time, there was a famous TCM practitioner in Nanyang called Shen Huai, who was over 70 years old and had no descendants. He was so melancholy because of no successor that he was unable to eat and sleep, and slowly became ill. Local TCM practitioners came to see Shen Huai but no one could find out the old man's disease, and he was getting worse. After Zhang Zhongjing knew about it, he went to Shen Huai's house. Zhang Zhongjing checked the condition and confirmed that it was a disease caused by worries. He immediately prescribed a prescription, made pills with one jin of flour from each of the five grains and coarse grains, coated them with cinnabar, and asked the patient to take it. Shen Huai learned it, and he thought it was ridiculous. He ordered his family to hang the pills made of grain flour under the eaves, and pointed at the pills to everyone and ridiculed Zhang Zhongjing. When relatives came to see him, he smiled and said, "Look! This is the prescription given by Zhang Zhongjing. Did you see that the grains can cure illness? Such a joke! Joke!" When his peers came to see him, he smiled and said, "Look! This is the prescription given by Zhang Zhongjing. I've been a TCM practitioner for decades. I haven't heard of any prescription like that." All his mind was the ridiculousness of the matter. He put all his anxieties behind him, and he was relieved of his illness unconsciously.

A few days later, Zhang Zhongjing came to visit him and said, "Congratulations on your recovery! Forgive me for my boldness." Shen Huai suddenly understood his intention, and admired him and felt ashamed. Zhang Zhongjing continued, "Sir, we are medical practitioners to benefit the people and dispel diseases and prolong their life. You have no children, but aren't these young people like us just like your children? Why worry about the issue of successor?" Shen Huai heard it and felt very reasonable. He was very moved. Since then, he taught all his medical skills to Zhang Zhongjing and other young TCM practitioners.

3. Medical ethics

Zhang Zhongjing was originally an official, but he was able to stop his pursuit of official rank to study medicine, and despised those who "competing for prosperity, chasing the powerful, and diligently fishing fame and fortune". He was not only famous for his medical skills at that time, but also had quite strict requirements for TCM practitioners' medical ethics and medical style. He criticized those TCM practitioners who did not practice medical ethics and had bad medical practices.

Zhang Zhongjing is modest and cautious and advocates lifelong learning. He said, "Confucius said, those who are born to know are the best, followed by those who learn to know. I've learned a lot, and belong to the second most knowledgeable person. I always like medical skills, and I'll tell you everything." Zhang Zhongjing quotes Confucius as saying that he is not a genius and can only acquire knowledge by studying hard. He has shown that he loves medicine since he was a teenager and has studied it in a down-to-earth manner according to Confucius' words.

Zhang Zhongjing has also established a simple, unsophisticated, diligent and down-to-earth style of study for later generations. The writing style of *Treatise on Febrile and Miscellaneous Diseases* is simple and concise, and has no empty words, which has a great impact on TCM works in later generations. When he encountered the slightest doubt during diagnosing and studying, he would immediately "examine and test", and never let go of them.

4. Evaluation of later generations

Zhang Zhongjing is one of the most outstanding medical experts in the Chinese history. He has made important contributions to the development of Chinese medicine and promoted the development of Chinese medicine. The principle of syndrome differentiation and treatment established in his book *Treatise on Febrile and Miscellaneous Diseases* is the basic principle of TCM clinical practice and the soul of TCM. This book is also a necessary classic work for later scholars to study TCM. Zhang Zhongjing's medical theory has made great contributions to the development of ancient Chinese medicine, as well as to modern medical research. In addition, he also has a great influence on Southeast Asian countries. Later generations study his medical science, admire his medical skills and medical ethics, and call him "Medical

Sage". In Nanyang City, Henan Province, people built a "medical shrine" for him and a "Zhang Zhongjing Memorial Hall" to commemorate the medical scientist who laid the therapeutic foundation of TCM.

2.2.4　Guo Yu

1. Brief biography

Guo Yu, born in Guanghan Prefecture of the Eastern Han dynasty (now Guanghan City, Sichuan Province), with the courtesy name Zhitong, was the most famous medical expert during Emperor He of Han dynasty. When he was young, he learned medical skills from Cheng Gao. He was the deputy imperial medical head during Emperor He of Han dynasty with sound medical skills and good medical ethics.

Guo Yu's master's teacher was a legendary medical scientist named Fu Weng. Like Jiang Ziya, Fu Weng fished on Fujiang River every day and led the life of a recluse. Fu Weng was a recluse who knows well the technique of medicine. He was good at treating diseases with acupuncture and moxibustion with immediate effect. Fu Weng also wrote medical books, such as *Acupuncture Classic and Pulse Diagnose Method* (both have been lost). Fu Weng had an outstanding apprentice named Cheng Gao, and Guo Yu was the apprentice of Cheng Gao. Under the earnest guidance of his master, Guo Yu got the essence of Fu Weng's teaching, and was proficient in pulse diagnosis and acupuncture.

2. Medical ethics

In the Emperor He of Eastern Han dynasty, Guo Yu served as the deputy imperial medical head, who felt the pulse to diagnose the disease very accurately. He treated the patient with acupuncture with very good effect. Emperor He appreciated his excellent medical skills and wanted to check Guo Yu's medical skills in person. Therefore, the Emperor He asked a man with delicate skin to put his wrist with a maid, and ordered someone to separate Guo Yu with a curtain, let him feel the pulse and ask what disease she has. After feeling the pulses, Guo Yu judged that it was not a same person's pulse, and told Emperor He. The emperor admired Guo Yu after listening to it, thinking his medical skills were indeed good. Guo Yu not only has excellent medical skills, but also speaks frankly and seeks truth from facts, which is the embodiment of his good medical ethics.

Guo Yu had excellent medical skills and was kind to patients. He was not arrogant. He said, "For those poor patients, I must do my best." However, when he was treating high officials and nobles, the effect was not good, so Emperor He visited him to find the reason. Emperor He asked several sick officials and nobles to put on the clothes of the poor and dress up as poor people to see Guo Yu. As a result, Guo Yu cured them with a single acupuncture. The Emperor asked Guo Yu why the acupuncture effects were different. He said, "When the nobles come to see me, I was nervous to diagnose them. There are four dilemmas in their cure. First is that they feel good for themselves and do not trust me. The second is that they are careless about their body. The third is that they have weak bones and cannot take many medicines. The fourth is that they are indolent and hate labor. With the mind of fear and cautiousness, I cannot do my best to cure the patient." Guo Yu believed that there were reasons in both TCM practitioners and patients for the poor therapeutic effects. Those dignitaries had good life, indolence, and poor physical fitness. However, TCM practitioners often use needles with different depth, which would be insufficient or excessive for different patients. Coupled with fear, the TCM practitioners would be prudent and cautious in the treatment. Therefore, in the fear of the high officials, TCM practitioners cannot exert their medical skills, and lead to bad treatment effect. After hearing what he said, the emperor praised him. Guo Yu's discussion correctly estimated the adverse effects of the life and thoughts of the nobles in the Eastern Han dynasty on the diagnosis and treatment of diseases, and also scientifically revealed the psychological obstacles existing in the diagnosis and treatment of patients with different social status.

Guo Yu is another TCM practitioner who has researched the social and psychological aspects of medical care after Bianque. Guo Yu's medical skills, medical ethics and contributions to acupuncture and diagnosis were admired by the imperial court and later died during his time in office.

2.2.5 Hu Gong

1. Brief biography

Hu Gong, whose name is not known, is also known as Xuanhuzi and Xuanhuweng. According to some records, "Hu Gong's name is Xie Yuan. He was a native of Liyang who sold medicine in the market. He allowed no bargaining and cured all his patients. He spoke to others that taking his medicine will make the patient vomit something and recover some day. Everything turned out to be true. He earned tens of thousands of coins a day, and gave the money to the poor and the hungry." It can be seen that Hu Gong is a hermit with medical skills and kindness. Since he often hung a pot as a medical sign when he diagnosed illness and sold medicine, he is called Hu Gong. There are many myths about him in folklore.

2. Medical allusions

The allusion of "hanging pot" comes from Fan Ye's *Book of the Later Han Dynasty* in the Northern and Southern dynasties and Ge Hong's *Legend of Immortals* in the Jin dynasty. There is an unknown old man hanging a pot selling medicine in the market. People call him Hu Gong ("Hu" means pot and "Gong" is a respectful term for elder male in Chinese language). The characteristic of Hu Gong selling medicine is never accepting counter offer. After diagnosing and dispensing medicine, Hu Gong often explains to the patient that "if you take this medicine, you will vomit something, and get healed on some day". Hu Gong's medicine is effective, and he could sell it for tens of thousands of copper coins a day, but he uses the money for the poor and hungry in city, leaving only 30 to 50 coins for himself. Hu Gong often hangs an empty pot on the roof. The story of "hanging pot" has been passed down, and "hanging pot to save the mass" has also become a synonym for "medical ethics and benevolence" in Chinese medicine. Today, when doctors opened their clinics, people would congratulate them with the saying "hanging pot to save the mass".

3. Medical ethics

Hu Gong is a hermit and famous TCM practitioner with exquisite medical skills in the Qin and Han dynasties. His erratic image is just a true portrayal of the uniqueness of ancient TCM practitioners. Hu Gong's magical medical skills, the honest quality and affordable prices for medicine, and the kindness are all his embodiment of medical ethics as a TCM practitioner.

2.2.6　Su Dan

1. Brief biography

According to legend, at the end of the Western Han dynasty, there was a person named Su Dan, with the courtesy name of Zi'an. Su Dan was talented and clever. He started to learn literature at five and learnt swords at seven. He became proficient in astronomy and geography when he grew up and was determined to fight evil for the world. At the end of the Western Han dynasty, the continuous war lasted for several years, the plague spread, the people suffered. Su Dan could not fulfill his ambition and was very worried. He heard that there was a Taoist immortal living in seclusion in Dasu Mountain. His Taoist name was Master Chaoyang, and his spiritual power was boundless. After telling his mother, he went all over the green mountains to find Master Chaoyang to be his student.

2. Medical allusions

Su Dan visited Master Chaoyang, got several pills and took them home. According to Master Chaoyang's instructions, he put the pius into water for people to take, and relieved the plague. After that, he quit his home and went up the mountain to learn immortal arts. Before the trip, he told his mother that there would be a great plague in the county two years later, and instructed her mother to teach people to plant orange trees and drill wells, and boil orange leaves with well water for drinking, which can treat the plague. Later, a plague broke out and spread in all adjacent regions. His mother treated the infected with the method of Su Dan, and the plague was quelled. The story was passed down to later generations as the allusion of "Orange Well Spring Fragrance".

Later, it is said that after his mother died, Su Dan performed filial piety for his mother. Dozens of yellow cranes flew to his home. After Su Dan knelt and bowed three time before his mother's tombstone, he climbed over the rock in front of the gate and went up to the back of the crane. He became an immortal, leaving only deep footprints on the rock, which still exist today. Later, people missed Su Dan and called the stone "the Stone Where Su Became an Immortal" and the cave where Master Chaoyang lived on Dasu Mountain was called "Chaoyang Cave".

Wang Wei, a poet of the Tang dynasty, wrote in his poem "*Send Master Fang Back to Songshan Mountain*": "I ask the two white cranes, they told me they had sent Su Dan to Songshan Mountain."

2.2.7　Han Kang

1. Brief biography

Han Kang, whose courtesy name was Boxiu or Tianxiu, was born in Baling,

Jingzhao (now Xi'an, Shaanxi Province). He came from a prestigious family, but he did not admire fame and fortune. He devoted himself to the pharmaceutical industry. He picked herbs from famous mountains and sold them in Chang'an market but he never change the price for more than 30 years. He did it to show that credit is paramount, and the drugs sold are genuine.

2. Medical allusions

Han Kang sold medicines in the market with fixed prices. Some woman bargained when they bought medicines from Han Kang. Han Kang kept the price unchanged. The woman said angrily, "Why do you allow no bargain? Are you Han Boxiu?" Han Kang sighed, "I wanted to be anonymous. Now everyone knows my name." Then he went into Baling Mountain for seclusion.

Later, the imperial court knew the knowledge and talent of Han Kang and titled him Boshi (learned scholar). The Emperor Heng of Han sent his envoys to Han Kang's house with imperial edicts. He had no choice but to agree. But instead of taking the court's carriage, he took his own ox cart. He drove first before dawn to a place. The police inspector was building roads and bridges with manpower and domestic animals. Seeing Han Kang's appearance, he thought he was a farmer, so he asked someone to take his ox. After the imperial envoy arrived, he saw that Han Kang's ox was snatched, so he wanted to put the inspector to death. Han Kang said it was his fault. He couldn't blame the inspector. Then he fled eastward into Baling Mountain and then lived in seclusion till his death.

Han Kang sold medicine with fixed prices for 30 years, which reflected his integrity and medical ethics. His noble character of not admiring fame and fortune and not willing to serve feudal rulers also reflected his honest nature.

2.3   Medical Education

The medical system of the Qin dynasty followed the blueprint of the Qin State in the Spring and Autumn Period and the Warring States Period. The medical level from the state to the local area was more distinct and the system was more rigorous. The books of medicine were not burned, which not only protects medicine and TCM practitioners, but also shows the world that the state attaches great importance to medicine. Burning books and burying Confucius scholars prompted more scholars to switch to medicine, which objectively promoted the development of medicine. In the early Western Han dynasty, the active and steady policies of recuperation were adopted, which made the national economy develop steadily and medical education develop fully.

During this period, TCM practitioners usually studied in government or private schools, and then passed the probation system, so that their talents could be recognized and played a role. Many official TCM practitioners in the Han dynasty were from Imperial College. Imperial College was the main place for the generation of official TCM practitioners in the Han dynasty. However, due to the limitation of people receiving education, many talents with great potential had lost opportunity, and the groups receiving education were very limited. Private education played an active role in supplementing and promoting the education of more people, including medical education, which had made the development of medical undertakings increasingly perfect.

Chapter Summary

In the Qin and Han dynasties, the unity of the state and the consistency of ideology accelerated the formation of the medical ethics system. The medical ethics in this period was mainly reflected in two aspects: the tendency and practice of official medical ethics, and the consciousness and practice of medical ethics of TCM practitioners.

In the Qin and Han dynasties, the medical ethics principle of "life first, practicing benevolence and saving people" was also established; many medical ethics norms to realize the medical ethics principle of "practicing benevolence and saving people" were put forward; the medical ethics education thought of "teaching the right people" was formed.

In this period, medical thoughts and medical ethics penetrated each other. Medical thoughts contained medical ethics, and medical ethics contained medical thoughts.

Application in Contemporary Times

1. The thought of "benevolence" is conducive to the establishment of the basic thought of medical ethics

This chapter tells the general situation of medical ethics in Qin and Han dynasties. The core value of China feudal society is "benevolence", which has a great influence on the medical ethics. Therefore, "practicing benevolence and saving people" became the core content and basic principles of ancient medical ethics in China. Physicians call medical skills "benevolent skills". The purpose of medicine is to "help the world and save people", and TCM practitioners should be "benevolent people". All later generations of TCM practitioners should regard the high spirit of benevolence as the basic virtues that they must possess. Starting from the moral concept of "practicing benevolence and saving people", it is very valuable to emphasize the excellent medical ethics and practices of treating patients equally, universally, fearless of hardship and dedicated to saving.

Medical students and medical workers should keep in mind the moral concept of "benevolence and saving people", and never forget the ancient precepts of "human life is paramount, as precious as countless gold" and "medicine is a benevolent skill". In the construction and development of Chinese medical ethics, we should inherit the foundation of Chinese traditional medical ethics and serve the construction and development of socialist medical ethics.

2. The emotional view of "providing liberal relief to the poor" is conducive to the improvement of doctor-patient relationship

All the medical representatives studied in this chapter take medical treatment as their ideal personality pursuit. In medical practice, they helped the poor and did not seek money, and also worked seriously and did not involve in dishonest practices. During the Three Kingdoms period, Dong Feng, a famous TCM practitioner in Jiangxi, had the story of "apricot forest in the warm spring", which was passed down to today. This noble medical ethics and practices have been eulogized for generations. Hua Tuo, a famous TCM practitioner in the Eastern Han dynasty, had excellent medical skills. The imperial court repeatedly recruited him to be an official, but he refused. This kind of dedication spirit of fearless against power, not pursuing fame and fortune, not caring for gains and losses, and live up to the spirit of medical practitioners has set an example for ancient and modern TCM practitioners.

Doctor-patient relationship is the relationship based on the trust of patients to TCM practitioners. The majority of medical students and medical workers need to start from the true feelings of patients and pay attention to the situation and experience of patients in the shoes of patients during the medical practice, so as to promote the development of harmonious doctor-patient relationship.

Medical Ethics Culture in the Wei, Jin, Southern and Northern Dynasties

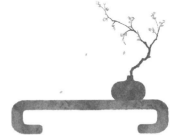

3.1 Overview of Medical Ethics

3.1.1 Social Background of Medical Ethics

The Wei, Jin and Northern and Southern dynasties were a period with the most frequent shifts of regimes in Chinese history, a period from "great governance" to "great chaos", including the Three Kingdoms, the Jin and Southern and Northern dynasties. From Cao Pi's establishment of the Wei after the Han dynasty in 220 AD to Emperor Wen of the Sui dynasty's overthrow of Chen and unification of the whole country in 589 AD, China was in a period of great chaos. It took 369 years in total for the division and unity, the nomadic people to invade the Central Plains and the residents of the Central Plains to move southward. During this period, the Han and nomadic peoples successively established multiple regimes in the north, and fight each other, while the south entered a relatively stable development stage. Due to long-term feudalism and continuous wars, class conflicts and national conflicts were very sharp and complex, which had a profound impact on politics, economy, culture, social thoughts, science and technology and other fields.

1. Influence of political environment

At the end of the Eastern Han dynasty, warlords fought in chaos, and the Central Plains dynasty gradually lost power. Since Cao Pi abandoned the Han dynasty and established the Wei dynasty in 220 AD, the Western Jin dynasty was the only dynasty that realized the temporary unity of the whole country. Other dynasties were basically in a state of division, and the whole society moved forward in turbulence. The social turmoil forced a large number of people in the north to migrate southward, and millions of nomadic people also invaded the Central Plains with the chaos of war. According to the *Book of Jin*, "Central Plains was in turmoil recently, the wars continued for years. Sometimes, there was great defeat leading to the killing of the whole army. Ninety percent of families lost their men." People lost their ability to resist disasters due to years of warfare. Wars and natural disasters left the people displaced and unable to settle. With years of war, the medical treatment of war injuries began to develop, and clinical experience and technology were continuously accumulated and improved.

2. Impact of ecological environment

From the end of the Eastern Han dynasty to the beginning of the Sui dynasty, the abnormal climate and serious natural disasters in China frequently caused epidemic diseases, resulting in a sharp decline in the population. Mr. Zhu Kezhen believes that the basic feature of China's climate during the Wei, Jin, Southern and Northern dynasties is cold. According to Qin Dongmei, "The climate in the Western Han dynasty was relatively warm, and changed from warm to cold between the two Han dynasties. After that, the temperature rose again, but became relatively cold in the Wei, Jin, Southern and Northern dynasties. One of the characteristics of the climate anomalies in the Wei, Jin, Southern and Northern dynasties was cooling. The main manifestations were an increase in the number of cold events and an increase in the frequency of extreme cold events. Another prominent manifestation of climate anomalies during the Wei, Jin, Southern and Northern dynasties was the change of climate from humidity to dryness." Mei Li and Yan Changgui pointed out: "Excessively cold climate can contract the mucosa of the upper respiratory tract, reduce the secretion of immune substances, reduce the ability to defend against diseases, and provide conditions for the invasion of pathogens. In winter, the room temperature is high with no smooth indoor air circulation, which is more conducive to the survival and infection of pathogens, so it is prone to infectious diseases." Therefore, during this period, there were frequent and wide epidemic outbreaks. In addition, the epidemics were very serious with high fatality rate.

In addition to the epidemic caused by abnormal climate, natural disasters at that time also frequently caused epidemic diseases. Mr. Deng Yunte believes, "The Three Kingdoms inherited the exhaustion of the Eastern Han dynasty, and the number of disasters had increased without abatement. During the two Jin dynasties, the situation was even worse. In the whole Wei and Jin dynasties, there were fierce disasters between the Yellow River and the Yangtze River in successive years, rarely stopping for one year. In all, there were 304 disasters in 200 years. Its frequency was much higher than that of the previous dynasties. Earthquakes, floods, droughts, winds, hail, locust, frost and snow, and epidemics all come in succession. The drought was recorded in history books for 60 times in 200 years, and the flood was recorded for 56 times during the same period. As for the wind disaster, there were 54 times in total; followed by earthquakes of 53 times in total with a high frequency; and hail disaster of 35 times in total. In addition, there were 17 epidemics; 14 locust plagues; and 13 poor yield and famines. For others, there were two frost and snow and 'ground boiling', which was not comparable to the former ones. At that time, the extent of the disaster was no less than, or even more than that of the previous generation." According to some historical records, there were at least ten outbreaks of famine during this period.

Whether due to climatic factors or natural disasters, the outbreak of epidemic diseases has prompted physcans to summarize the research and treatment methods of epidemic diseases in this period to a certain extent, and medicine has been developed.

3. Influence of social ideological trends

With the collapse of the system of the Eastern Han dynasty, the dominant position of Confucianism was greatly impacted, its influence was continuously weakened, and the Taoist re-emerged. In the Wei, Jin, Southern and Northern dynasties, Confucianism, Taoism and Buddhist thoughts of ancient India introduced through the Western Regions were intertwined, resulting in metaphysical thoughts prevailing in the whole era.

Metaphysics became the manifestation of this era, and then influenced the social atmosphere at that time. In the upper society, people had the hobby of talking of mystery and metaphysics; in the lower society, the Taoist mystic techniques were also widely accepted by the people. And metaphysics thought also brought profound influence to the TCM practitioners of this period. In Taoist thoughts, learning and practicing medicine was a matter of virtue and meritorious service. Therefore, people who believed in Taoism would also practice medicine and save people, so that medicine and Taoism can be integrated and complement each other. For example, Ge Hong of the Wei and Jin dynasties, who came from a scholar family of the South of Yangtze River, was deeply influenced by Taoism and wrote many books throughout his life. He was not only a Confucian-Taoist theorist, but also a medical master who saved a lot of people. Tao Hongjing, who resigned and lived in seclusion during the Qi and Liang dynasties of the Southern dynasties, was also good at medicine and health preservation.

4. Impact of scientific and technological development

During the Wei, Jin, Southern and Northern dynasties, science and technology have also developed and advanced to a certain extent due to the emancipation of ideas and the diversity of culture. Liu Hui, Zu Chongzhi, He Chengtian, Pei Xiu, Li

Daoyuan, Jia Sixie, Ma Jun, Ge Hong, Tao Hongjing and other scientists were all born in this era. They have made great contributions to the development of science and technology such as ancient mathematics, astronomy and calendar, geography, cartography, agronomy, mechanical invention and medicine.

Liu Hui, a mathematician in the Wei and Jin dynasties, put forward "Liu Hui's π algorithm" and used it to calculate π. He was one of the founders of Chinese classical mathematical theory. Zu Chongzhi, a mathematician and scientist of the Southern dynasties, further calculated π accurately, and was the first scientist in the world to calculate π to the 7th decimal place. Pei Xiu of the Western Jin dynasty drew the Regional Maps of Yugong, and put forward the principle of "Six Principles of Mapping", which clarified the relationship of scale, orientation and distance in mapping, and had a profound impact on the development of mapping technology. In the Northern Wei dynasty, Li Daoyuan wrote the *Water Classics Commentary*, which records more than 1,000 rivers and related historical sites, anecdotes of historical figures, myths and legends in China. It is the most all-round and systematic comprehensive geography monograph in ancient China. It also records some inscriptions and fishing songs, so it also has certain literary value. Wang Shuhe compiled two books, *Treatise on Febrile and Miscellaneous Diseases* and the *Synopsis of the Golden Chamber*, which have made important contributions to the specific treatment and theory of infectious diseases and various miscellaneous diseases. Wang Shuhe's *Pulse Classic*, Huangfu Mi's *Canon of Acupuncture and Moxibustion*, and Tao Hongjing's *Annotations of Shennong's Herbal Classic* are all of great significance to the development of TCM pharmacy. In order to meet the needs of war, production and life, the mechanical technology in Wei, Jin and Northern and Southern dynasties was further developed, and a number of mechanical inventors such as Ma Jun, Du Yu and Geng Xun emerged. In terms of agronomic achievements, *Important Methods to Condition the People's Living (Qimin Yaoshu)*, a comprehensive agricultural book written by Jia Sixie, an agronomist in the Northern Wei dynasty, was the first to be introduced. The cultivation methods of various crops, the growth rules of economic trees, and how to use wild plants are recorded in detail in *Qimin Yaoshu*, which is of great significance to agricultural research.

In general, the Wei, Jin and Southern and Northern dynasties were not only an era of long-term division and confrontation between the north and the south, but also an era of unprecedented national integration. It was not only an era of ideological emancipation and cultural diversity, but also an era of connecting the past and the future and occupying a special position in history.

3.1.2 Main Contents of Medical Ethics Culture

During the Wei, Jin, Southern and Northern dynasties, famous TCM practitioners such as Dong Feng, Wang Shuhe, Huangfu Mi, Ge Hong, Tao Hongjing, Yao Sengyuan and Chu Cheng emerged. Adhering to the "practicing benevolence", they further improved and expanded the TCM on the basis of inheriting the predecessors and medical skills. In addition, the medical ethics in this period was deeply influenced by Confucianism, Buddhism and Taoism. In the practice of medical treatment, TCM practitioners took the humanitarian spirit of "helping the world and saving people" as the starting point, aimed at saving human life, and made the "exquisite of evidence" as the medical ethics and norms, reflecting the noble feelings of TCM practitioners in medical practice. The medical ethics culture in this period is mainly reflected in the following four aspects.

1. Advocating medical science, saving patients

During the Wei and Jin dynasties, the influence of Confucianism on TCM practitioners' moral concepts became deeper. During this period, famous TCM practitioners such as Wang Shuhe, Huangfu Mi, Ge Hong and Tao Hongjing emerged successively. In turbulent times, they were determined to practice medicine, took the responsibility of helping the world and saving people in medical practice, reflecting the sense of "benevolence". Ge Hong put forward the concept of health preservation and medical ethics; Yang Quan first put forward the conditions that medical practitioners should have, emphasizing the importance of morality; Chu Cheng put forward medical practice norms in combination with medical practice; Tao Hongjing put forward the positive and enterprising concept of life of "cultivating nature and dominating one's own life". From the whole view of medical ethics, the concept of "benevolence" as the core is increasingly emerging.

2. Focus on medical ethics and be rigorous and responsible

Although Wang Shuhe was in a social environment advocating metaphysics and impractical talk, he could be immune from the effect of metaphysics, but focused on medicine, sorted out *Treatise on Febrile and Miscellaneous Diseases*, made it more suitable for clinical application, and wrote the *Pulse Classic* combing his own clinical experience. He pointed out in the preface of the *Pulse Classic* that TCM practitioners should pay attention to the physical factors of patients when diagnosing pulse, and should be rigorous and cautious, because he believed that "the pulse is delicate and it is difficult to distinguish" and a slight carelessness would lead to medical accidents. Therefore, in the review of the diseases, it requires TCM practitioners to "examine for testing whenever there is doubt". In the era of metaphysics, Wang Shuhe's rigorous and responsible attitude focusing only on medicine embodied his humanistic spirit of advocating medicine.

3. Indifferent to fame and fortune, learning from hundreds of schools

During the Wei and Jin dynasties, Huangfu Mi, who was diligent and devoted to farming and studying, reached the peak of his contemporary era in literature, history, philosophy, medicine and other aspects. He not only compiled *Canon of Acupuncture and Moxibustion*, but also wrote many literary and historical works such as *The Imperial Lineage, Annals, Noble Characters, Virtuous Characters and Annals of Feudal Ethic Code*. Wen Changlu commented that he was "a typical comprehensive scholar with all-round knowledge". He refused to be employed by the imperial court four times, did not serve the court throughout his life and took writing books as his career.

In the Jin dynasty, Ge Hong was once honored as Marquis of Guannei and later lived in seclusion in Luofu Mountain. He had read nearly 10,000 volumes of books from classics to articles. He wrote *The Emergency Prescriptions Kept in One's Sleeve* for the purpose that "the mortals can see it and use it".

Tao Hongjing, who studied hard since childhood, was a famous scholar with profound knowledge in Confucianism, Taoism and Buddhism. In the spirit of medical humanity, he was determined to save the people from diseases. At the age of 36, he resigned and lived in seclusion in Maoshan Mountain. In order to solve the problem of no medical treatment in poor and remote areas, he compiled the *Annotations to Shennong's Herbal Classic*.

4. Exquisite examination and life first

Chu Cheng, author of *Chu's Manuscripts* in the Southern Qi dynasty, believes that for TCM practitioners, exquisite examination is not only a professional requirement, but also a responsibility. Only by the "four diagnoses" of observing, smelling, inquiring and palpating, and carefully identifying the symptoms and mechanisms of the diseases can they treat the diseases accordingly. Chu Cheng stressed, "A small difference would lead to the damage to life." Every behavior of the TCM practitioner is related to the life of the patient and must be cautious.

During this period, based on the achievements of former scholars, TCM practitioners not only sorted out and wrote various classical works, but also developed various departments within medicine. They also combined the principles and norms of medical ethics with medical methods and skills, which has made medical ethics more implementable and improved the practice of medical ethics by TCM practitioners.

3.1.3　Characteristics of Medical Ethics Culture

On the one hand, TCM practitioners in the Wei, Jin, Southern and Northern dynasties were influenced by metaphysical thoughts, on the other hand, the characteristics of TCM practitioners' medical ethics were gradually revealed.

1. Cultivating Taoism to lengthen life and accumulate virtue in medical practice

Most of the TCM practitioners in this period were influenced by Taoist thoughts, and most of the pill-makers were TCM practitioners, who combined the realization of their own life value with the study of medicine.

Ge Hong advocated the combination of Taoism and medical practice. He said in the *Main Chapter of Bao Pu Zi*: "If you do not practice virtue in medicine, you cannot lengthen your life." If you don't learn medical skills, you may not be able to diagnose and treat yourself once you get sick. You cannot lengthen your life, even cannot save your own life. Therefore, he believes that learning medicine is the prerequisite for immortality. At the same time, he also stressed: "The Taoist saves people from dangers and disasters, protects people from diseases, and keeps people away from disease-led death." This reflects his belief that practicing medicine is an important way for Taoist to accumulate virtue. For the practice of medicine itself, he also practiced the "benevolence" as a TCM practitioner in the medical rescue out of compassion and care for life.

2. Practice medical filial piety and promote morality through medical treatment

Throughout the Chinese history, the moral code of "being kind to parents" is an important manifestation of filial piety. In the Wei, Jin, Southern and Northern dynasties, studying medicine is also one of the ways to show filial piety.

Huangfu Mi once said, "People are born to have a body of eight feet. If they do not know about medicine, they can be called wandering soul. If you are not good at medicine, although you have the loyalty and filial piety and kindness, there is no way to help your father and your son in danger. This is what the sages tell us and is extremely right." Huangfu Mi believes that if you don't understand medicine, even if you have the loyalty and filial piety and kindness, how can you be regarded as filial piety when your parents are ill and painful and you can't do anything to help them? From Huangfu Mi's concept of medical practice, we can clearly understand the value and the importance of filial piety in medical practice.

3. Emphasize moral cultivation

Medical ethics cultivation is the essential moral qualities of TCM practitioners. In the traditional concept of TCM practitioners, moral cultivation plays a very important role and is the basic premise directly related to the ability to learn medicine and master medical knowledge. In the Jin dynasty, Yang Quan first clearly put forward the moral cultivation standard of "benevolence, wisdom and integrity". Yang Quan believed that as a TCM practitioner, if he was not a kind and loving person, he could not be entrusted; if he was not a smart and reasonable person, he could not be appointed; if he was not an integrated and kind person, he could not be trusted. This emphasizes the need for moral accomplishment as a medical practitioner.

4. Transition from "Benevolent Man" to "Good Medical Practitioner"

According to traditional medical ethics, we often describe sophisticated TCM practitioners with noble medical ethics as "miracle-working TCM practitioners", "commonly respected TCM practitioners", "immortal TCM practitioners" and "famous TCM practitioners". These evaluations are more than the identity of "TCM practitioners" but exemplify "humans". In the Western Jin dynasty, Yang Quan clearly put forward the concept of "good TCM practitioner" and said in his book *Theory of Things*: "As a medical practitioner in ancient times, he must be selected from a famous family with virtues of forgiveness and fraternity, and intelligence to understand difficult things; so as to know heaven, earth, gods, and lives; differentiate symptoms, know the direction, understand the severity, and determine the amount of the medicine. They can understand the most trivial things in medical practice and never get lost in details. This is called a good TCM practitioner." From the quality of "good TCM practitioner" in his words, we can see that good TCM practitioner is no longer related to the value pursuit beyond the identity of TCM practitioner, but is understood from the medical activities of practitioners themselves. The traditional medical ethics began to change from "physician's morality" to "medical ethics".

3.2 Representative Medical Practitioners and Their Medical Ethics

3.2.1 Dong Feng

1. Brief biography

Dong Feng had the same reputation as Zhang Zhongjing in Nanyang and Hua Tuo in Qiao County. The three were called "Three Divine Medical Practitioners in Jian'an Period". Dong Feng practiced Taoism and medicine in Lushan Mountain and helped the people. With superb medical skills and selfless dedication, he won people's heartfelt love. Taoism respected him as "immortal" and "master", and people respected him as "Great Doctor of the Mass" and "Jian'an Immortal Doctor". Emperor Hui of Song dynasty conferred the title of "Shengyuan Zhenjun" on Dong Feng, and people in Jin dynasty, Southern Tang dynasty, Northern Song dynasty and other dynasties all constructed "Taiyi Taoist Temple" for Dong Feng. Dong Feng was born in the late Eastern Han dynasty and witnessed the social turmoil and the hardships and sufferings of the people. Therefore, he had been committed to studying medicine since childhood and to saving the people from suffering. After years of hard work, he finally achieved study success, and was famous for his noble medical ethics and exquisite medical skills, resulting in an endless stream of patients.

2. Medical ethics

According to the *Biography of the Immortals* written by Ge Hong, "Shi Xie was dying of toxin, and Dong Feng was there. He prescribed three pills of oral medicine for Shi Xie with water, and let others held his head up to swallow the pills. After a while, his hands and feet seemed to move, and the color of the face gradually recovered. He could sit up in half a day, and could speak in the next four days."

The special article for Dong Feng in the *Legend of Immortals* highly affirmed

Dong Feng's medical ethics, "He lived in the mountains and treated diseases, but he did not take money and other benefits. If patients with serious disease were cured, he would ask them to plant five apricot trees, and if the disease is mild, he would ask one apricot tree be planted. After so many years, more than 100,000 apricot trees have been planted to form a forest." Dong Feng never received money for the cure of diseases. He never received gifts from those with serious illness, and only asked them to plant one to five apricots according to the severity of their diseases. A few years later, there were more than 100,000 apricot trees, forming an apricot forest. According to the different effects of apricot flowers, leaves, roots, barks, fruits and cores, he picked leaves and flowers to prepare medicine, cores to relieve cough and reduce phlegm, and roots and barks to connect bones and dispel rheumatism. After the apricot trees bear fruit in autumn, he picked fruits and made them dry for food, and exchanged fruits for grains to relieve the poor. Later generations praised Dong Feng's noble medical ethics and exquisite medical skills with "apricot forest in the warm spring" and "famous apricot forest". The famous "apricot forest" also came from this story, and Dong Feng's residence was also known as "apricot altar" by later generations.

The above records all reflect the noble medical ethics of Dong Feng. The spirit of selfless dedication, great love and fraternity of Dong Feng has sublimated with the development of TCM and become the main theme of traditional Chinese medical ethics.

3.2.2　Wang Shuhe

1. Brief biography

Wang Shuhe, with the name Xi, was born in Gaoping, Shanyang (now Zoucheng, Shandong Province), during the Wei and Jin dynasties. According to *Theory of Health Preservation*, he "specialized in the left texts, collected group theories, compiled ten volumes of *Pulse Classics*, and compiled thirty-six volumes of *On Zhang Zhongjing's Prescriptions*, which were spread widely in the world". According to the *Biography of Famous Doctors*, he "was calm in nature, knew classics and histories, thoroughly studied prescriptions and pulses, carefully diagnosed and understood the way of nourishing and health preservation, and had a deep understanding of treating illness". These two medical achievements of Wang Shuhe give him a special place in Chinese medical history.

2. Medical ethics

(1) Exquisite research on classics.

During the Wei and Jin dynasties, metaphysics and religious thoughts were in full swing. It was prevalent to have unpractical talks and take stone medicines. Wang Shuhe served as the head of imperial TCM practitioners, and worked together with the scholars and officials, but he was not affected by metaphysics and did not follow the unpractical talks. Instead, he studied medicine hard and advocated practice, which was valuable.

During the Wei and Jin dynasties, the society was turbulent. Zhang Zhongjing's *Treatise on Febrile and Miscellaneous Diseases* was lost due to wars. Wang Shuhe, as the head of imperial TCM practitioners, tried his best to collect, sort out and edit it, and supplemented it with his own achievements in medical research, as well as his own academic opinions to compile the book which was passed down to today, making great contributions to the development of TCM. At the beginning of the Ming dynasty, Wang Andao commented, "Wang Shuhe collected the scattered chapters of the old theories of Zhang Zhongjing, which is a great contribution." Lü Zhenming of the Qing dynasty also said in *Searching for the Sources of Treatise on the Cold Pathogenic and Miscellaneous Diseases*: "The contribution of Wang Shuhe to the book circulation is indispensable."

(2) Study the *Pulse Classics* carefully.

Wang Shuhe once commented on pulse theory, "The pulse is delicate, and is difficult to distinguish." He deeply felt the importance of pulse theory in clinical diagnosis. If the conditions of some pulses are not carefully distinguished and carefully studied, they will lead to misdiagnosis and even serious consequences.

Before the Western Jin dynasty, although some medical achievements about pulse studies were inherited by TCM practitioners in the past dynasties, the materials were complicated and disordered, and the contents were not consistent, and not conducive to the study and mastery of TCM practitioners. On the basis of the medical achievements of predecessors, Wang Shuhe learned from others and studied the prescriptions, thus summarizing 24 pulses and writing the *Pulse Classics*. Wang Shuhe's *Pulse Classics* not only collected and sorted out the materials of sphygmology at that time, but also summarized them systematically. It is a book that integrates the achievements of previous sphygmology and plays a conclusive role in sphygmology. *Pulse Classics* not only plays an important role in the history of medical development, but also connects the preceding and the following history of TCM literature. It is respected by later generations of TCM practitioners as "the guide of medicine and the reference of diagnosis and treatment". Chen Bangxian commented in the *History of Chinese Medicine*: "Wang Shuhe is more than just the head of imperial TCM practitioners, he is actually a clinical TCM practitioner. He attaches great importance to sphygmology and symptoms for the diagnosis of diseases. He felt that Zhang Zhongjing's *Treatise on Febrile and Miscellaneous Diseases* was not enough to distinguish the pulses, so he added some pulse differentiation methods to it so that later scholars could 'follow pulses over symptoms', 'follow symptoms over pulses' or 'refer to both the pulses and symptoms'. He also sorted out the pulses in the *Canon of Medicine* or the *Classic of Difficult Issues* and compiled them into ten volumes of *Pulse Classics*. Before and after Wang Shuhe, there were many authors writing *Pulse Classics*, but Wang Shuhe's existed till today. It can be seen that this book was left after a long test."

(3) Rigor and responsibility forging the medical spirit.

Wang Shuhe said in the preface to the *Pulse Classics*: "Medicine is a matter of life. Even great TCM practitioners such as Bianque would still think carefully on pulses. With Zhang Zhongjing's clear examination, he would still need to refer to the symptoms and check for verification if there is any doubt." As a TCM practitioner, Wang Shuhe attaches great importance to the way of medical treatment, advocates more careful examination of symptoms and prudent medication, and emphasizes the great responsibility of TCM practitioners. He would check for verification if there is any doubt. This highly responsible medical practice attitude was followed and practiced by Wang Shuhe throughout his life, and was also a clear manifestation of his noble medical ethics.

3.2.3　Huangfu Mi

1. Brief biography

Huangfu Mi, with a courtesy name of Shi'an, was born in Chaona County of Anding (now Pingliang or Lingtai, Gansu Province) in Wei and Jin dynasties. As a representative figure of scholarship in Wei and Jin dynasties, Huangfu Mi not only made achievements in medicine, but also had great attainments in literature and history. In addition to *Canon of Acupuncture and Moxibustion*, which is regarded as a treasure book of TCM acupuncture and moxibustion, he has also written many literary and historical works, such as the *Imperial Lineage*, *Noble Characters*, *Virtuous Characters*, *Principled Women* and *Annals of Feudal Ethic Code*. Professor Wen Changlu once said, "Among the many TCM practitioners in ancient China, Huangfu Mi is probably the most unique one. As the best philosopher, historian, writer and medical scientist of his time, he is a typical comprehensive scholar with all-round knowledge. He can do well in both the humanities of values and the medical field."

2. Medical ethics

(1) Determined to study hard with strong will.

Huangfu Mi was born in the turbulent Wei and Jin dynasties. During his teenage years, he had no intention of learning. He had no respect of teachings at all, and never get into the way of learning. Later, after being taught by his aunt, he awakened and changed to devote himself to learning. As his family was poor, he did farming and took care of the crops with classic books. He carefully arranged the time for farming and studying, working hard during the day and studying hard at night. Huangfu Mi said in *Annals of Feudal Ethic Code*: "My family was poor. I work in the daytime and get tired at night. When the farming work began, my book would have dust, and the book box would be kept closed. Only in later winter, I could study for ten days, when I would study during my sleeping time at night, forgetting to eat, or not being aware of the time. He was determined to study hard and worked hard, and was called "nerd" at that time. Huangfu Mi showed his determination and perseverance in studying with the words that "if I learned the truth in the morning, I could be content to die in the evening".

Huangfu Mi later had gout and suffered a lot from the illness. Instead of being depressed, he wrote twelve volumes of *Acupuncture and Moxibustion Classic* based on the essence of three books, *Plain Conversation*, *Acupuncture Classic* and *Acupoints* (*Ming Tang*). He was honored as the originator of acupuncture and moxibustion in TCM by later generations.

Huangfu Mi was not knocked down by the miseries all his life. Instead, he studied hard and finally became a intellectual celebrity of his time. His talents and morality were highly praised by people of later ages.

(2) Indifference to fame and fortune.

Huangfu Mi is not only knowledgeable, but also noble. According to *The Book of Jin: Biography of Huangfu Mi*, Huangfu Mi "has ambition of being noble and focuses on writing". In the early years, Huangfu Mi was persuaded to cultivate his name among the dignitaries, but he wrote *Xuan Shou Lun* to answer the person who persuaded him. "Being poor is the common situation of scholars, and being lowly is where the way resides. With this, I would have no worries till my old age. Why would I have my spirit and essence disturbed and consumed for being rich and distinguished?" "If I can be strong and true, not counting benefits and losses, I will have my way perfect." Huangfu Mi believes that poverty is a common thing for scholars. For moral people, although they are often underestimated, they have no worries for a lifetime. Compared with the men that are often worried in pursuit of wealth, poverty is definitely more suitable for him. He believed that if he could maintain a strong body and put aside fame, wealth and status, it would be "complete" for him.

In his lifetime, Huangfu Mi experienced three dynasties and seven emperors. The imperial court repeatedly invited him to become an official, and he refused to accept it with the excuse of chronic disease. His noble morality of indifference to fame and fortune, his morality of refusing the emperor, and his behavior of putting aside wealth, fame and fortune should be learned by later generations.

3.2.4　Ge Hong

1. Brief biography

Ge Hong, whose courtesy name is Zhichuan and literary name is Bao Pu Zi, is known as "Immortal Ge". He was born in Jurong County, Danyang (now Jurong County, Jiangsu Province). He was a famous Taoist teacher, medicine expert and pill-maker at the intersection of the Jin dynasty and the Han dynasty. He was good at pill-making and medical skills. He was once honored as Marquis of Guannei, and later lived in seclusion in Luofu Mountain to refine pills. He has written works such as *The Emergency Prescriptions Kept in One's Sleeve* and *Bao Pu Zi*.

2. Medical ethics

(1) Earnestness to learn with tirelessness and persistence.

Ge Hong was born in a large family and was keen to learn since childhood. After his father passed away, his family declined and lived in poverty. In the Ming dynasty, Li Zhi wrote in *Chu Tan Ji* that "Ge Hong was poor and had no child servants. He weared hazels to go out and disperses grass before entering into his room. His home suffered from repeated fires, and all the books and records had all been burnt. So he had to go a long way on foot to borrow books and copy by hand. He needed to sell firewood to buy paper, and light a fire to read." The poverty of his family did not prevent Ge Hong from studying. In order to study, he walked a long way to borrow books and copied them with his bookcase on his back. He sold firewood to buy paper to copy by hand and then lit firewood to read. Ge Hong believed that learning can make sense and enlighten people, both for oneself and for the country. He also encouraged people with the allusions of Ni Kuan, Lu Sheng, Huang Ba and Ni Zi. He believed that as long as we persist in learning, we can understand the profound knowledge and insight into the profound and subtle words. Ge Hong not only attached great importance to learning, but also advocated in *Bao Pu Zi: Critics* that "we should accumulate our knowledge to reach a higher understanding, like using feathers to sink dragon boat." He believed that only by persistence and accumulation can we complete the transformation from quantitative change to qualitative change and finally achieve something.

In addition to advocating the persistence in learning and accumulate our knowledge to reach a higher understanding, Ge Hong also warned the world against the prejudice of taking the ancients as gods, and thinking of the works of the present life as superficial. He believed that a learner must remove the false and preserve the truth, take its essence and remove its dregs, so as to learn the truth and achieve results.

(2) Write medicine book after learning all schools of thoughts.

Ge Hong collected and screened some convenient prescriptions and diagnosis and treatment methods in medical practice, summarized many first aid measures in life, and wrote China's first emergency manual *The Emergency Prescriptions Kept in One's Sleeve* (referred to as *Sleeve Prescriptions*). The title of *Sleeve Prescriptions* means that the book can be carried around to respond to emergency and cure people, because it records pragmatic, highly adaptive and operable measures for acute diseases. The book records the symptoms, causes and treatments of tuberculosis, rabies, smallpox, tsutsugamushi disease (which Ge Hong calls "chigger infection") and other diseases found by Ge Hong, as well as emergency treatment methods such as the use of acupuncture.

According to *Bao Pu Zi*, when Ge Hong practiced medicine, he found that although there were many former medical books and prescriptions, "they are not operable, and the various urgent diseases is mixed with mistakes, which were not systematic and difficult to find. When it comes to the cure of serious emergency illness, the TCM practitioners would use precious medicines of dozens of kinds. Only those wealthy families who lived in the capital city could afford it. Most TCM practitioners treat diseases with acupuncture, but the moxibustion is not clear in details, only saying the names of acupuncture points." In order to change this chaotic situation, he classified all names of diseases, put them in order in case of misunderstanding in his book *Sleeve Prescriptions*.

When Ge Hong wrote *Sleeve Prescriptions*, he adhered to the principle of simplifying the prescription in order to "let mortals see it and use it". *Sleeve Prescriptions* are mostly single prescriptions and prescriptions commonly used in the folk, with simple compositions. According to the statistics of 8 volumes and 70 articles of *Treasures* of *Taoism*, there are 1,060 prescriptions in the book, including 510 single prescriptions composed of one medicine, and 494 compound prescriptions composed of two medicines and more than two medicines. It can be seen that the number of one medicine prescriptions used is greater than that of compound prescriptions. In order to take care of the poor family patients, he deliberately selected some very common drugs in the prescription, which were very cheap. In his prescriptions, garlic, ginger, green onions, salt, fermented soya beans, bitter wine, raw oil, grains, six livestock and other common products are most commonly used; the tools used are mostly reed pipes, bamboo tubes, swabs, cotton and silk fabrics and other easily available utensils; the therapies used are simple methods such as decocting orally, smoking, applying, wiping and blowing. In addition, in view of the changeable actual situation, the use of multiple prescriptions for one diseases has greatly improved the effectiveness in coping with various situations. *Sleeve Prescriptions* has changed the disadvantages of difficulty in understanding the prescriptions, difficulty in finding the medicine and expensiveness of the medicines. In addition, Ge Hong's *Sleeve Prescriptions* explains the specific positions of various acupuncture points in simple and easy-to-understand language, so that people who do not know acupuncture skills can also use it. *Sleeve Prescriptions* let the people at the bottom of society treat most diseases without a medical practitioner's help.

3.2.5 Tao Hongjing

1. Brief biography

Tao Hongjing, whose courtesy name was Tongming and self-made literary name was Huayang Yinju, was born in Moling, Danyang (now Nanjing, Jiangsu Province), posthumously named Zhenbai. He lived in seclusion in Juqu Mountain (now Maoshan Mountain) of Jurong due to the frustrations of his official career in the Southern Song, Qi and Liang dynasties. Tao Hongjing's thoughts originated from Laozi and Zhuangzi and were influenced by Ge Hong, mixing some views of Confucianism and Buddhism.

He is good at calligraphy, medicine, calendar calculation, geography, pill-making, literature, history, etc. He is a knowledgeable Taoist thinker, pharmacist, spagirist and litterateur with both Confucianism, Taoism and Buddhism. He is a famous all-round figure in the Qi and Liang dynasties.

Tao Hongjing is highly valued and appreciated by Emperor Wu of Liang dynasty. In case of national events, the emperor would discuss with Tao Hongjing. In the Tang dynasty, Li Yanshou once commented, "Every time the country has big events, Tao would be consulted. There are often several letters in merely one month, and he was called the prime minister in the mountains."

Tao Hongjing was born in a medical family. His grandfather and father both learned medical skills and martial arts skills. He has been smart since childhood and loves reading. It was the spirit of seeking knowledge and learning that had made him a representative figure who integrates Buddhism, Taoism and Confucianism.

2. Medical ehics

(1) Save the patients and write herbal medicine books.

In terms of medicine, Tao Hongjing was one of the earliest figures who contributed the most to the development of Chinese herbal science. After he lived in seclusion in Maoshan Mountain, he found that people in poor places were often ill without medical treatment. Some people could not get timely treatment after getting sick, so he set a goal of saving the patients. He said, "People have great concern about diseases. If you do not save them, it is like you do not use water to put down the fire." He felt that since he had lived in seclusion, although he cured many patients and accumulated virtues, it would only be temporary. To spread the knowledge, it was better to write books. Therefore, Tao Hongjing devoted himself to the compilation and research of medical classics. In his lifetime, there were more than ten herbal works, but there was no unified standard. In particular, ancient herbal works were inconvenient for clinical application due to their age, scattered contents, not distinguishing grass and mineral medicines, insects and animals. He compiled various versions of herbal books at that time into *Shennong's Herbal Classic* and *Famous Medical Practitioner's Bibliography* respectively, and added materials to them, added personal experience in medical research, and finally formed *Annotations of Shennong's Herbal Classic*. This is a masterpiece that systematically sorts out the classic of ancient pharmacology in China. It is a masterpiece with high scientific value. It preserved many ancient pharmaceutical books before the Liang dynasty of the Southern dynasties, and invented the method of classification according to the nature of drugs. It indicated the names, places of origin, characters, indicating diseases, configuration and storage methods of various drugs, with rich contents and clear regulations, which had an important impact on the development of herbal science after the Sui and Tang dynasties. Tao Hongjing said in the auto-preface of the *Annotations of Shennong's Herbal Classics*, "Nowadays, we often combine all kinds of classics and study them in a timely manner. Based on the 365 kinds of herbals in three categories of the *Shennong's Herbal Classic*, there are another 365 kinds of herbals, with 730 in total."

Tao Hongjing changed the classification method of upper, middle and lower grades of drugs in the *Annotations of Shennong's Herbal Classics*, and creatively divided 730 kinds of drugs into seven categories according to the natural source and nature of drugs: stones, grass and trees, insects and fishes, birds and animals, fruits and vegetables, rice and foods and those with only names but no descriptions. This new drug classification has a profound influence on the development of pharmacology in China. In terms of taxonomy, a methodology for the classification of therapeutic effects on different diseases, namely "generic drugs for various diseases", has also been created. This is a classification that brings together several drugs with the same effect for clinical reference and selection, which is obviously another improvement over the previous classification. As Tao Hongjing put it, "According to all kinds of medicines, although one herbal medicine can cure several diseases, there is still some bias in nature. On the day of prescription, this could lead to doubts and questions, and could not be studied. Now it is appropriate to list the main curing herbal names under different diseases for treatment, which is easy for searching and understanding." His method of classification according to the clinical function of herbals provides many conveniences for later generations to learn and use drugs clinically.

(2) Be rigorous and focus on investigation.

Tao Hongjing is very rigorous in his studying. When he encounters doubtful problems, he would definitely try every means to investigate and study them to understand them. This is a habit he developed in the process of studying.

Tao Hongjing's *Annotations of Shennong's Herbal Classic* can reflect his rigorous academic attitude. When he wrote, he attached great importance to the literature, and strictly noted the original source of all literature sources, while small annotations for new or annotated contents. In addition, in order to distinguish the new contents from the original texts in the *Annotations of Shennong's Herbal Classic*, and prevent readers from confusing it, he also deliberately distinguished it with red and black ink. The new content was written in black, while the original content from the *Shennong's Herbal Classic* was written in red. Therefore, later generations called them "Shennong's Herbal Classic in black" and "Shennong's Herbal Classic in red".

In addition to being rigorous, he pays great attention to investigation. There was such a story. One day, Tao Hongjing read *The Book of Songs·Xiaoya·Xiaowan* and read that "the lacewings have sons, and the Anterhynchiums would carry them". He found in the old notes to *The Book of Songs* that the Anterhynchiums are all males, and the male Anterhynchiums bring the larvae of the lacewings back to their own nests, so that the larvae become their own shapes, thus becoming their offspring (the ancients also often use the metaphor of lacewings to refer to adopted child). A friend of his happened to mention this question and wondered why. Tao Hongjing went to other books to find out the reasons, and the results were the same as the explanation of the old notes to *The Book of Songs*. But he was still confused, so he decided to investigate and see the truth. Therefore, Tao Hongjing went to the courtyard to find a nest of Anterhynchiums. After several careful observations, he finally found that the larvae of lacewings were not used by Anterhynchiums to become their offspring, but they took the lacewings back to their nests, stabbed the lacewings with the poison needles on their tails, and then laid eggs on them to reproduce their offspring. Tao Hongjing finally unveiled the mystery. He believed that the saying in *The Book of Songs* was a "fallacy, and Confucius has not examined it. Why does the master make the mistake?" "Saints are not perfect, as this is the case", bluntly criticizing the fallacy of ancient saints. From the above examples, we can see that Tao Hongjing focuses on investigation, thinks comprehensively and does not blindly follow the saints.

3.2.6　Yang Quan

Yang Quan, whose courtesy name was Deyuan, was a native of Liang (now Shangqiu, Henan Province) in the Western Jin dynasty. He was a philosopher who studied philosophy, astronomy, calendar calculation, medicine and agronomy, paid attention to the production and practice activities of ordinary people, and attached importance to the national economy and people's livelihood. Yang Quan lived in an era of increasingly declining Confucianism. Faced with the development of metaphysical thought and its impact on Confucianism, he neither advocated Confucianism nor metaphysics. Therefore, he refused to be an official and lived in seclusion. He wrote a lot of books in his life, but they were mostly lost. His *Theory of Things* inherited the simple materialism traditions of Yang Xiong, Wang Chong and Zhang Heng in the Han dynasty, and promoted the simple materialism theory based on the traditional natural science of Taoism. In medicine, he said in *Theory of Things*: "Doctors can only be those with benevolence, intelligence, reasoning ability, integrity, innocence and trustworthiness." He is the first person in Chinese history who clearly proposed that TCM practitioners should meet three standards: benevolence, wisdom and integrity. He also said: "As a medical practitioner in ancient times, he must be selected from a famous family with virtues of forgiveness and fraternity, and intelligence to understand difficult things; so as to know heaven, earth, gods, and lives; differentiate symptoms, know the direction, understand the severity, and determine the amount of the medicine. They can understand the most trivial things in medical practice and never get lost in details. This is a good TCM practitioner." He believes that "good TCM practitioners" have virtues, "famous TCM practitioners" have skills, each has their own strengths, and the employment of TCM practitioners needs to "refer to both".

3.2.7　Yao Sengyuan

Yao Sengyuan, whose courtesy name was Fawei, was born in Wukang of Wuxing (now Huzhou, Zhejiang Province). He was a famous TCM practitioner in the

Northern and Southern dynasties. He lived through four dynasties, including Qi, Liang, Northern Zhou and Sui, with nine emperors. He held official positions in Liang, Northern Zhou and Sui successively. He had excellent medical skills and was one of the few aristocrats in the Chinese history who had won the title of aristocrat with medical skills. He authored 12 volumes of *Proved Recipes* and 3 volumes of *Travelling Records*.

The Book of Zhou: Biography of Yao Sengyuan recorded two things about his use of rhubarb to treat diseases, which proved his excellent medical skills. His use of medicine varied excellently and properly according to different patients and syndromes.

Emperor Wu of Liang dynasty once wanted to take rheum officinale because of fever. Yao Sengyuan told Liang Wudi after diagnosis that rheum officinale was a purgative, and the emperor was too old to take it. The emperor did not listen, resulting in critical illness.

Emperor Yuan of Liang dynasty once suffered from heart and abdominal diseases, and he called all TCM practitioners to discuss the treatment plan. Other TCM practitioners believed that the emperor's status was noble, and should not take medicine rashly. It was best to use a mild treatment method, and use the peaceful medicines to slowly dredge the viscera. However, Yao Sengyuan said after diagnosis: "The pulse is large and solid, which is a sign of food accumulation. If you don't use rheum officinale, there is no way to heal." In the end, Emperor Yuan adopted his opinion, taking in decoction of rheum officinale, which dredged his accumulated food, and recovered his health.

The case of Yao Sengyuan treating Emperor Wu and Emperor Yuan reflects his excellent medical skills, and his spirit of being blunt and fearless of imperial power is also worth learning by later generations of TCM practitioners.

3.2.8 Chu Cheng

Chu Cheng, whose courtesy name is Yandao, was born in Yuzhai (present day Yuzhou, Henan Province). He was a TCM practitioner in the Southern and Northern dynasties. He wrote *Chu's Manuscripts*. In the Jianyuan Period of the Southern Qi dynasty, he was appointed as the governor of Wu Prefecture, and later became the left minister. *Chu's Manuscripts* is a medical work with only theory but no prescriptions. The whole book is divided into 10 parts: body, chi, wind, body parts, essence and blood, anti-disease, careful examination, discussion and questioning. Chu Cheng's medical ethics thoughts are mainly reflected in "careful syndrome differentiation to reach norms".

Chu Cheng believes that TCM practitioners must be based on "four diagnosis" (observation, smelling, questioning and pulse taking). When differentiating the symptoms, they must be careful, and carry out diagnosis and treatment according to the disease, people and local conditions. Medication is like fighting a war and a trivial mistake would mean life and death. His knowledge and requirements for medical practitioners reflect his understanding of medical ethics responsibilities of medical practitioners.

3.3　Evaluation of Medical Practitioners and Their Medical Ethics

During the Wei, Jin, Southern and Northern dynasties, the long-term division of the country caused social unrest and frequent wars, thus giving birth to people's sense of disillusionment in life. In the scholar-official class, metaphysics is popular, while the people at the bottom are suffering from endless war disasters, famine and disease epidemics. Under such a social background, all kinds of religious thoughts are increasingly popular in society. Medical thoughts are influenced by Confucianism, Buddhism and Taoism. On the basis of inheriting the simple humanitarian thoughts of former sages, medical theories advocating medical humanitarianism are further advanced. During this period, TCM practitioners such as Wang Shuhe, Huangfu Mi, Ge Hong, Tao Hongjing, Yang Quan, and Yao Sengyuan advocated medical ethics, rigorous academic learning, careful diagnosis and treatment, and helped the world and saved people. They took "saving the world and helping people" as their duty in medical practice, reflecting the noble feelings of the benevolence of TCM practitioners. Ge Hong, for example, wrote the *The Emergency Prescriptions Kept in One's Sleeve to* relieve the poor from the suffering of diseases. The book introduces many simple treatment methods. Medicines are also cheap, easy to obtain and effective, which greatly eases the difficulty of poor people in seeking medical treatment. For example, Wang Shuhe said in the preface of *Pulse Classic* that he would "examine for testing whenever there is doubt". For example, Chu Cheng said in his *Chu's Manuscripts* that one should have "exquisite examination" and "only a small difference would mean life and death". However, Yang Quan clearly put forward the concept of "good TCM practitioner", which not only has clear medical practice standards, but also clarifies the moral qualities, so that TCM practitioners begin to transition from "morality" to "medical ethics", and the identity of TCM practitioners begins to be established. Their professional quality fully reflects the professional awareness, attitude and sense of social responsibility that TCM practitioners should have.

3.4   Medical Education

3.4.1   Education for TCM practitioners

The Wei, Jin, Southern and Northern dynasties were a period from great governance to great chaos. Due to the special political and ecological environment, the influence of wars, ethnic integration and social ideological trends, the cultural diversity was formed, which promoted the transformation of the cultural education trend in this period from only Confucianism ideology to the coexistence of multidisciplinary education, and successively emerged specialized education in history, Buddhism, calligraphy, medicine, law, literature and arithmetic, which promoted closer ties between specialist education and society. With the rise of education in different disciplines, medical education has received more attention. During this period, medical education was mainly inheritance from teachers or parents, and official medical education was only in its infancy.

According to the *Records of Officials in the Book of Wei*, in 399 AD, "at the beginning, all the five classics established the post of doctoral officers and 30 imperial students respectively"; in 400 AD, "a post of immortal doctoral officer was established to refine hundreds of medicines". *The Notes of Six Classics of the Tang Dynasty* shows: "Medical apprentices after the Jin dynasty should be taught by teaching assistants." It indicates that TCM practitioners had been taught officially as early as the Jin dynasty, which was the beginning of official medicine education. According to the *Notes to Volume 14 of Six Classics of the Tang Dynasty*, in 443 AD, Qin Chengzu, the head of imperial TCM practitioners, suggested to set up medical education institute to enroll medical students. The institute was dismissed 453 AD

According to *The Book of Wei: Records of the Officials*, in the Northern Wei dynasty, there were doctoral officers among the imperial TCM practitioners ranked the lower seventh, and teaching assistants ranked the lower ninth. "Doctoral officers" and "teaching assistants" should be selected from those who were taught by the official medical education institute. The imperial court specially set up teaching posts for the purpose of promoting medical education. According to *Book of Wei: Records of Emperor Shizong*, in 510 AD, Emperor Xuanwu of the Northern Wei dynasty issued an imperial decree on the popularization of medical education and the assessment of the ability of learners, "It is ordered that the Chief Etiquette Officer set up an additional place, so that people with diseases inside and outside the capital can live there. It is strictly ordered that the medical institutes treat them in different categories and reward and punish them after examining whether they could cure the patients. With different learning period and specialties, different diseases could need acupuncture and stone therapy, or Bianque's words which are testified till today. In addition, there are a great many of prescriptions which spread widely, making it hard to trace the use of medicine. So it is ordered that all medical workers are collected to simplify the essentials, with a total of more than 30 volumes, to be distributed to the world. The counties and prefectures would write post noticing the countryside so that the people have the knowledge." It can be seen from the imperial decree that the imperial court aims to widely carry out medical education and examine the moral integrity of medical learners.

During the Wei, Jin, Southern and Northern dynasties, although the official medical education did not form a scale in the initial stage, and even got interrupted due to the unstable political ecological environment, the development of the official medical education system in this period laid the foundation for further development in the Sui and Tang dynasties to a certain extent.

During this period, the medical knowledge was relatively popularized. Firstly, frequent wars require a large number of doctors. Secondly, the custom of "taking stone medicines" prevails. Those who take stone medicines need to know some medical knowledge. Thirdly, medical practice is one of the necessary conditions for filial piety at that time. Fourthly, influenced by Taoist thoughts, there are many Taoists, who take medical practice to save people as the way of "accumulating virtue". Therefore, the popularization of medicine is inevitable, and medical skills are also known as "skills for the convenience of the people". Mr. Lv Simian commented in the

History of Jin, Northern and Southern Dynasties, "Although Taoism and Buddhism were mutually exclusive at that time, it doesn't mean that they did not know each other's creeds at the beginning. However, since both intended to spread their doctrines, they studied medicine and drugs and other skills conducive to people's life."

During this period, in addition to official medical education, medical skills were gained mainly based on the teachings from masters and from the old generations of the family. Thus, the majority of medical learners then were from the feudal aristocracy. Fan Xingzhun described them as "TCM practitioners from the aristocracy" in the *Brief History of Chinese Medical Sciences* and they were often renowned as TCM practitioners due to working as officials in successive dynasties.

Despite political turbulence, the diversified medical education model has taken shape during this period, which is characterized by multi-disciplinary teaching and multi-channel school-running. Only a few words and phrases about specific contents of medical education in the Northern and Southern dynasties can be found in history books. It can be inferred from the flourishing medical education in Sui and Tang dynasties, however, that medical education became popular and developed well in this period, laying a foundation for its prosperity in Sui and Tang dynasties.

3.4.2 Medical System

During Wei, Jin, Northern and Southern dynasties, in spite of simple descriptions of medical education and medical system in history books, we can still know from historical sources that the internal settings of medical officials at that time were more specific than those in previous dynasties, forming a top-down hierarchical system.

During the Three Kingdoms period, the medical official system in Wei, Shu, and Wu basically inherited the system of the Han dynasty, setting up official positions such as Prefect of the Grand Physicians, Assistant Prefect of the Grand Physicians, and Shang Yao Jian (an officer in charge of medical products administration). The development of medicine and the improvement of clinical technologies required more detailed duties of medical officials and brought new official positions such as the Yao Chang Si Ren Jian (a position for drug administration) and Ling Zhi Yuan Jian (supervisor of the Glossy Ganoderma garden). According to the *Records of the Three*

Kingdoms: Book of Wei, "Emperor Wen of Wei asked Palace Attendant Liu Ye to take an imperial physician to diagnose Zhang Liao. A succession of imperial guards was ordered to seek information along the roads."

Western Jin determined the ranks for medical officials on the basis of the system used in the Han and Wei dynasties and the nine rank system. Medical officials were subordinate to Director of Imperial Clan, and were awarded "a bronze seal with black ribbon" (a symbol of certain ranks). It is recorded in *The Book of Jin: Treatises Government Service* that "The Director of Imperial Clan is an official that manages the genealogical documents of the imperial members, supervises Imperial Physician Lingshi, and takes charge of Si Mu Yuan (officials for livestock rearing)." Prefect of the Grand Physicians and Assistant Prefect of the Grand Physicians were subordinates of Director of Imperial Clan. According to *The Book of Jin: Treatises Travel and Dress*, "The following is a large carriage that runs in the middle of the path. Prefect Grand Provisioner and Assistant Grand Provisioner are on the left and Prefect of the Grand Physicians and Assistant Prefect of the Grand Physicians are on the right." This reflects the status of imperial physicians in Western Jin. According to *Tongdian: Government Office: Officials*, the Imperial Medical Bureau was equipped with "a bronze seal with black ribbons, a one-ridge Jinxian crown, and crimson court dress, and was subordinate to Director of Imperial Clan". According to *Tongdian: Ranks of Officials*, "In Western Jin, Prefect of the Grand Physicians is a seventh-rank official, granted a bronze seal with black ribbon." The origin and ranks of the imperial physicians in Western Jin reflected that the official ranks of the imperial physicians were established according to the nine rank system.

In Western Jin, the imperial physicians and their subordinates provided medical services for the royal family. Imperial physicians were generally divided into Dianzhong Imperial Physician (imperial physicians serving in the palace), Imperial Physician Colonel, Imperial Physician Commander, Jinchuang Yi (surgeon in ancient China), Shang Yao Jian, and Yao Chang Si Ren Jian. It is recorded in *The Book of Jin: Biographies Jia Chong*, "The emperor asked an imperial courtier holding the imperial edict to enquire about Jia Chong's condition, and requested a Dianzhong Imperial Physician to deliver decoction." It can be inferred that Dianzhong Imperial Physicians served the emperor in the palace, and hence, they could be regarded as a close attendant of the emperor and enjoyed a high status. *The Book of Jin: Biographies Imperial Affines* says, "Liu De, born in Pengcheng, learned medicine by studying prescriptions at a young age, and was finally promoted to the position of Imperial Physician Colonel." In *The Book of Jin: Annals Emperor Wu*, "On November 16th in the lunar calendar, Imperial Physician Commander Cheng Ju offered a pheasant feather coat." Since Colonel and Commander were military officials, Imperial Physician Colonel and Imperial Physician Commander were physicians who served in the army. According to *The Book of Jin: Records Liu Yao*, "Yao was imprisoned in Chengxie, Henan, and was treated by Jinchuang Yi Li Yong." Jinchuang Yi mainly treats wounds, a common injury in the army; so Jinchuang Yi could also be physicians working in the army. Shang Yao Jian could be a position in charge of the medical products used by the royal family. During the reign of the State of Wei, eunuchs served as Yao Chang Si Ren Jian, whose responsibility was equivalent to that of Yao Cheng (an official for managing medication) in the Eastern Han dynasty.

According to *The Book of Jin: Treatises Government Service*, "After crossing the river, Emperor Ai made Director of Imperial Clan the subordinate to Minister of Ceremonies, and thus, imperial physicians were incorporated in Chancellery (Menxia Sheng in Chinese)." After the eastward river crossing, during the reign of Emperor Ai, the Director of Imperial Clan was put under the charge of the Minister of Ceremonies and become the subordinate to Chancellery. The imperial medical official system started to transform from the Three Lords and Nine Ministers system to the Three Departments and Six Ministries system. Palace attendants were responsible for all matters of Chancellery. It is since Eastern Jin dynasty that Prefect of the Grand Physicians began to become subordinate to Palace Attendants.

Throughout the Northern and Southern dynasties, the medical system was mostly modeled on the system of the Han and Wei dynasties. Nevertheless, the changes in the subordinate relationship of imperial physicians had their own characteristics in different dynasties.

The medical system in the Wei, Jin, Northern and Southern dynasties basically followed the system adopted in the Qin and Han dynasties. However, it had more subordinate officials with more specific and detailed duties compared with the Qin and Han dynasties, forming a top-down hierarchical management system. This reflected that the orderly management of physicians by rulers was conducive to physicians' career development and professional ability improvement. This also laid a foundation for the development of the medical system in the Sui and Tang dynasties.

Chapter Summary

During the Wei, Jin, Northern and Southern dynasties, TCM practitioners not only advocated and adhered to medical humanitarianism but also linked medical ethical principles and norms to people's life safety in a more systematic and deeper manner, on the premise of predecessors' medical ethical principles and norms. This, thus, better reflected the professionalism and the professional qualities of TCM practitioners and emphasized their professional and social responsibilities as well as professional attitudes.

During this period, TCM practitioners integrated medical ethical principles and norms with medical theories and skills. Holding a benevolent heart, a strict code of conduct and a rigorous personality, and being dedicated to medical skills and indifferent to fame and fortune, these TCM practitioners emphasized moral cultivation and endeavored to realize their values through medical learning and practice. The theoretical works of TCM collated and complied during this period prompted the sprouting of the theoretical system of traditional Chinese medical ethics. In addition, the medical system in this period had a more detailed and specific division of duties based on the system of the Qin and Han dynasties. This facilitated physicians' career development and professional ability improvement and meanwhile laid the groundwork for the development of the medical system in the Sui and Tang dynasties.

Application in Contemporary Times

1. Medical ethics of "putting yourself in the place of others", passed down by doctors in the new era

This chapter describes the main contents of medical ethics culture in the Wei, Jin, Northern and Southern dynasties. The long-term political division brought about social unrest, war, famine, and disease. In such a social context, various religious thoughts gradually prevailed. Chinese medical ethics culture in this period is also marked by the features of the times. Influenced by Confucianism, Buddhism, and Taoism, the theory of medical humanitarianism was put forward on the basis of naive humanitarianism of the predecessors. The TCM practitioners of this period loved others as themselves and made it their mission to save patients and benefit mankind in that turbulent times. Wang Shuhe, a TCM practitioner lived in the Wei and Jin dynasties, carefully studied the pulse and wrote *The Pulse Classic* to standardize the principle of pulse diagnosis and treatment. Also, he held the attitude of "if there is something indeterminate, research and compare documentation to verify it" in medical practice throughout his life. These aspects clearly embodied how he felt for patients. Ge Hong, a notable TCM practitioner in the Jin dynasty, wrote *The Emergency Prescriptions Kept in One's Sleeve* to provide cheap, easily available, and effective prescriptions for the poor people living in hunger and war, thus exempting them from the difficulties in seeking medical treatment.

In the new era, TCM practitioners should develop the value of "putting yourself in the place of others" and the human-centered spirit demonstrated in it. When TCM practitioners provide medical services for patients, it is necessary to weigh medical professional technical problems alongside the economic conditions of patients, so as to adjust treatment according to patients' circumstances and achieve precise medical treatment that features TCM practitioners' benevolence. Medical practice is the art to express love, loving others and loving oneself.

2. Carrying forward modern medical professionalism, with "benevolence, wisdom, and integrity" as the standard medical ethics

This chapter elaborates on famous TCM practitioners and medical ethics in the Wei, Jin, Northern and Southern dynasties and reviews the characteristics of medical ethics culture in this period. The Wei, Jin, Northern and Southern dynasties witnessed the transformation from "great governance" to "great chaos". The long-term feudal separatist rules and continuous wars had a profound impact on politics, economy, culture and social ideological trends, and other fields. The core of medical ethics culture has also transformed from "virtue of people" to "medical ethics". According to traditional medical ethics, we often describe sophisticated TCM practitioners with noble medical ethics as "miracle-working TCM practitioners", "commonly respected TCM practitioners" and "immortal TCM practitioners". These evaluations are more than the identity of "TCM practitioners" but exemplify "humans". In the Western Jin dynasty, Yang Quan proposed the concept of good physicians in his book *Wu Li Lun* and clearly pointed out that physicians should abide by the three standards "benevolence, wisdom, and integrity". Thereby, traditional medical ethics began to concentrate on "good physicians" instead of "benevolent men". The concept of a good TCM practitioner is illustrated based on the medical activities of TCM practitioners rather than the value beyond the identity of a medical practitioner.

The code of conduct of a "good medical practitioner" is the very source of modern medical professionalism, which fully reflects the professional consciousness, the attitude towards medical practice, social responsibility, and the sense of mission that medical practitioners should have. In a career of licensed medical practice, TCM practitioners should keep in mind "preventing and curing diseases, healing the wounded and rescuing the dying" and take professional medical technologies as the basis for health care services. We should not only behave with integrity but also have a sense of social justice, taking the first priority of benefiting patients' lives. Medical students and healthcare workers should take "benevolence, wisdom, and integrity" as professional ethics, make themselves benevolent, wise, and righteous TCM practitioners, and strive to become medical practitioners who are worthy of being entrusted by people, recognized by the community, and trusted by patients.

4

Medical Ethics Culture in the Sui and Tang Dynasties

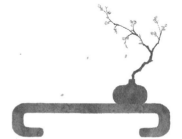

4.1 Overview of Medical Ethics

4.1.1 Social Background of Medical Ethics

The Sui dynasty and the Tang dynasty were collectively known as the Sui and Tang dynasties. Ancient China had strong strengths during these periods and there appeared golden ages such as "Reign of Kaihuang", "Reign of Zhenguan" and "The Flourishing Kaiyuan Reign Period". The Tang dynasty was a unified dynasty following the Sui dynasty. It is the heyday of feudal China and one of the most prosperous dynasties in ancient China. After the Anshi Rebellion, the Tang dynasty went into decline. Separatist regimes and eunuchs grabbing power weakened the strength of the Tang dynasty.

1. Influence of the politics of the Sui and Tang dynasties on medicine and medical ethics

During the Sui and Tang dynasties, the great reunification brought about political stability. The ruling class made great changes in politics, economy, and other aspects. In view of the sharp population decline after wars, the ruling class reduced labor services and taxes to rest and build up national strengths. Medical and healthcare development became an important guarantee and boost of social production and national thriving. Therefore, medicine was valued by the rulers and grew steadily, and medicine and medical ethics evolved under this background. Both the Sui and Tang dynasties set up institutions in charge of medical affairs and medical education and attached importance to cultivating medical talents. During this period, medicine flourished and famous physicians such as Sun Simiao and Chao Yuanfang sprang up, coming with typical medical classics, for example, *Treatise on Causes and Manifestation of Diseases*, *The Thousand Golden Prescriptions*, and *The Arcane Essentials from the Imperial Library*, etc.

The opening-up policies enabled the Sui and Tang dynasties to interact more with other nations. The Silk Road strengthened the exchanges between the East and the West and the connection among different ethnic groups in China. Plus the prosperity of the market, the pharmaceutical trade in Sui and Tang dynasties achieved great progress. In the early days of the Sui and Tang dynasties, open political and economic systems were formulated, making the nation enjoy a period of prosperity. Further, economic recovery and boom awakened public moral consciousness, and aspirants appealed for the emphasis on morals. The laws of the Sui and Tang dynasties gradually improved, which restricted and guided moral behaviors to some degree. In addition, the prosperous and stable society cannot come into being without growing moral consciousness. However, the medical sector also experienced moral chaos. Immoral behaviors, such as selling fake drugs, charging high prices, and treating patients differently based on status and wealth, greatly dissatisfied officials and commoners, and high-standard medical ethics were urgently needed. In short, economic and social development has laid a foundation for the growth of moral consciousness.

2. Influence of cultural education in Sui and Tang dynasties on medicine and medical ethics

The establishment of the Sui dynasty ended the division. However, influenced by the perennial war, the new nation badly needed talents to build it. During the reign of Emperor Yang of Sui, the imperial examination system was established. Examinations were held by category to objectively select outstanding talents in various fields. The selected medical talents also contributed to medical and healthcare development. During the Sui and Tang dynasties, medical education was highly valued. The central government and prefectures established medical education institutions to train medical students. Also, the central government set up Imperial Medical Bureau, the highest medical administration and medical education management institution, to manage medical administration affairs and engage in medical education and medical services. The bureau had sound rules and regulations and determined clear duties for different positions. In addition, the Sui and Tang dynasties adopted more comprehensive and strict systems to manage and assess medical practitioners. The emphasis on medical education raised the training quality of medical students. Accordingly, medical talents were required to improve excellent medical techniques and foster medical ethics.

The Sui and Tang dynasties were ideologically and culturally inclusive and willing to learn from others' strengths. In the early reign of the Sui and Tang dynasties, the rulers advocated Confucianism, creating the coexistence of Confucianism, Buddhism, and Taoism. Despite mutual exclusion, Confucianism,

Taoism, and Buddhism integrated their doctrines with each other's and together affected people's thoughts and spirits at that time. While researching medical skills and studying medical classics, TCM practitioners also learned the main ideas of Confucianism, Buddhism, and Taoism from their classics. This may affect their medical thoughts and morality. "Benevolence", the core of Confucianism, is consistent with the sympathy and mercy stressed in medical ethics. The medical moral thoughts influenced by Buddhism such as "great compassion", "universal equality", and "humans and animals equally cherishing their lives" reflect the medical ethics of treating patients equally and compassionately relieving people in need. Taoist principles such as "ways of life" and "spiritual cultivation" coincide with the codes of conduct for TCM practitioners of integrity and indifference to fame and fortune. In addition, medical ethics was also influenced by the morals and medical techniques of TCM practitioners of the past. In brief, the medical ethics of the Sui and Tang dynasties grew in such cultural backgrounds.

4.1.2　Main Contents of Medical Ethics Culture

1. Professional principles of saving people with benevolence and benefiting mankind with sincerity

Establishing the principle of medicine is a benevolent skill in medical practice. Medicine is a benevolent skill. Medicine has been called "a kind of benevolence" since ancient times, so "benevolence" is the core of medical ethics. Medicine is a discipline full of benevolence, a scientific technology to save lives. TCM practitioners are committed to relieving patients' sufferings. Hence, in addition to treating patients' physical illnesses, they should also respect their personalities and dignity, putting them first, caring for them, and sympathizing with them. Medicine is a science beneficial to humans, and treating patients is a noble profession in human health services. Only by adhering to the purpose of saving people with benevolence and benefiting mankind in sincerity can TCM practitioners truly protect human health. Sun Simiao stressed that medical practitioners must "first feel great compassion and vow to ease the sufferings of living creatures". This means medical practitioners have a kind heart and save people in distress. Sun Simiao also said, "When seeing the sufferings of patients, take it as yours." It suggested that medical practitioners sympathize with patients to understand their pains and try the best to treat them.

Yutuo Yundeng Gongbu, an outstanding medical master in the Tang dynasty, said that medical practitioners should excel in virtue, which specifically is to treat patients equally and help those in distress, regardless of their status and wealth; to seek no personal gain, leaving selfishness, greed and cunning behind.

Life is the priority of medical practice. "People's lives are of vital importance, as valuable as a thousand pieces of gold. Thus, if physicians could cure patients with prescriptions, what we gained is worth more than gold." The above saying of Sun Simiao interprets the preciousness of life and the importance of medical ethics. The clinical symptoms are complex and changeable. As the old saying goes, "Diseases may have the same causes but differ in symptoms and vice versa." Therefore, diagnosis and treatment are so "delicate tasks" that medical practitioners should carefully examine patients. They should "diagnose diseases attentively, checking physical conditions in detail and not losing anything. The acupuncture and medication used should be accurate." Since life is paramount, physicians should scrutinize patients, meditate on their symptoms, accurately identify the disease, and efficiently select treatment in the process of diagnosis, to save the life of patients. "The act of prolonging human's life at expense of animals' life and the purpose of saving lives are opposite poles." The two sayings express that the lives of animals including livestock matter. Thus, killing animals to save humans deviates from the original intention to save lives. This is also why Sun Simiao never used live animals as medicinal guides, which showed his greatest respect for lives.

"Universal equality" is the principle of medical practice. Starting with the moral concepts of "making medicine a humane art" and "saving people with benevolence", TCM practitioners emphasized "the practice of treating patients equally" and "wholehearted dedication to saving lives". Sun Simiao pointed out that a medical practitioners is expected to "equally treat whoever came for medical treatment, even like families, regardless of their status, wealth, age, appearance, relationship, ethnicity, and intelligence". The hierarchical system of feudal society made it rare to treat patients equally, regardless of their identity. "Animals equal human beings" also emphasizes that both human and animals are living creatures, reflecting that all lives in the world are of equal value. Yutuo Yundeng Gongbu believed that "people should treat others kindly as their own parents". He also insisted on "loving others more than yourself, whether they are your friends or enemies, especially not holding a hostile attitude to the latter". These thoughts demonstrate his moral qualities of eradicating prejudices about others, kindly treating patients, and loving others more than himself.

2. Holding attitude of wholehearted dedication to saving lives and careful treatment during medical care

Be wholeheartedly dedicated to saving lives. According to the basic principle of medical ethics of "saving people with benevolence", medical practitioners are required to deeply sympathize with patients and have a strong sense of responsibility for them. Medical practitioners should give priority to protecting patients' life and health, and endeavor to treat diseases. Sun Simiao advised that while treating patients, medical practitioners "should not be overtaken by misgivings and worry too much about their safety. They should take patients' distress as theirs. With sorrow at their sufferings, physicians should be wholeheartedly dedicated to saving them, not afraid of challenges and obstacles, and wasting no time on unimportant things. Only in this way can they become a commonly respected medical practitioner. Otherwise, they would be a killer of creatures." A great physician is someone who can be highly responsible and dedicated to saving lives, neglecting personal safety, risks, and gains and losses. A physician who cannot do would harm others and himself.

Carefully treat patients in medical practice. The *Absolute Sincerity of Great Physician* says, "Take pity for people with sore ulcers and diarrhea and the patients who stank. Do not disdain them. This is what I'd like to fulfill during my lifetime." This means that good TCM practitioners should not hate or complain about patients with ulcers, diarrhea, and unpleasant smells. Instead, they should be immensely sympathetic to those patients and endeavor to save them, not afraid of filth and stink. Medical practitioners are expected not to be overtaken by misgivings and worry too much about themselves even if they are likely to be infected. They should first carry out their duties to save lives. That was what Sun Simiao did. He once took six hundred leprosy patients to the deep mountain forests and lived with them there to relieve their pains. Not afraid of being infected, he personally took care of those patients and carefully treated them.

3. Study attitude of extensively exploring medical theories and diligently researching theoretical basis

Study diligently. In ancient times, medicine was regarded as "the skill of saving lives" and "a career about life", thus being more important than wealth. The complex human body and obscure diseases make treatment "a delicate task". Therefore, TCM practitioners should have excellent medical skills that can be acquired only with hard work and an inquisitive mind. Diligence and inquisitiveness are not only study attitudes but also important parts of medical ethics. Sun Simiao criticized those who had poor command of medical skills but were self-righteous. He asked physicians to "extensively explore medical theories and diligently research the theoretical basis of medicine". Sun Simiao was diligent and studious since his childhood and continued studying tirelessly until his twilight years. In addition, the saying that "I was never deterred from learning by harsh winters and scorching summers" is a portrayal of how Wang Bing devoted himself to his studies. Wang Tao spent twenty years on Hongwen Library reading a large number of books, acquiring the thoughts of sages and learning the essence of theories raised by previous talents. Yutuo Yundeng Gongbu traveled far to study medicine, away from his comfortable home. He successively traveled around Tibet, Nepal, India, and other places for five years or more. He went to India twice and even visited Mount Wutai. In the process, he studied and accumulated comprehensive medical knowledge. He practiced medicine in various countries and founded Tibetan medicine schools, finally becoming a well-known medical expert in ancient China. The intestinal anastomosis, induced abortion, tooth extraction, and other operations recorded in *Treatise on Causes* and *Manifestation of Diseases*, which was compiled by Chao Yuanfang, are the first operations in the surgery history of the world, which demonstrates his spirit of research and innovation.

Keep rigorously studying while being dedicated to working. In order to spread medicine and benefit common people, Sun Simiao wrote *The Thousand Golden Prescriptions* through painstaking effort during his twilight years. Having lived in seclusion in mountain forests, he picked up herbs and made medicines for patients, as well as personally tested medicines. He collected proven prescriptions and secret prescriptions from local areas, learned medical theories, and summarized his clinical experience. Sun Simiao enthusiastically treated diseases and saved lives for most of his life. In his later years, he wrote books and presented them to later generations. Zhang Lu, a physician in the Qing dynasty, commented on *The Thousand Golden Prescriptions* that "the 30-volume book showed me great medical methods, numerous medical strategies, and Sun Simiao's kind intention. The book analyzed the methods of diagnosis and treatment in detail and introduced the treatment strategy of Fan Ji Ni Cong (treating a disease with medication whose properties were opposite to the syndrome of the disease). How can he make such a miraculous book without the total mastery of medical theories and skills?" The prescriptions recorded by Sun Simiao show particular intentions and have unique efficacy, which would last for generations. Many prescriptions in the book are effective and easy to use, and can treat multiple syndromes at the same time. These prescriptions have tremendous medical value and deserve the reputation of "priceless medical classic". Sun Simiao's spirit of researching and rigorous study attitude is self-evident here. Wang Tao held a rigorous attitude towards medical practice. He criticized quacks for lacking in both medical knowledge and practical skills, not examining prescriptions, neglecting common diseases that possibly develop into terminal diseases, and treating patients recklessly. When it comes to the experience of his predecessors, he said he would "repeatedly 'research' it", because "the misunderstanding of a single word may harm human life". Therefore, his book *The Arcane Essentials* from the Imperial Library indicated all the sources of materials cited in it. And a rigorous attitude is required to list such a great number of references. Although deeply impressed by the exquisiteness of *Plain Conversation*, Wang Bing found that some contents were too obscure to understand. Hence, he tried to annotate it in combination with his own medical thoughts and experience. It took him 12 years to finally complete the book *Annotated Plain Conversation*. He reorganized, classified, collated, and annotated the contents of *Plain Conversation*, making them clearer. Later generations studied *Plain Conversation* mostly on the basis of Wang Bing's research.

4. Decorous behavior and modest manner

With the emphasis on medical ethics and practices, great TCM practitioners pay much attention to their own manners and behaviors in front of patients and their peers. Sun Simiao insisted that "great medical practitioners should clear their minds and introspect. They should have a solemn look and a generous mind. Also, they ought to be neither humble nor pushy". What he meant is that physicians should be full of spirit, righteous and generous, kindly treat patients but also keep a right distance from them. Physicians should not keep a watchful eye on the beautiful clothes (of patients' families) and not be immersed in recreations, delicacies, and alcohols. When in the patients' homes, medical practitioners should be totally absorbed in medical treatment, preventing themselves from immersion in music, delicious foods, and so on. It is because it is not reasonable that TCM practitioners enjoy themselves while patients are suffering. This principle reflects that physicians have great empathy with patients and understand the hardships that patients' families are encountering. Medical practitioners should hold their tongues. They should not joke around, gossip about patients, or boast about their reputation. It is further not allowed to advertise themselves by defaming other physicians. As stated above, medical practitioners should be cautious about their words and it is inappropriate for them to tease or judge others, and even belittle peers' achievements for self-praise. Yutu Yundeng Gongbu said that medical practitioners should care for their teachers and respect them like gods. They are also expected to maintain a good relationship with their classmates, respecting and caring for each other.

5. Moral qualities of indifference to fame and fortune and being honest and upright

Medical practitioners shoulder the responsibility of healing the wounded and rescuing the dying. Such being the case, they should put life first and have a benevolent heart in the practice of medicine. When serving patients, they should be honest and upright, neglect personal gains and losses and not seek fame, benefits, and privileges. Similarly, Sun Simiao advocated that "when treating diseases, great physicians should clear their minds and get rid of desires". Wang Bing also said, "If you are not greedy for benefits, fame, and other things, you can easily get what you want and things may go as you wish. It is because you want nothing special." Through *On the Absolute Sincerity of Great Physician*, Sun Simiao warned that "physicians should not be preoccupied with making benefits with their medical skills but hold the belief of helping people in distress" and "physicians should not prescribe patients, who may be wealthy though, unnecessary precious and hard-to-get ingredients to flaunt their capabilities". Sun Simiao repeatedly refused to enter the court and served as an official. Instead, he would rather seek ingredients and research medicines in the mountain forests and treat patients from the local areas. He practiced the medical morality of being indifferent to fame and wealth and wholeheartedly dedicated to saving lives. According to Liu Yuxi's *Chuan Xin Fang*, Zhang Tingshang paid a lot of money to recruit capable physicians to treat his subordinates. Though facing Zhang Tingshang's financial incentives, the physician who came for treatment said, "this prescription is donated just to save people's lives." This shows that the unknown physician took it as his duty to relieve the patient's illness, not caring about the monetary reward. Yutuo Yondeng Gongbu also emphasized that physicians should leave concupiscence, personal gains, selfishness, and greed behind. He said, "Having observed physicians' behaviors, I found that most of them tend to have prescriptions in reserve to demonstrate their outstanding medical skills and earn more money in later treatment. Why not prescribe more medications to produce a more powerful effect." Liu Yuxi, though recognized the achievements of physicians, criticized the physicians who seek improper benefits from patients by virtue of his medical skills. Not only physicians but also medicine merchants are deeply influenced by the culture of integrity. Song Qing was right a great medicine merchant with noble medical ethics in the Tang dynasty. Song Qing had a medicine shop in Chang'an. He usually bought medicines at an attractive price from sellers who came from remote places. Physicians praised Song Qing for the high quality of his medicines. The medications made from Song Qing's ingredients sold well and had an appreciable effect. The people also tend to buy medicines from Song Qing to treat common diseases such as scores. He even sold good medicines to those who did not bring money and accepted IOUs they wrote. However, at the end of the year, Song Qing would burn the IOUs from those who did not pay the money back, no longer mentioning or claiming his money afterward. It can be seen that Song Qing was not for money. He was a man of chivalry who helped people regardless of pay.

4.1.3　Characteristics of Medical Ethics Culture

1. Medical ethnics principles based on benevolence

The medical ethics culture in the Sui and Tang dynasties developed on the basis of the practice of the TCM practitioners represented by Sun Simiao at that time. During this period, the medical ethics goal of saving people with benevolence was formed, and the medical ethics concept of "life first" developed. The concept combines the medical ethics of sacred life with clinical practice and inherits and develops the medical humanitarianism tradition, which promotes the all-around development of medical ethics.

On the Absolute Sincerity of Great Physician, the first volume of The Thousand Golden Prescriptions, is an essential document on medical ethics, which spreads widely and has far-reaching effects. In the concept of "absolute sincerity" (Jing Cheng in Chinese) advocated by it, the first word is Jing (absoluteness), which means that physicians are required to have excellent medical skills. They should consider the medical career to be "a delicate task", so medical practitioners must "extensively explore medical theories and diligently research the theoretical basis of medicine". The second word is Cheng (sincerity). Specifically, the TCM practitioners should save lives with benevolence, respecting the life values of patients, wholehearted dedication to saving lives, indifference to fame and wealth, and being honest and upright. Short as it is, *On the Absolute Sincerity of Great Physician* fully demonstrates the big picture of traditional Chinese medical ethics and is regarded as the essence of medical ethics. Its widely-covered contents display the high standards and strict requirements for physicians. These medical ethics and norms should be followed by contemporary and later-generation medical practitioners. In the Sui and Tang dynasties, *On the Absolute Sincerity of Great Physician* deeply affected the medical thoughts and behaviors of physicians, the medical ethics and practice of the whole society, the education and evaluation of medical ethics, and the medical ethics culture at that time.

2. Establishing a good medical practitioner-patient relationship

In view of problems between physicians and patients, TCM practitioners in the Sui and Tang dynasties proposed to establish a good medical practitioner-patient relationship through communication and coordination. This is beneficial for close cooperation in diagnosis and treatment, so as to cure diseases. Both Wang Tao and Sun Simiao attached great importance to the improvement of a medical practitioner-patient relationship. In *The Arcane Essentials from the Imperial Library*, Wang Tao quoted the analysis of beriberi from *The Thousand Golden Prescriptions*. He was in favor of Sun Simiao's views that "there are good medicines and good words everywhere, but not everyone will accept the words and use the medicines. Therefore, we should provide medical treatment for those who trust us, but needn't explain much to those with an unbelieving attitude." He emphasized that physicians should respect patients' autonomy and adjust treatments according to situations and patients' conditions. It is important to build mutual trust between physicians and patients. According to his analysis, there are three reasons for dying from beriberi: "being diagnosed as the terminal stage, being too arrogant to follow medical advice, and being doubtful about physicians' skills". At that time, patients' health often deteriorated as they were hesitant about accepting medical treatment or doubtful about physicians. As is often the case, relatives and friends came to visit patients. They had no idea of the disease and corresponding prescriptions but pretended to be knowledgeable about it and talked nonsense. Some believed it was deficiency syndrome while others considered it excess syndrome. Some may think the disease was caused by wind, yet others called the disease Gu (a kind of disease marked by prolonged duration, emaciation and depression just like being consumed by parasites inside the body). Some would say the disease was about water but others insisted it was about phlegm. As opinions varied, patients were confused about the real causes. Thus, they hesitated to receive treatment until they missed the best time for medical care. Startled by the unexpected calamity, those visitors scattered without trace. This indicated how others' words affect patients' minds and conditions. Both patients and their relatives and friends should be fully confident in TCM practitioners. Patients should trust the TCM practitioners they have chosen, no matter what others say.

In addition, the noble medical ethics of TCM practitioners provides a foundation for a good medical practitioner-patient relationship. For example, TCM practitioners ought to treat patients "equally" and wholeheartedly dedicate themselves to saving lives. Medical practitioners should not be preoccupied with making benefits with their medical skills, that is, they are not allowed to abuse power to collect money. Also, as the saying goes, "medical practitioner should have a solemn look and a generous mind and be neither humble nor pushy." Thus, TCM practitioners should speak and behave properly while treating patients... Only by improving their morals can TCM practitioners win the trust of patients, which will help build a harmonious and mutual-trust medical practitioner-patient relationship.

The Tang dynasty also stressed the management of medical practitioner-patient disputes and medication affairs, for which it issued the first Chinese pharmacopoeia *Newly Revised Cannon of Herbal Classic*. As recorded in Tang Code (a penal code established and used in the Tang dynasty), special provisions were made to deal with medical accidents. For example, "provided that physicians make errors in medicine dispensing, medication instructions, and acupuncture out of their poor medical skills or carelessness, making them inconsistent with the prescription and thus bringing death to patients, the physicians will be sentenced to two years and a half in prison." "Provided that physicians make an intentional inconsistency and hence injure or kill the patients, they are to be convicted under the charge of assault or intentional homicide. Even though their behaviors caused no harm to patients, they will be also sentenced to a flogging of 60 strokes." "Physicians who run counter to prescriptions for the purpose of seeking improper benefits will be charged with larceny." These provisions standardize physicians' behaviors and responsibilities and help improve the morals of medical practitioners, which could contribute to a harmonious medical practitioner-patient relationship.

3. Life ethics of caring for vulnerable groups

In the Sui and Tang dynasties, the ruling class attached importance to the life and health of vulnerable groups, and thus, established the "Yang Bing Fang" (an area for urban residents' healthcare activities), the "Bei Tian Fang" (an area for aiding the poor), and "Shang Ren Fang" (a place to accommodate leprosy patients). "Shang Ren Fang" was one of the original forms of charities. Women, children, and the elderly are the key groups concerned by TCM practitioners.

The Prescriptions for Women and *The Presciprions for Children and Infants* are listed before all other parts in *The Thousand Golden Prescriptions*. Childrearing is the centerpiece of population increase. Children can develop into adults only with careful attention and early health preservation. That's why *The Book of Changes* stresses that from little things, big things grow. *The Commentary of Zuo* records that Sheng Zi gave birth to Duke Yin. Those classics all emphasized the same thing, that is, many a little makes a mickle; humans grow from a little embryo. Everybody knows the importance of parenting before being informed by classics and history books. Therefore, prescriptions for women, children, and infants came first in this book, followed by those for men and the elderly, to stress the protection of the fundamentals of population increase. That indicates the awareness of attaching importance to women and children and emphasizes the significance of providing maternal and child specialist medical services, which is conducive to establishing the specialties of pediatrics, obstetrics, and gynecology. *The Thousand Golden Prescriptions* systematically describes the dietary care for women in regulating menstruation, nourishing the fetus, and postpartum care, and elaborates on the care of newborns, the causes and treatment of exogenous febrile diseases, cough, epilepsy, and other diseases in children. In addition, *The Cases of the Elderly in Qian Jin Yi Fang* (a supplement to *The Thousand Golden Prescription*) introduces the physical and mental characteristics of the elderly, such as "physically and mentally failing", "deteriorating eyesight", "volatile temperament" and "sleeplessness". It also proposes that descendants "should carefully attend to the elderly, quickly giving them whatever they want and not making them unhappy and discontented. This is called the way of filial piety". This shows that people should respect the elderly and consider their needs. In addition, it also instructs the elderly in health care. "Influenced by their temperament, the elderly tend to rely on their ages and make demands unscrupulously. They are usually arrogant and wilful and do not follow common rules. Even their sudden desire must be satisfied. Knowing these facts, it is advisable to be mentally prepared and treat them cautiously." "Shut ears to things that do not conform to rites, prevent talking nonsense, avoid reckless actions, and perish improper thoughts." That is, a healthy diet, good words and deeds, as well as a peaceful state of mind can make the elderly maintain health and prolong their life.

4. Social responsibility with emphasis on disease prevention

Disease prevention is the guiding principle of the medical ethics. In the Sui and Tang dynasties, the medical thought of "preventing micro-diseases at the outset" was emphasized. Doctors put forward the significance and methods of preventing epidemic diseases after long-term observation and clinical practice as well as the exploration of the causes. As mentioned in *Treatise on Causes and Manifestation of Diseases*, infectious diseases are influenced by seasons and climate, and it is possible to take medicines in advance to prevent infections. Thus, taking medicines in advance is a way to prevent an infection. It also warns people off eating half-cooked fish to prevent parasitic diseases such as tapeworm infection. It further proposes that moxa-moxibustion can be used to treat sores for killing sarcoptic mites because the sarcoptic mites cause scabies. Dermatitis rhus is a disease caused by an endogenous allergic reaction to lacquer, and thus allergies vary from person to person. Mountain goiter is caused by drinking "sandy water". If spring water flows out from black mountains, rivers, and black soil, it is necessary to avoid residing there and drinking local water for the long term. In late spring and early summer, dogs may go mad and attack people, so the vulnerable group such as children and the elderly should be warned of taking a stick just to be safe. *The Thousand Golden Prescriptions* and *The Arcane Essentials from the Imperial Library* introduce the prevention and treatment of rabies in detail. Doctors have also left profound insights into health preservation. In *Health Preservation Recipes Daoyin Methods*, Chao Yuanfang discusses 1,727 symptoms, establishes the method of "nurturing and guiding" to replace drugs, and widely uses the guidance method in medical treatment. Also, he proposed that brushing teeth was the key to ensuring tooth health. Sun Simiao put forward the "Four Less" health preservation method, "speaking less, thinking less, eating less, and sleeping less". He believed "whoever does like that will live a healthy and comfortable life". Besides, he also suggested other health preservation methods such as gargling after meals, kneading, and strolling. Liu Yuxi, a writer in the Tang dynasty, criticized the thought of belittling health preservation and put forward the idea of "prevention beyond treatment". The above contents reflect the medical thought of "putting prevention first and combining prevention with treatment" and the sense of social responsibility of caring for the masses.

4.2 Representative Medical Practitioners and Their Medical Ethics

4.2.1 Chao Yuanfang

1. Brief biography

Chao Yuanfang, who was said to be born in Jingzhao Huayin (now Huayin City, Shaanxi Province) of the Sui dynasty, was a famous medical scientist. He once served as Imperial Physician Scholar and Prefect of the Grand Physicians. He received an imperial edict to preside over the compilation of *Treatise on Causes and Manifestation of Diseases*, a monumental work about etiology in Chinese history. The book elaborates on the etiology and pathology of diseases in internal medicine, surgery, gynecology, pediatrics, ENT, and other departments from the perspective of source and symptoms. It also discusses diagnosis, prognosis, prevention, health preservation, guidance, massage and surgery, and other treatment methods for certain diseases. Chao Yuanfang broke through previous theories and his new ideas developed the etiology theory. *Treatise on Causes and Manifestation of Diseases* features widely-ranged contents, detailed descriptions, and accurate analysis. It is the first Chinese text that deals with etiology and symptomatology of TCM. It is also the first medical theoretical work written by a team and organized by the imperial court. It plays an important role in the history of Chinese medicine and has a far-reaching impact on later generations. That's why Chao Yuanfang goes down in the history books.

2. Traditional Chinese medicine stories

Excellent medical skills bring about immediate effects. According to *Records of Opening the Canal During the Time of Emperor Yang of Sui*, Ma Shumou, the canal commander, who administered the construction of the Great Canal, contracted wind disease and suffered from joint pain. Therefore, Emperor Yang of Sui ordered Chao Yuanfang to treat him. After diagnosis, Chao Yuanfang found that the wind penetrated the skin and attacked the chest. So, all the patient needed to do was to have the steamed tender lamb together with medicines. Ma Shumou prepared the medicine according to the prescription and ate it with the lamb. Surprisingly, the disease was cured before the medicine ran out. Chao Yuanfang asked him to continue to take medicinal cuisine for nurturing his body, to prevent the recurrence of the disease. This story shows that Chao Yuanfang had so excellent medical skills that his prescriptions can make instant relief.

Chao Yuanfang presided over, in an imperial edict, the compilation of *Treatise on Causes and Manifestation of Diseases*, China's first monograph on the etiology of TCM. He made enormous efforts and finally achieved the expectations. This book has a far-reaching influence on TCM. Medical practitioners of later dynasties considered it a necessary reference to the practice of medicine. The views in the book were accepted by famous physicians of later dynasties and were included in medical classics, which could benefit later generations. For example, *The Thousand Golden Prescriptions* by Sun Simiao in the Tang dynasty included many contents from *Treatise on Causes and Manifestation of Diseases*. In Tang dynasty, Wang Tao's *The Arcane Essentials from the Imperial Library* also quoted the views from the book. Among the 40 volumes of *The Arcane Essentials from the Imperial Library*, its contents were quoted in 28 volumes, totaling 341 places. In the Song dynasty, *Taiping Holy Prescriptions for Universal Relief* authored Wang Huaiyin et al. also recorded the contents in the book. In addition, in the Song dynasty, this book was listed as one of the "Seven Classics of Medicine" and became a required textbook for TCM. It was also a compulsory examination subject to assess the ability of physicians in the Song, Yuan, and Ming dynasties. During the Ming and Qing dynasties, more copies of the book were printed, which made it spread widely.

Physicians save lives with benevolence forgetting about their own. Stone medicines, which came into fashion among the aristocratic class in the Wei and Jin dynasties, still prevailed among the nobles and scholar-officials in the Sui dynasty, in order to "brighten" their decadent and corrupt life and fill the emptiness in their mind. Stone medicines would make the users have a fever, in which case Cold-Food Powder is needed. However, Cold-Food Powder produces serious side effects. Chao Yuanfang specially discussed this in his *Treatise on Causes and Manifestation of Diseases*, taking the example of how Huangfu Mi suffered from the Cold-Food Powder to exhort the masses. However, to save those suffering from Cold-Food Powder, physicians need to do something unreasonable or uncommon. These things may irritate the sufferers easily. This is the case with Wen Zhi, who wanted to save the Emperor of Qi but was killed. That's why physicians usually have some concerns while treating nobles and high officials, fearing to bring a fatal disaster. However, Chao Yuanfang said, "Life and death are of supreme importance. It is not benevolent for physicians to refuse to save those who could have survived. On the contrary, a benevolent physician, unwilling to give up, will treat those sufferers despite being subject to their outrage." With a benevolent heart, Chao Yuanfang seldom cared about his safety but to save people in danger. He also tried to relieve those suffering from Cold-Food Powder, though opposed to stone medicines taking.

4.2.2　Sun Simiao

1. Brief biography

Sun Simiao, Who was born in Jingzhao Huayuan (now Yao County, Shaanxi Province), is a prestigious medical scientist in the Tang dynasty. He is known as "Sun Zhenren" and is respectfully called "King of Medicine" by later generations. Sun Simiao used to get sick frequently in his early years, so he was determined to study medicine later. He assiduously studied medical theories and accumulated practical medical experience in local areas. His *The Thousand Golden Prescriptions* is described as China's earliest encyclopedia about clinical medicine, which profoundly affected the development of medicine in later generations. Sun Simiao also made outstanding achievements in medical ethics. In *The Thousand Golden Prescriptions*, he placed the medical ethics of "absolute sincerity of great physicians" at the beginning and made a detailed illustration. Sun Simiao himself is also a representative of physicians with excellent medical skills and noble medical ethics.

2. Traditional Chinese medicine stories

Write *The Thousand Golden Prescriptions* diligently and tirelessly. Sun Simiao took "extensively exploring medical theories and diligently researching theoretical basis" as a principle of medical ethics. He clearly pointed out that a great physician should digest the content of books such as *Plain Conversation*, *Canon of Acupuncture and Moxibustion*, and *Yellow Emperor Acupuncture Canon*, master the twelve meridians, the internal organs of the body, the exterior and interior, acupuncture points, and understand the classical prescriptions by Zhang Zhongjing, Wang Shuhe, and other medical experts. Perusing these classics and understanding pharmacology and prescriptions will lay the foundation for the mastery of excellent medical skills. He advised that apart from learning medical knowledge, practitioners should also "read widely and miscellaneously", for example, broadening the knowledge of humanities and social sciences through "Five Classics", "Three Histories", "Hundred Schools of Thought", etc. This reflects his emphasis on TCM practitioners' humanistic qualities. There once was a fool who engaged in medicine. After studying prescriptions for three years, he believed that no disease cannot be cured by those prescriptions. However, after practicing medicine for three years, he found that no prescriptions can be directly used to cure diseases. Sun Simiao criticized physicians who had poor command of medical skills but were self-righteous. He emphasized medical learners should "extensively explore medical theories and diligently research theoretic basis; and should not consider the half-baked knowledge gained from others as the complete picture of medicine". Sun Simiao researched hard himself, modestly learned from the masses and his peers, collected and verified secret prescriptions, and traveled a long distance to seek prescriptions, practicing the attitude of extensive exploration he preached. It can be seen that Sun Simiao focused on the study of theoretical knowledge and the summary of medical practice in local areas. Sun Simiao studied medicine hard and finally wrote the comprehensive clinical medicine masterpiece *The Thousand Golden Prescriptions*, which has a far-reaching impact on medicine in later generations.

Help people in distress but disregard the fame and benefits. Sun Simiao was very clever when he was a child. He could recite articles of a thousand words at the age of 7. When he was 18 years old, he was determined to be a physician and showed great perception in learning medicine. At the age of 20, he began to treat his neighbors. He was proficient in Taoist classics and talked much about the thoughts of Laozi and Zhuangzi, which brought him to the title "Genius Child". Sun Simiao was fully appreciated and was invited to become an official many times. Nevertheless, he declined due to his keenness on studying medicine and eagerness to treat people. Emperor Wen of Sui once asked him to be the director of the top education institution, but he refused, pleading illness. Tang Taizong wanted to grant him the title of nobility, and he also declined it. Later, Tang Gaozong ascended to the throne and invited him to work as Grand Masters of Remonstrance, but he turned down again. He stressed that "physicians should not be preoccupied with making benefits with their medical skills", and denounced the behavior of "seeking high positions, great wealth, power, and fame in haste". To obtain a prescription or treatment method, he usually trekked over hills and through rivers to visit the holders and learned from them even at great expense. He never refused to see a patient. He once personally cured more than 600 leprosy patients. His stories circulated among the people, such as "urinating with scallion", "diagnosing the pulse with strings", and "saving a woman in childbirth with a needle". These stories have shown his good morals of being indifferent to fame and wealth and wholeheartedly dedicated to saving lives.

Medical ethics are passed down forever. Why did Sun Simiao title his medical work as *The Thousand Golden Prescriptions*? "People's lives are of vital importance, as valuable as a thousand piece of gold. Thus, if physicians could cure patients with prescriptions in this book, what we gained is worth more than gold." He believed that life was more valuable than gold, and that the value of prescriptions lied in the ability to save people in danger. This reflects that he attached great importance to human life. "Absolute Sincerity of Great Physicians" is the opening chapter of *The Thousand Golden Prescriptions*, which puts forward the essential qualities of "great physicians". They are required to keep improving their medical skills and treat patients sincerely. It also expounds the connotation of "great physicians", including erudition, diligence, benevolence, compassion, and determination, which is regarded as a model of medical ethics in later generations. "Absolute Sincerity of Great Physicians" emphasizes the concept of equally treating patients like relatives, and proposes the standard of risking their own lives to save others, which was described as "not being overtaken by misgivings, not worrying overmuch about their own safety, and taking patients' distress as theirs", and stressed the principle of "fostering their morality first". The "Absolute Sincerity of Great Physicians" promotes medical ethics and practice and is honored with "the Hippocratic Oath of the East". Sun Simiao is also known as the "Master of All Generations" in the history of Chinese medical ethics for his excellent medical skills and noble medical ethics.

4.2.3 Wang Tao

1. Brief biography

Wang Tao, who was born in Shaanxi Mei (now Meixian County, Shaanxi Province), was a famous medical practitioner in the Tang dynasty. Wang Tao came from a family of officials. His great-grandfather was Wang Gui, a famous Grand Chancellor of the early Tang dynasty. His grandfather Wang Chongji served as Zhujue Yuanwailang, a low-level official at the ministry of civil service affairs. His father was Wang Maoshi, a poet and the Wulin Magistrate during the reign of Tang Gaozong. Wang Tao had an extraordinary life. He once worked as Investigating Censor and the Commander of Xu Prefecture. He was exposed to medicines at a young age because of his illness, which initiated his interest in medicine. Wang Tao had been in charge of Hongwen Museum for 20 years, which gave him the opportunity to read lots of medical books. After decades of research and collation, he wrote the medical masterpiece *The Arcane Essentials from the Imperial Library*, which spread to later generations. This book has a high medical and historical value and thus is called "a world treasure" in the *New Book of Tang*.

2. Traditional Chinese medicine stories

Wang Tao became a physician out of filial piety. Suffering from illness at a young age sparked Wang Tao's interest in medicine. But his mother's illness made him realize that "filial duty is hard to fulfilled without medical skills". Therefore, he decided to study medicine to understand diseases, take care of his mother, and provide treatment. As a dutiful son, Wang Tao personally took care of his sick mother for a long time. He had contacts with famous physicians. The connection with those physicians allowed him to gain a thorough understanding of medical skills. In the process, he gradually realized the key to medicine and mastered medical skills. His original intention to compile *Arcane Essentials from the Imperial Library* was to give the people easy access to the treatment of diseases and pass medical skills down from generation to generation, and to know the way of filial piety and fulfill his duty as a son. Wang Tao mentioned the dedication of filial sons Zengzi and Min Sun in the preface of *Arcane Essentials from the Imperial Library*. He emphasized that filial sons should "understand medical skills", "investigate disease sources" and "explore prescriptions"; otherwise, they are not dutiful. Wang Tao's compilation of *Arcane*

Essentials from the Imperial Library is a portrayal of his spirit of meeting filial duties with medical skills and benefiting the people.

During his tenure as Supervising Secretary of Chancellery, Wang Tao was in charge of books collected in the Hongwen Library. Thus, he was able to read, collect and sort out medical books, classical prescriptions, and documents of the past dynasties. To write *Arcane Essentials from the Imperial Library*, he perused thousands of volumes of medical literature of previous dynasties and extracted and edited useful information. As said in the preface of *Arcane Essentials from the Imperial Library*, "He acquired the thoughts of sages and learned the essence of theories raised by previous talents." When it comes to the experience of his predecessors, he said he would "repeatedly 'research' it", because "the misunderstanding of a single word may harm human life". He carefully selected the knowledge and learned the strengths from different scholars, practicing what he preached.

More than 60 medical classics of the past dynasties were cited in this book and more than 6,900 prescriptions were recorded, with the sources of all the cited materials being indicated. Many recorded treatment methods and prescriptions finally proved practical. The "elaborate" compilation fully demonstrates Wang Tao's rigorous academic attitude and extraordinary academic courage.

Mutual trust between TCM practitioners and patients benefits the treatment of diseases. Wang Tao said in *Arcane Essentials from the Imperial Library* that "good medicines and good words are everywhere, but not everyone will accept the words and use the medicines. Therefore, we should provide medical treatment for those who trust us, but needn't explain much to those with an unbelieving attitude". It means that good medicine and good words can be identified at the first sight, and there is no need to force others to accept them. Just treat whoever trusts us, and not explain to those that do not. This shows that he attached great importance to the mutual trust and sincerity between TCM practitioners and patients. He believed that only in this way can they cooperate closely. On the contrary, mutual suspicion will destroy the basis of cooperation, which is detrimental to the treatment of diseases. His viewpoints are of reference significance for building a harmonious medical practitioner-patient relationship currently.

4.2.4　Jianzhen

1. Brief biography

Jianzhen, with the surname of Chunyu, was born in Jiangyang, Guangling (now Yangzhou, Jiangsu Province). He was a Buddhist master in the Tang dynasty and the founding master of the Ritsu school of Buddhism in Japan. Jianzhen's family was poor in his early years. At the age of 14, he became a disciple of Dayun Temple in Yangzhou. At the age of 25, he became a prominent monk and served as the abbot of Daming Temple in Yangzhou. During the Kaiyuan period, monks from Japan were sent with diplomats to study in China. Jianzhen was invited to Japan to promote Dharma and transmit precepts. After difficulties and obstacles, he finally arrived in Japan at his sixth attempt and was heartily welcomed by the Japanese monks. Jianzhen is knowledgeable, especially in medicine. His voyage to Japan not only spread Buddhism but also brought Chinese medical knowledge to Japan. He thus enjoys high prestige in the Japanese medical community.

2. Traditional Chinese medicine stories

Jianzhen showed his perseverance when voyaging eastward. In 742 AD, Jianzhen accepted the invitation of Japanese monks and decided to go to Japan to preach Buddhism. In the second year, Jianzhen and his disciples Xiangyan, Daoxing and others began to cross the ocean to Japan. Within ten years, they tried to cross the sea five times. Due to arduousness of the journey, they didn't succeed. After the fifth failure, the 62-year-old Jianzhen lost his eyesight. His first disciple Xiangyan passed away and the Japanese monk who invited him died of illness. However, Jianzhen still did not change his hope of crossing the sea to Japan and insisted on going. In 753 AD, he led more than 40 disciples to cross the sea for the sixth time and successfully arrived in Japan. *The Biography of Master Jianzhen* recorded: "It's for Buddhism. Why should I cherish my life! Even if others don't go, I will go." It can be seen that in order to preach Buddhism and medicine, with the courage to take risks and dare to sacrifice, Jianzhen never give up. Jianzhen crossed eastward also promoted the exchange of Chinese and Japanese medicine.

Jianzhen had high prestige in Japan and was called Shennong of Japan. Jianzhen, with profound medical knowledge and proficiency in herbs, brought Chinese medicine identification, manufacturing, formulation, storage, use and other techniques to Japan. Jianzhen crossed the ocean to Japan and brought Chinese medicinal materials weighing more than 600 Jin (300 kilograms), as well as Chinese classical medical books and wonderful prescriptions. He performed good deeds, imparted medical knowledge and techniques, applied medicines to save people, and diagnosed and treated patients enthusiastically. He was quite famous and prestige in Japan, loved by the people, known as the originator of Chinese medicine and the Shennong of Japan. Jianzhen died in Japan, and was buried in the Japanese Yakushi-ji Temple. Later generations designed his tower, inscribing "Jianzhen Great Monk".

4.3 Evaluation of Medical Practitioners and Their Medical Ethics

4.3.1 Evaluation on Chao Yuanfang's Thinking on Medical Ethics

Chao Yuanfang's prescriptions and works were highly praised in *The Catalog of Imperial Collection of Four Kinds*: "It was not far from ancient times, and there were still many classical prescriptions in the theory of pulse since the Han dynasty. Furthermore, TCM practitioners gathered their strengths on medicines and discussed with each other. Therefore, their theories were deep and profound, beyond the reach of later generations. Following *Yellow Emperor's Canon of Medicine*, this is the most oldest book, except for several letters written by Zhang Ji, Wang Shuhe and Ge Hong. Investigate its purport, it can also say that the book is the bridge of diagnosis and treatment." Hu Bing summarized Chao Yuanfang's medical ethics as follows: "He is innovative in inheriting traditional medicine, and focuses on prevention, proficient in medical theory. And he has good medical skills, gathering TCM practitioners' strengths on medicines. His work *General Treatise on the Causes and Symptoms of Disease* has detailed contents." Professor Wang Yulai wrote a poem for Chao Yuanfang in his book *Poetry Biography of Famous TCM Practitioners of All Dynasties* to summarize his medical ethics thought: "As a Director of the Imperial Medical Bureau, his benevolence is even more amazing. He compiled the source and so on in an imperial edict, and exhausted his heart to clarify the cause of disease. He prepared in every aspects and detailed analysis on various diseases. Looking back on the etiology, Chao's book was the number one."

From the above evaluation, it can be seen that *General Treatise on the Causes and Symptoms of Diseases* has the characteristics of quoting ancient books and learning from others' strengths. It was full and accurate in content, which enabled many ancient precious medical materials to be preserved. It had high historical value and academic value in the development history of TCM. Chao Yuanfang showed the combination of medical skill and benevolence. He was not only proficient in medical theory, but also careful in thinking. He has lived up to the expectations of the public and organized the compilation of the medical masterpiece of etiology, which has a profound impact on later generations.

4.3.2 Evaluation on Sun Simiao's Thinking on Medical Ethics

Sun Simiao stayed away from bureaucratic system all his life and led a seclusive life in the mountains. He collected herbs and created medicines by himself to cure people. He collected folk prescriptions and secret prescriptions, summarized the clinical experience and medical theory of previous generation, and made important contributions to medicine and pharmacology. Later he was honored as "King of Medicine" and "Sage of Medicine". As Chen Jiamo in the Ming dynasty said in the book, *Materia Medica Companion*, "Sun Zhenren in the Tang dynasty have incomparable prescriptions, which can help the weak and dangerous patients, and their prescription should be as effective as a god." Xu Dachun in the Qing dynasty said in the *Currents of Tradition in Chinese Medicine*, "The *Thousand Golden Prescriptions* is not the case. To some extent, his theory of disease has based on the *Internal Canon*, and there have been speculations by the later generations. All the prescriptions in it were ancient prescriptions, which included some rare methods from later generations. All the herbs in it were not necessarily based on Shennong, and all the miscellaneous prescriptions and dredging herbs were adopted. Therefore, there were several prescriptions for one disease, and there was also one prescription for treating several diseases." It can be seen that Sun Simiao's prescription is based on the experience of his predecessors, and it is really valuable and can play a role in curing diseases and saving people. His work, *Thousand Golden Prescriptions*, was the epitome of medical prescriptions before the Tang dynasty. It was known as the earliest clinical medical encyclopedia in China's history and had a profound impact on the development of medicine in later generations.

Li Shimin, highly praised Sun Simiao, "Therefore, those who are skilled in medicine can be truly respected. How can Xianmen and Guangcheng said false! He was a famous medical practitioner who carved out the medical path. He was a master of all generations." Gan Zuwang reviewed on Sun Simiao, "Sun Simiao was strange, fantastic, wise, knowledgeable, despised wealth and honour. As an old man, a famous medical practitioner, a Confucian scholar, a monk and a Taoist, he was a rare legendary figure of TCM for two thousand years. So when anyone mentions 'Sun Zhenren', everyone knows." As the saying goes, "Sun Simiao in Tang dynasty was a magic and unpredictable figure." Sun Simiao was a legendary figure, and also a typical representative of the famous medical practitioner of the Tang dynasty. Professor Wang Yulai wrote a poem for Sun Simiao in order to sum up his medical ethics thought: "Sun Zhenren was a great medical practitioner, and humanity went through the past and present. He was knowledgeable, and he treated diseases quietly and diligently. Even when he met the poor, he would have compassion and did not cheat patients. He just wanted people to be healthy and not obsessed with interests." Hu Bing summarized Sun Simiao's medical ethics thought as follows: "He was a medical practitioner who studied Confucianism, Taoism and Buddhism. He treated patients with charity and compassion. He wrote his work *Thousand Golden Prescriptions* diligently and tirelessly. As a great medical practitioner, his work *The Absolute Sincerity of a Great Physician* showed his noble ethics."

Sun Simiao not only had excellent medical skills but also had high medical ethics. He emphasized that TCM practitioners should take relieving patients' pain as their bounden duty and have compassion for others. Based on his clinical practice and his understanding of medicine, he extracted the medical ethics standard of *The Absolute Sincerity of a Great Physician*, which is hailed as the "Hippocratic Oath of the East". Sun Simiao was also hailed as the "teacher of a hundred generations" in the history of Chinese medical ethics due to his excellent medical skill, noble professional ethics, strong social responsibility and deep feelings for his country.

4.3.3   Evaluation on Wang Tao's Thinking on Medical Ethics

Regarding Wang Tao's medical ethics thinking, Hu Bing summarized it as follows, "Knowing medical filial piety for a long time, seeing the secrets of Aosheng Hall, he was meticulous in his scholarly research and made great efforts to become a world treasure." "A world treasure" was a high praise of *Medical Secrets of an Official* written by Wang Tao in *New Book of Tang*, which had extremely high medical value and historical value. Wang Yulai commented on Wang Tao, "When he was a child, he was confined to illness and suffered hardships, and when he was older, he devoted to medicine and compiled history books. He had lived in the border town of Hubei and Shanxi for fifteen years and in the Hong Wen Pavilion for twenty years. Despite the disease in summer, he still read books and believed that ancient books contained wisdom. *Medical Secrets of an Official* gathered the medical theories of the past dynasties, and it was wonderful."

Wang Tao devoted himself to studying for 20 years and read extensively, which can be said that "from Shennong to the Tang dynasty, all books were selected to read by him". He collected and sorted out the medical books and documents of the ancient classics and prescriptions day and night, comprehended the beauty of them, studied repeatedly, eliminated the false and retained the true, and made a large number of extracts and catalogs. He learned extensively, noted clearly, and studied rigorously. He was praised by Mr. Li Jingwei as a "master of medical literature". Many TCM practitioners in past dynasties believed that "if one did not observe the prescriptions in *Medical Secrets of an Official* or read the theory of *Thousand Golden Prescriptions*, the TCM practitioners' medical knowledge would not be extensive and the medication would not be magic". This showed the high status of the book in the medical field and its outstanding achievements are self-evident. The original intention of Wang Tao's study of medicine and painstaking compilation of medical tomes was to "know medicine and fulfill filial piety", which was a reflection of the realization of the idea that "those who have no knowledge of medicine are not allowed to be filial sons".

4.3.4 Evaluation on Jianzhen's Thinking on Medical Ethics

Jianzhen practiced medicine in Japan to rescue patients. Because of his excellent medical skills, he enjoyed high prestige in the Japanese medicine community and was known as the founder of Chinese medicine and Shennong of Japan. When Jianzhen died, the Japanese people called it "the Demise of Tenpyō", meaning that his achievements were enough to represent the roof of the Tenpyō era in Japanese history. Fujigawa You, a Japanese medical historian, pointed out in *The History of Japanese Medicine* that "although there were many famous ancient Japanese TCM practitioners, only Jianzhen and Tashiro Sanki were commemorated by building statues". For a foreign medical practitioner, this is a very high evaluation.

4.3.5 Evaluation on Wang Bing's Thinking on Medical Ethics

"When he was young, he pursued medical ethics, and liked to study health preservation. After retirement, he met the Sutra. He annotated *Yellow Emperor's Canon of Medicine: Plain Conversation* (including proofreading, annotation, translation and development), making the book complete and clear. He was famous for annotation of the book." This was a portrayal of Bing Wang's life. Wang Bing was famous for his annotation of the famous ancient Chinese medical work *Yellow Emperor's Canon of Medicine: Plain Conversation*. *Plain Conversation* was written in the Spring and Autumn Period and the Warring States Period. Although the content was exquisite but obscure, it often led to misdiagnosis and tragedies. Out of TCM practitioners' conscience and considerations for patients, Wang Bing decided to study the book carefully. He went to the Taoist temple to worship the teacher. After rigorous learning and assessment, he completed the *Sub-note of Plain Conversation*, adjusting the original 9 volumes to 24 volumes, and the content discussed was very abundant. He made outstanding contributions to the medical career. The later generations studied *Plain Conversation* mostly on the basis of Bing Wang's study.

4.3.6 Evaluation on Yutuo Yundeng Gongbu's Thinking on Medical Ethics

Yutuo Yundeng Gongbu was an outstanding master of Tibetan medicine. He wrote *The Four Medical Tantras*, which is the founder of the theoretical system of Tibetan medicine. He went to Nepal, India and other countries with an open mind to study. He had also visited various parts of his motherland many times and accumulated rich medical knowledge. With a benevolent heart, he saved lives in risk and was invited to treat the disease of the foreign royal families many times. He was scientifically creative in clinical treatment and was recognized and respected for his superb technology and pioneering spirit. He also selflessly dedicated himself to the cultivation of medical talents and founded the Tibetan Medical School. Yutuo Yundeng Gongbu had combined the theoretical study and clinical experience and devoted more than 20 years to writing books. The contents of *The Four Medical Tantras* were clear and detailed, with strong practicability. It was a necessary book for Tibetan medical scientists in past dynasties to learn medicine. Some people claimed that this book can be compared with *Yellow Emperor's Canon of Medicine*. Due to its outstanding achievements, Yutuo Yundeng Gongbu has been regarded as "medical saint" and "medicine king" by the Tibetan people. Many words and deeds of Yutuo Yundeng Gongbu reflected his noble medical ethics of keeping improving medical skills, treating patients equally regardless of rank and treating teachers with reverence and respect.

4.3.7　Evaluation on Song Qing's Thinking on Medical Ethics

The Supplement to the History of the Tang Dynasty recorded that people in Chang'an City preached the great righteousness of Song Qing as a medicine merchant for the people. As a businessman, Song Qing had such a high reputation among the people because of his noble quality of not being greedy for money and giving medicine with benevolence.

4.4　Medical Education

4.4.1　Medical System in Sui and Tang dynasties

Since the Western Zhou dynasty, an official system has been established for medical affairs. Since then, each dynasty and each generation have its own development and evolution. During the Sui and Tang dynasties, a relatively specific and perfect, large-scale and standardized medical system had been formed. Medical organizations in Sui and Tang dynasties included medical administration, medical treatment and medical teaching. Compared with the medical system in the Sui and Tang dynasties, the medical officers in the Sui dynasty were simpler to set up, the classification of medical personnel was more extensive, and the number of TCM practitioners and TCM practitioners was huge, more than that in the Tang dynasty. The establishment of medical organization personnel in the Tang dynasty not only continued the Sui dynasty system, but also made some innovative changes. The setting of medical officers in the Tang dynasty was more detailed. The ranks of medical officers were more complex. The duties of the personnel were relatively clear and the division of labor was more precise. The medical system in Sui and Tang dynasties mainly had three systems: the Palace Dispensary and Dietetic officer for serving the Emperor; the Medicine Reserve Bureau and special medical practitioner for serving the Heir Apparent; The Imperial Medical Bureau for managing medical officers and medical education, and local medical institutions.

1. Central medical institutions

(1) The Palace Dispensary.

The Palace Dispensary was a medical institution specially set up for Emperor, which was responsible for the daily diagnosis, treatment and health care of Emperor and other royal families. Generally, without the permission of the Emperor, officers and ministers had no legal requirements for medical treatment from the officers of the Palace Dispensary. The Palace Dispensary had a post named Chief Steward with Rank 5, which was held by experts who were proficient in medical skills. This was the top executive of Imperial Medical Bureau. Foreman in the Imperial Pharmacy was its assistant, and the deputy chief executive was a Rank 7-2 chief executive. The Chief Steward of the Imperial Pharmacy's duty was to "take charge of and treat the Emperor". In other words, they must personally feel the pulse, make prescriptions, make medicine and taste medicine for the Emperor. Foreman in the Imperial Pharmacy cooperated with Chief Steward of the Imperial Pharmacy to cure diseases and manage the Palace Dispensary. The Imperial Physicians participated in the treatment of the Emperor, but the main responsibility was to serve the Emperor, observe his illness in time, and prepare medicine. Chief Herb officer and apprentices were mainly responsible for herb processing and medicine preparation. The physician with lower ranks and their assistants were responsible for the medical treatment of other members of the royal family. The medication maker was responsible for making some beauty products and the storage keeper was in charge of the drug storage. The Palace Dispensary had strict regulations on taking medicine for the Emperor when he was ill, and every procedure should be recorded in detail. When making medicine for emperor, Chief Steward of the Imperial Pharmacy and Director of the Palace Administration supervised together until the medicine was finished. Then the personnel above the medical assistants tried to seal it, wrote the name and composition of the medicine, and indicated the time when the system was formed. The supervisor also needed to sign before they can play. Before the Emperor took the medicine, the Chief Steward of the Imperial Pharmacy needed to taste it, then Director of the Palace Administration and the Heir Apparent, and finally the Emperor took it. The medicines that the Palace Dispensary gave to Emperor should be checked regularly by Master of Ceremony every season and returned to those who have rotten and mildewed. In addition to the Palace Dispensary, the Dietetic officer of the Imperial Food Bureau and Academician Awaiting Orders in the Hanlin Academy were all dedicated to the Emperor's medical and health services. Dietetic officer, who was Rank 9-2 chief executive, was similar to today's nutritionist. They were in charge of the Emperor's nutrition according to the seasonal changes. Academician Awaiting Orders in the Hanlin Academy were called Medical Officers in the Hanlin Academy, who were selected from the Imperial Medical Bureau or the people with superb medical skills and special skills. Some people have been appointed to the imperial edict according to the Emperor's preferences.

(2) The Medicine Reserve Bureau.

As the crown prince, he had his own independent medical and health care institution. The Medicine Reserve Bureau was a medical institution in the Eastern Palace dedicated to serving the crown prince. The functions of the Medicine Reserve Bureau were similar to those of the Palace Dispensary, with different official positions. The chief executive of the Medicine Reserve Bureau, the drug collection supervisor, with the top title of Rank 6, only inferior to that Chief Steward of the Palace Dispensary. The Assistant Director in the Medicine Reserve Bureau, a senior official with the top title of Rank 8, was the deputy of the drug collection supervisor. The work nature of Director in the Medicine Reserve Bureau and Assistant Director in the Medicine Reserve Bureau was similar to Chief Steward of the Imperial Pharmacy and Foreman in the Imperial Pharmacy. When the crown prince was ill, court doctors and classical medicine officers were in debt to diagnose, serve, and feed medicine. The Apprentice Pharmacist in the Imperial Pharmacy shook and screened the medicine. The storage keeper was responsible for taking charge of the medicine storage. They were jointly responsible for the crown prince's medical care. Among the eunuchs serving the crown prince, there was also the position of medical practitioner in charge with Vice Rank 8 to the main medicine, who was responsible for treating other people's diseases in the Eastern Palace. Same as the Emperor, the crown prince had a complete system of tasting medicine. First of all, the Medicine Reserve Bureau diagnoses and made prescriptions. It was responsible for refining medicines and delivering them to TCM practitioners. Then it tested medicines from the food department of the Eastern Palace officials. Finally, the crown prince consumed the medicine.

(3) The Imperial Medical Bureau.

The Imperial Medical Bureau was established in the Sui dynasty. The system in the Tang dynasty inherited the system of the Sui dynasty and established the Imperial Medical Bureau, which was under the jurisdiction of the Court of Imperial Sacrifices. The Court of Imperial Sacrifices acted as the general agent of the state's medical policy to master medical resources. The Imperial Medical Bureau was responsible for medical administration and medical education throughout the country. It was a medical institution integrating scientific research, medical treatment and education.

In terms of administration, the Director of the Imperial Medical Bureau, which was in charge of the medical treatment method, was set up as the supreme administrator of the Imperial Medical Bureau. The assistant officers included the Assistant Director of the Imperial Academy of Medicine and the Director of the Imperial Medical Bureau, who were in charge of the overall arrangement of work, and issued and implemented the orders on medical treatment, medical education and other aspects nationwide. In terms of treatment, there were Director of TCM practitioners, medical workers and TCM practitioners, who mainly serve the Emperor, dukes, officials and the harem, and were also responsible for the medical treatment of the army in the palace, official craftsmen and palace people. In addition, in the event of a major epidemic, the Imperial Medical Bureau also treated the average people. In terms of education, the Imperial Medical Bureau was responsible for providing talents for the royal court and the government, including education management, administrative facilities, and course examinations. In addition to medical treatment, Scholars and Instructors mainly taught students with medical skills. In terms of staffing and equipment, the Tang dynasty strengthened the responsibility of medical policy management and education. The Imperial Medical Bureau clearly set up four departments, namely, medical department, acupuncture department, massage department and incantation department. The acupuncture department was a new department, and there was also a drug learning department. There were Scholar and Instructors in each department, medical professionals and TCM practitioners to guide teaching assistants to learn, and Director of the Imperial Medical Bureau and officials to take responsibility for assessment, which strengthened the educational responsibilities of the Imperial Medical Bureau.

2. Local medical affairs management

In the Sui and Tang dynasties, the local medical systems also developed. However, there was no special medical institution. Local medical administration and medical education were indistinguishable. Local medical affairs in Tang dynasty were paid more attention than those in Sui dynasty, and a set of institutions were established to determine the medical settings according to the local population. There were regulations on the number and rank of teachers and learners in medical schools in all provinces and prefectures. Medical Scholars, Medical Instructors and Medical Students were set up in the administrative units at the local state level, and Medical Scholars were also responsible for medical treatment and education. The Medical Instructors, together with the Medical Scholars, carried the medical affairs with debts, and the Medical Students were responsible for the itinerant medical service throughout the state.

The local state department shall implement treatment, the competent department in charge shall timely ask for a medical practitioner to deliver medicine, and the chief medical officer shall also timely provide treatment. Dereliction of duty is not allowed, and dereliction of duty shall be punished according to the law. According to *The Tang Law Explanation*, the director and chief drug officer who were negligent in treatment were sentenced to forty flogs; one who caused death was sentenced to one year in prison. Gong Cao or Si Gong were responsible for medicine collection and pharmaceutical matters in all prefectures under the military jurisdiction, and medicines were used to treat people's diseases, which also reflected that the official was responsible for the daily medical treatment of the local people.

Bingfang run by the government was an important part of the local government's efforts to save people's suffering, because it was an important part of the medical system and played an important role in public medical charity. The predelessor, of the Bingfang was the Beitian Nursing Home. In the early Tang dynasty, the Beitian Nursing Home was founded by the Buddhist temple, which was used to adopt the poor and treat diseases. Later, it was specially managed by envoys. The beggars in the capital were managed by the Bingfang. As the Bingfang was assisted by the officials of the temple office, the necessary funds and expenses were allocated by the state and presided over by the monk. The official government indirectly led and supervised Bingfang. Bingfang were a little similar to government-run hospitals, where patients and homeless people could rest and recuperate. Bingfan made up for the deficiencies of folk medical care, were beneficial to the poor and sick patients, and played a certain role in assisting the official medical system in the Tang dynasty.

4.4.2 Education and Management of Medical Practitioners

Medical education was divided into government-run school education and traditional folk education. Folk medical education mainly included the form of teacher apprentice teaching, family inheritance, self-study, etc. The early forms of folk medical education in China played an important role in training medical students. Such as Bianque, a famous medical practitioner in the Warring States Period; Zhang Zhongjing, a famous medical practitioner in the Eastern Han dynasty; Hua Tuo, a famous medical practitioner in the Three Kingdoms; Xu Zhicai, a famous medical practitioner in the Northern and Southern dynasties, whose family practiced medicine from generation to generation; Huangfu Mi learned to become a famous medical practitioner in the Western Jin dynasty. With the development and progress of medicine and pharmacology, the demand for medical talents in society has increased, and the traditional education methods have gradually failed to meet the social needs, which has also brought difficulties to the assessment and management of the government. Therefore, the official medical education system came into being. The central government established a medical education system and carried out personnel training, which made up for the shortcomings of fewer medical students and limited knowledge in folk education. Starting from the demand of the ruling class, the medical education system was an educational model integrating politics and education. The government organized the education in terms of talents, money and materials. The official medical education in ancient China began in the Jin dynasty, and was formed and perfected in the Sui and Tang dynasties. The Sui dynasty set up the "Imperial Medical Bureau", which was not only a medical institution, but also the largest medical education institution in China. The system in the Tang dynasty had a greater development on the basis of the Sui dynasty. In addition to the central government, medical schools were widely established in all regions. School-based education was popularized throughout the country. Medical education made great progress in terms of school system, education scale, setting of education majors, teaching content, teaching methods, and so on. For the first time, medicine was accepted into the imperial examination system. During the Sui and Tang dynasties, while the official medical education had developed greatly, the folk medical education also enjoyed some development.

1. Medical education in the Sui dynasty

After the unification of the Sui dynasty, a special institution in charge of medical education, the Imperial Medical Bureau, was established and improved. In addition to engaging in the royal medical business, the Imperial Medical Bureau also taught students various medical skills and was responsible for the training of specialized medical talents, which created a new situation for school-style medical education. Medical education in the Sui dynasty had relatively complete provisions in terms of setting, scale and system. At that time, it began to carry out branch education, with three departments: medical practitioner department, massage department, incantation department, and pharmacy specialty. At that time, the acupuncture department was included in the medical education. In addition, there was the Veterinary Department. Although there was a position as Scholar, as long as it did not belong to the Imperial Medical Bureau, it attached to the Court of imperial stud and was not in the general medical education system.

There were 2 Scholars, 2 Instructors, 200 TCM practitioners and 120 medical students in the medical education department. The medical Scholars were in charge of teaching students the methods of diagnosis and treatment. There were 2 massage Scholars, 120 masseurs and 100 massage students in the massage department. The massage Scholars and masseurs mainly taught students the "message guided" massage method of meridians and acupuncture points. The massage department received the most attention in the Sui dynasty. *General Treatise on the Causes and*

Symptoms of Diseases written by Chao Yuanfang also introduced many methods of curing diseases through massage guidance. The incantation department taught students various folk exorcisms, footwork and incantations. The pharmacy specialty had 2 chief drug officers, 2 pharmacists and a number of students, and the pharmacists, chief drug officer, director of drugs, etc. They were responsible for drug teaching and management, mainly teaching students to identify the origin, quality, medicinal properties and planting methods of various medicinal materials. The good teachers, medical officers and medical workers of the Imperial Medical Bureau should not only be responsible for educating and training TCM practitioners, but also participate in medical work. They should also take medical achievements as the basis for the examination of medical education courses. Although the reign of the Sui dynasty was short, its medical education was highly valued, with 580 medical teachers and students at most. The continuous development of medical education in the Sui dynasty had a profound impact on the medical education in the Tang dynasty, both in teaching organization and specialty settings, and laid a solid foundation for the prosperity of medical education in the Tang dynasty.

2. Medical education in the Tang dynasty

(1) Central medical education.

The medical system in the Tang dynasty inherited official medical education in the Sui dynasty, carried out reform and development, and improved and standardized the specific institutional settings. The Imperial Medical Bureau of Tang dynasty was still the highest medical education management organization, but its scale, educational system, assessment and other systems had undergone major changes.

(2) Specialties setting and staffing.

The Imperial Medical Bureau of Tang dynasty was divided into a medical department and a pharmaceutical department. Under the medical department, there were four departments: medicine department, acupuncture department, massage department, and incantation department. Among them, the medicine department was the largest, and it was also the focus of the Imperial Medical Bureau's education. Under the medicine department, there were five specialties: physical therapy, sore and swellings, youngster, ear, eye, mouth and teeth, and horn cupping therapy. The length of schooling was seven years, five years, and two years respectively. Physical therapy specialty was equivalent to internal medicine, sores and swellings specialties was equivalent to surgery, youngster specialty was equivalent to pediatrics, ears, eyes, mouth and teeth specialties was equivalent to today's ENT and Stomatology Departments, and the horn cupping therapy was the external physical therapy such as cupping. The Imperial Medical Bureau of Tang dynasty had a medical Scholar, an acupuncture Scholar, a massage Scholar, an incantation Scholar and a Scholar Instructors, enrolling 85 students, including 40 medical students, 20 acupuncture students, 15 massage students and 10 incantation students. In addition, the government had a pharmacy specializing in pharmacy. There were 8 students in the pharmacy, who had studied medicine for up to 9 years. They specialized in cultivating medicines, collecting medicinal materials and preparing medicines.

As a matter of fact, the Imperial Medical Bureau of Tang dynasty can be regarded as the Central Medical University, which was headed by the Court of Imperial Sacrifices. In terms of administration, there were two directors from the Imperial Medical Bureau, equivalent to the president, who was responsible for the overall leadership. In addition, there were 2 assistants, equivalent to vice principals, assisting Director of Imperial Medical Bureau. There were 2 archive officers, 2 official historians, 4 directors of the Imperial Medical Bureau, 8 medical supervisors, and 4 storage keepers, assisting the Imperial Medical Bureau in the work of academic affairs, documents, archives, and daily affairs. Educational institutions had more staffs and clearer responsibilities.

(3) Admission requirements for medical students.

In the Tang dynasty, there were strict requirements on the admission qualifications and order of admission. First, they were people with hereditary medical positions and pharmacist titles; second, they came from hereditary families with more than three generations of medical profession; third, for common people, only those who were quite smart and aged 13 to 16 and were children of officials above Rank 5. In addition, for the children of officials above Rank 8, those with outstanding qualifications can also be admitted exceptionally.

Medical students who were new to school need to practice discipline with their teachers. *The Medical Disease Order* clearly stipulated that "all new medical students and acupuncture students should give tuition fee to the teacher. The medical students and acupuncture students should give a piece of silk respectively, and the massage students, incantation students and other students should give a piece of silk. All students should send wine and dried meat. It set the tuition fee standard for students in the Directorate of Education." About the distribution of tuition fees, "Students in Directorate of Education and the Imperial College, three pieces of silk for each; four schools, two pieces of silk for each; Junshi, Lüshu, and Suanxue (student types), one piece of silk by prefecture and county respectively. All students should send wine and dried meat. The tuition fee was divided into five parts, and three parts for Scholars and two parts for Instructors.

(4) The content of medical education.

After entering the Imperial Medical Bureau, medical students should first learn the basic courses such as *Mingtang*, *Plain Conversation*, *Shennong's Herbal Classic*, *Pulse Classic*, and *Canon of Acupuncture and Moxibustion*, understand the knowledge of acupuncture, vasculology, and pharmacology, and then study for physical therapy, wound, youth, ear, eye, mouth and teeth, and angle method respectively. Each major had different years of study, which were seven, five, five, two, and two years. There were 40 medical students, including 22 students learning for physical therapy, 6 students learning for sores therapy, 6 students learning for young people therapy, 4 students learning for ears, eyes, mouth and teeth therapy, and 2 students learning for the cupping therapy. In the medical department, there was one Scholar, with the position of Rank 8-1, and one or two Instructors. The medical Scholars and medical Instructors taught students to learn medicine. In addition, there were 20 TCM practitioners and 100 medical workers, who assisted in education and teaching.

The acupuncture department was newly established in the Tang dynasty and was independent from medical department. There was one acupuncture Scholar in the acupuncture department, whose position was slightly lower than medical Erudite, and it was the top title of Rank 8. Acupuncture teaching was mainly in the charge of acupuncture Scholar, who taught students acupuncture skills. In addition, there was 1 acupuncture Instructor, 10 acupuncture therapists, 20 acupuncture workers, assistant acupuncture Scholars and acupuncture Instructors to carry out teaching. The learning contents of acupuncture students mainly include *Plain Conversation*, *Yellow Emperor's Acupuncture Classic*, *Ming Tang*, and *Pulse Technique*. They also learnt *Liu Zhu*, *Yan Bian* and *Chiwu God's Acupuncture*.

The position of massage department in Tang dynasty was inferior to that in Sui dynasty. The department had one massage Erudite, whose position with vice title of

Rank 9 was lower than medical Scholars. They were in charge of massage students from the ninth grade, using the method of information guidance to eliminate the eight diseases of human wind, cold, heat, dampness, ridicule, satiety, fatigue, and leisure, and to treat those who were injured or fallen. There were 4 masseurs and 16 massage workers in the massage department to assist massage students in their study. In addition to basic courses such as medical theory and medicine, massage students also needed to learn "the method of information guidance", "the stretching of bears and birds, the art of prolonging life", bone setting, etc.

Although the scale of the incantation and prohibition discipline was small in the Tang dynasty, it was professional and well-developed. There was one incantation Scholar, who taught the method of removing evil spirits with vice title of Rank 9. There were also 2 incantation teachers and 8 incantation workers to assist the teaching of the incantation Scholars. The courses of incantation and prohibition mainly included the road prohibition of mountain dwelling alchemists, the forbidden incantation in Buddhism, etc. The contents were superstitious, but Qigong and psychotherapy were among them.

Pharmaceutical education and medical education in the Tang dynasty were separated, but were still managed by the Imperial Medical Bureau. There were 2 archive officials, 4 official historians, 4 storage keepers, 8 chief drug officers, 8 main drug administrators, 2 teachers in the pharmacy, 8 students in the pharmacy, and 24 Apprentice Pharmacist in the Imperial Pharmacy. In addition to planting and collecting medicinal materials, the teachers of the pharmacy were also responsible for the education, as well as undertaking the teaching of herbal medicine courses for students of other disciplines, providing medical students of various disciplines with practical opportunities to identify medicines.

(5) Assessment and appointment of TCM practitioners.

In order to improve the level of medical education, TCM practitioners, acupuncturists, masseurs, and incantations should also follow medical Scholars to study. The assessment of educators was attached great importance in The Tang dynasty. The evaluation rank of Scholars and Instructors was based on the amount of teaching. The government paid attention to the actual medical practice of TCM practitioners, medical workers and other teaching auxiliary personnel, and took the number of people being cured as the assessment index of TCM practitioners, medical officers and medical workers. And medical officials in medicine, acupuncture, massage, incantation and worker, among which the outstanding ones were selected as teaching Instructors and Scholars, or the outstanding ones among teaching Instructors were further selected as Scholars.

For medical students, there were three kinds of examinations: routine examination, completion examination and employment examination. The routine examination was divided into monthly examination, quarterly examination and year-end examination. The monthly examination was presided over by the Scholar in charge of teaching, the quarterly examination was presided over by the Director of the Imperial Medical Bureau and Assistant Director of the Imperial Academy of Medicine, and the annual examination was conducted by Chief Minister or Vice Minister of the Court of Imperial Sacrifices. The examination forms were trial reading and experimental research. The trial reading was that students memorize the scriptures, then filled in the blanks by silent writing, and examine the student's memorization of the scriptures, while the trial lecture examined the students' understanding of the scriptures. The examination results were divided into upper, middle and lower grades, and the students will be dismissed for three consecutive years of lower grade. After nine years of study, if students cannot meet the standard they will also be expelled.

Only after the students have completed the prescribed courses and years of study can they have the opportunity to participate in the career success test hosted and supervised by the Palace Dispensary and Assistant Director, and their examination results should be reported to Department of Imperial Affairs in detail. After passing the test, they had the opportunity to participate in the selection examination of Department of Imperial Affairs, namely the medical examination, and then fill the post of medical officer. Those who failed to pass the medical examination will be returned to the Imperial Medical Bureau for further study. If the students had mastered medical skills and were able to perform them, they will compete with TCM practitioners and acupuncturists to test their medical skills. The winner will be the complementary TCM practitioners, followed by the complementary TCM practitioners. The massage and incantation students can not take part in the imperial examination. After graduation, they can only work as masseurs, massage workers, incantations and incantation workers.

In addition, the Tang dynasty also set up a separate education system for female TCM practitioners, who had to study for five years. A total of 50 female TCM practitioners were selected from officer servants who were 20 to 30 years old, without husband, child and without sexual experience, and the responsible professors of female TCM practitioners were medical Scholars from the Imperial Medical Bureau. The teaching content was abortion and the methods of treating dystocia, sores, injuries, and acupuncture, which were orally taught by text. The year-end examination for female TCM practitioners was presided over by the medical supervisor and medical officer of the Imperial Medical Bureau.

(6) Local medical education.

Before the Tang dynasty, the official medical education was only carried out in the central level. During the Zhenguan Period, local medicine was established, which was the earliest record of local medical education. In the Tang dynasty, national medical education was valued, and local medical education was also valued. It spread the scale of medical education to all states and counties in the country, making medical education more popular. In addition to carrying out education and training medical talents for all needs, local medical schools were also responsible for the medical treatment and medicine application of the people. Medical Scholars, medical Instructors and medical students all had dual responsibilities of medical education and disease treatment.

In terms of teaching staff, there were great differences between local and imperial medical offices. Except for medical Scholars, medical Instructors and a small number of TCM practitioners, there were no other official medical personnel in the local area, and TCM practitioners can only be selected from civilian TCM practitioners. If there were qualified TCM practitioners in the military, they should be ordered to leave the military and join the medical education industry. The selected TCM practitioners shall pass the examination and the local government shall report the selection results to Department of Imperial Affairs, and then fill the position of medical Scholars or medical Instructors. The selection of medical students must come from the jurisdiction where they were located. Students with medical pedigrees or from medical families, or those who study medicine themselves, were preferred. *The Medical Disease Order* in the Tang dynasty indicated that "the years for medical students to be taught and teaching methods in every states should in accordance with the training law of the Imperial Medical Bureau." During the Kai Yuan Period, the Imperial Medical Bureau promoted the central medical education system to the local governments. In terms of teaching materials, teaching methods, examination and selection, the local medical education has been connected with the central medical education. Local areas also had their own cultivation characteristics. Outside of the prescribed textbooks, TCM practitioners of the Imperial Medical Bureau have chosen to copy ancient prescriptions and read them aloud. Besides that local education has carried out some effective treatment methods. In terms of the assessment of TCM practitioners in prefectures and counties, there were quarterly tests and year-end examinations. The quarterly tests were presided over by medical Scholars, and the year-end examinations were more formal, presided over by the officers and the Division, and the test registration was established. Like the Imperial Medical Bureau, those with poor exam results will be punished or even dismissed.

Although the establishment of local medicine in the Tang dynasty was intermittent, and the education scale was small, the staffing was simple, and the implementation of teaching was not very stable, the government always maintained the importance of local medicine, and did not slaken its efforts. Its effectiveness and promoting effects in local medicine development were worthy of recognition, and many measures were conducive to the development of medical and health undertakings.

Chapter Summary

The Sui and Tang dynasties were a prosperous period of China's feudal society. With national unity, economic development and cultural prosperity, medicine also developed unprecedentedly and became mature. This was mainly reflected in attaching importance to the collection and collation of medical achievements; Establishing medical institutions and establishing medicine; Developing medicine, standardizing medicine and improving medical level; Combining professional education with medical ethics education; Passing legislation to protect public health interests.

The TCM practitioners in Sui and Tang dynasties attached great importance to the understanding and practice of medical ethics, and formed quite perfect views on various aspects of medical ethics, which made the feudal medical ethics mature in theory and practice. First of all, the principle of sacred life and healing the wounded and dying has become a voluntary principle for TCM practitioners; Secondly, a fairly comprehensive medical ethics standard have been formed; Third, TCM practitioners have a deep understanding of the medical practitioner-patient relationship; Furthermore, the basic idea of medical ethics education and medical ethics evaluation has been formed; Finally, TCM practitioners should pay attention to vulnerable groups and practice social responsibility.

Application in Contemporary Times

1. Medical education and medical ethics evaluation are consistent with the goal of cultivating medical talents in the new era of "high moral and medical excellence"

This chapter describes the education, assessment and appointment of TCM practitioners in the Sui and Tang dynasties. The Imperial Medical Bureau was established in the Sui dynasty. The Tang dynasty followed the Sui dynasty system and established the Imperial Medical Bureau. The Imperial Medical Bureau was responsible for medical administration and medical education throughout the country. It was a medical institution integrating scientific research, medical treatment and education. In terms of education, the Imperial Medical Bureau was responsible for providing talents for the royal court and the government, including education management, administrative facilities, and course examinations. In terms of personnel allocation, the management and education responsibilities of medical administration have been strengthened. There were clear divisions, specialized professors and auxiliary teaching staff in each department, and special personnel was responsible for the assessment. There were also certain requirements for the admission conditions of students. The curriculum arrangement of medical students after admission, the length of study in each major, the form of examination, persuasion and employment had been clearly stipulated. The educational responsibilities of the Imperial Medical Bureau were strengthened. In addition, a relatively perfect medical examination system was established in the Tang dynasty, and medical department was included in the imperial examination system for the first time, which was conducive to the selection and appointment of excellent medical talents. Moreover, the laws of the Sui and Tang dynasties were also gradually completed, which had a certain role in restricting and guiding the morality of medical practitioners. During the Sui and Tang dynasties, the emphasis on medical education and strict management and assessment system improved the training quality of medical talents, and the requirements for medical talents were also constantly improved, not only limited to medical skills, but also medical ethics.

Medicine is a noble cause to safeguard human life safety and health, and medical students are the main force and reserve talents in China's medical and health undertakings. The goal of medical education is to train medical students to become future TCM practitioners with superb medical skills, high professional quality and both ability and morality. To achieve the goal of medical talent training in the new era, it is necessary to have a systematic medical talent training program and accelerate the construction of a medical talent training system with Chinese characteristics. Medical students can improve their medical professional ability by learning theoretical knowledge and practicing skills. Medicine is benevolence, and morality is medicine based. Medical students must establish noble professional ethics as the goal of their own development and career pursuit. We should strengthen medical ethics, integrate medical humanistic education into professional education, constantly explore and practice, strengthen medical ethics and medical ethics education, cultivate humanistic feelings, form good moral customs and professional values, further improve the quality and level of medical and health teams, and promote the development of medical and health undertakings and social progress in China.

2. Promoting the spirit of the Absolute Sincerity of a Great Physician is consistent with cultivating and practicing socialist core values

The culture of medical ethics in Sui and Tang dynasties was practiced and developed by TCM practitioners represented by Sun Simiao. Sun Simiao was the founder of medical ethics in China. The idea of "the Absolute Sincerity of a Great Physician" advocated by him was widely spread and has far-reaching influence. The Absolute Sincerity of a Great Physician systematically expounded the moral requirements of TCM practitioners and fully displayed the panorama of traditional medical ethics in China. It was the essence of medical ethics, and became the medical ethics standards and norms followed by practitioners at that time and later generations.

General Secretary Xi Jinping pointed out in the reports of the 19th National Congress of the Communist Party of China, to cultivate and practice the core socialist values, we should focus on cultivating new people of the times who are responsible for national rejuvenation. Medical personnel shoulder the important mission of saving the dying and healing the wounded and promoting the development of modern medical and health undertakings, and more importantly, they need to cultivate and practice socialist core values. The promotion of the spirit of "The Absolute Sincerity of a Great Physician" can help practitioners to establish noble professional ethics, cultivate medical humanistic feelings, and fulfill their social responsibilities and historical missions. Therefore, the two meet the requirements in terms of talent training content.

Absorbing the ideological essence of "The Absolute Sincerity of a Great Physician" medical ethics culture and combining with the socialist core values, it has certain reference significance for contemporary practitioners. First, at the personal level, high professional ethics should be established. Doctors should set up correct values, not practice medicine as a means to control property, to obtain reputation, regardless of personal gain and loss. Doctors should attach importance to the value of life, adhere to the concept of people-oriented service, human life is at stake, and the responsibility is great. Doctors should highly respect and doubly cherish people and life and treat them with caution. Doctors should never act rashly or treat them lightly. Patients should be treated with care, empathy, no fear of dirt and odor, and painstaking care with all efforts. The behavior of doctors should steady and dignified, and maintain a modest and courteous appearance. Doctors should treat patients' families with civility, warmth and friendship, and treat colleagues with sincerity, friendship and solidarity. Second, at the social level, a strong sense of social responsibility should be cultivated. Doctors should maintain equality between doctors and patients, respect the dignity of patients, and protect the health privacy of patients. Doctors should establish the awareness of fair distribution of medical and health resources, treat patients equally, treat patients according to disease, diagnose and treat fairly, and use drugs rationally. Doctors should establish legal awareness, abide by the law, and practice medicine with integrity. Third, at the national level, profound feelings of family and country should be cultivated. In diagnosis and treatment services, doctors should build a harmonious doctor-patient relationship through superb medical skills and quality services. They should study hard, explore and practice, serve patients by improving scientific research ability and practical skills, promote the development of medical and health care, and benefit the people.

5

Medical Ethics Culture in the Northern and Southern Song Dynasties

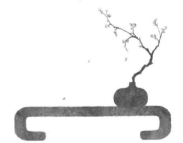

The Northern and Southern Song dynasties ended the social turmoil and division during the Five dynasties and Ten Kingdoms Period, and the political, economic, scientific and technological, cultural, artistic and other aspects were recovered and developed. It was another peak period of development following the great prosperity of the Tang dynasty. During this period, there was the prosperous and stable social environment, the enlightened and honest political style, the policy of emphasizing civil administration at the expense of national defense, and the rapid development of science and technology, which greatly promoted the development of politics, economy, culture, medicine, society, and foreign exchanges at that time and had a profound impact. Chen Yinke, a master of Chinese culture, said, "After thousands of years of evolution, the culture of the Chinese nation reached its peak in Song dynasty." That is to say, in such a period, the development of traditional medicine and medical education in China has also reached a peak. There are also many famous TCM practitioners, such as Qian Yi, Pang Anshi, Tang Shenwei, Song Ci, Chen Ziming, who explained and acted with the noble virtues of practicing medicine. TCM practitioners' benevolence, insidious study, valuing justice over profit, and rigorous pursuit of reality reflect the important value of medical ethics.

5.1   Overview of Medical Ethics

5.1.1   Social Background of Medical Ethics

The development of medical ethics was closely related to the development of medicine. The development of medical ethics and medicine in the Northern and Southern Song dynasties was deeply influenced by the political, economic, technological and social trends of thought at that time.

1. Political factors

The rapid development of TCM in the Northern and Southern Song dynasties was greatly influenced by its political environment. Before the establishment of the Song dynasty, it experienced about 205 years of social upheaval. The separatist regime of the vassal states and the eunuch's seizure of power led to social chaos and people's livelihood. In the more than 200 years of turmoil, China's traditional virtues have almost disappeared, and even been replaced by the law of the jungle. The political environment was complex and changeable, wars were rife, and people's lives were miserable. Even the most basic food, clothing, housing and transportation were difficult to guarantee. In addition, the continuous wars have caused serious damage to the productivity. Whether the wound or disabled soldiers in the battlefield or the civilian plague patients, they can not be effectively treated. It was precisely in this medical situation that the demand for the number of medical practitioners and the level of medical skills were more urgent. As Zhao Kuangyin, the Emperor Taizu of the Song dynasty, ended the long chaotic situation and established a unified Song dynasty, the people were able to live and work in peace and contentment. Under the background of the times, medical practitioners also devoted themselves to studying, improving medical skills, practicing medicine to help the world, and inheriting medical ethics, which promoted the rapid development of TCM and formed the medical ethics culture of the Northern and Southern Song dynasties.

After the establishment of the Song dynasty, the government paid more attention to medicine. Throughout the history of China, the emphasis on medicine and practitioners reached its peak in the Song dynasty. The Song dynasty was established in the era of feudal separatism. The rulers learned from the previous generation, greatly weakened the military authority at all levels, and at the same time increased centralization, forming a political environment that emphasized culture and military power. The rulers of the Song dynasty, who established political power after the war, knew that the development of medical treatment could promote the people to receive good treatment, which would stabilize the people's hearts, show the world a benevolent government, and stabilize social development. Therefore, all the rulers of the Song dynasty attached importance to medical science. At that time, on the one hand, many edicts were issued to promote the development of medicine. According to Han Yi's statistics in the article "Medical Edicts in the Song Dynasty and Their Influence on Medicine in the Song Dynasty", the Song dynasty issued more than 830 edicts related to medicine. On the other hand, many medical institutions have been specially set up to take charge of medical affairs, such as the Imperial Academy of Medicine in the Hanlin Academy, the Palace Dispensary, the Imperial Academy of Medicine, the Office of Revising Medical Books, and the Medical Institute of Benevolence, which were beyond any dynasties before the Song dynasty and incomparable for later generations. In addition, some emperors of the Song dynasty, such as Emperor Taizu and Emperor Taizong, were extremely fond of medicine. In addition, the rulers of the Song dynasty organized specialized personnel to collect, correct, and sort out medical books before and at the time of the Song dynasty on a large scale. At the same time, medical books were issued rigidly, which played an important role in the dissemination of medical knowledge, the study of TCM practitioners, and the public's understanding of diseases. The emphasis on medical education in the Song dynasty promoted the development of traditional medicine, especially the "three parts method" advocated by Wang Anshi in the Shenzong period of the Song dynasty, which was to treat medical education and university education equally in the education system. Under the political background of putting mental pursuits above martial arts, TCM practitioners in the Northern and Southern Song dynasties, with the strong support of the imperial court, learned medical skills, studied medical science, and honed their moral character, which promoted the development of traditional medicine. TCM practitioners were inherited and carried forward in this period.

2. Economic factor

The Northern and Southern Song dynasties can be said to be another prosperous period after the Tang dynasty, with outstanding achievements in agriculture, commerce, handicrafts, transportation and foreign trade. The political tendency in the Northern and Southern Song dynasties to put mental pursuits above martial arts, and the strategy of advocating "peaceful surrender" in the face of minority regimes, to a large extent, provided a good environment for social stability, productivity development, and economic prosperity. The economic development not only improved the living standard of the people in the Song dynasty, but also promoted the further development of China's traditional commercial trade, and further promoted the convenient dissemination of various medical books, medical skills, famous medicines and ancient prescriptions, famous TCM practitioners and famous cases. For example, Tang Shenwei, a famous TCM practitioner in central Shu area in the Northern Song dynasty, collected famous herbal medicines from all over the world and regularly participated in the drug fair held in Chengdu every year. The drug fair was held in Chengdu at a fixed time every year. At that time, TCM practitioners, medicine sellers and farmers' families from all over the country would display, exchange and sell their medicines. The fair attracted a large number of medical practitioners to participate, which greatly promoted the communication among the TCM practitioners. Not only in Shu, the commercial development in various places in the Northern and Southern

Song dynasties, promoted the exchange of medical materials, technology, famous treatment cases, etc., which greatly facilitated the spread of medicine and medical ethics. At the same time, the medical exchange with foreign countries was the closest during this period. The invention of science and technology and the development of southeast coastal ports made the exchange of foreign trade more frequent. A large number of overseas trade also brought a lot of overseas drug resources and medical technology, which not only enriched China's medical resources during the Song dynasty, but also spread China's traditional medical culture. In a prosperous and stable social and economic environment, people's living and working in peace and contentment put forward higher requirements for keeping their health. The Medical Institute and the Medical Institute of Benevolence were set up by the government in various places. Those promoted the development of medical culture in the Song dynasty, and created a group of famous TCM practitioners with high moral integrity.

3. Technology factor

The development of science and technology in the Northern and Southern Song dynasties played an important role in the long history of China and even the world, and promoted the inheritance and development of traditional medical ethics culture and medical technology in China. In particular, Bi Sheng in the Northern Song dynasty invented clay typography in the 11th century, which was a major leap in the history of human civilization. The invention of typography and the continuous improvement of paper-making techniques provided unprecedented convenience for the collation, correction and publication of ancient medical books in the Northern and Southern Song dynasties, as well as the dissemination of various books at that time and the exchange of Chinese and Western medical culture. At that time, a large number of medical books were widely printed and distributed in engraved editions, which made the number of medical books increase greatly and the price was relatively affordable. It gave TCM practitioners the opportunity to improve their own medical ethics by absorbing and drawing on the experience of predecessors, and at the same time, compile their own practical experience, widely disseminate it, and benefit others. The improvement and wide use of the compass in the Northern and Southern Song dynasties and the development of the shipbuilding industry also created conditions for the dissemination and exchange of TCM practitioners or biochemical and medical materials at home and abroad. During this period, many foreign medicines were also studied and used by TCM practitioners. In addition, the development of science and technology had promoted the emergence of various medical theories and the creation of different medical disciplines and academic schools. For example, the Yongjia School of Medicine, established by Chen Wuze, a medical scientist in the Southern Song dynasty, based on the "Sanyin Theory", had a profound impact at that time.

4. Social ideological trend factor

The medical ethics culture in the Northern and Southern Song dynasties was also deeply influenced by social ideological trend. In the Northern Song dynasty, a new social ideological trend, Neo Confucianism, emerged in the society. It integrated some viewpoints, including Confucianism, Taoism, Buddhism and Xuan-Xue philosophy in the Wei and Jin dynasties. Neo Confucianism paid more attention to the study of classical works in Confucian culture, and absorbed and spread the ideas and cultures that adapt to the social development at that time from the classics. Its representatives were mainly Cheng Yi, Cheng Ying, Zhu Xi and other Neo Confucianism scholars. During this period, the development of Neo Confucianism was highly praised by the rulers and local officials, so the development of TCM practitioners' morality was also deeply affected by it, providing a cultural ideological trend background for the emergence of "Confucian medical practitioners". Confucian medical practitioners are a group of medical experts with rich Confucian cultural learning background. The appearance of Confucian medical practitioners has greatly changed the situation that former subordinate TCM practitioners were not valued. Fan Zhongyan even put forward the view that "if one can't be a good prime minister, he should be a good TCM practitioner". Confucian medical practitioners have greatly demonstrated the "benevolence" of medical practitioners, and further enriched the theoretical basis for the development of medical ethics culture. In addition, the thoughts of Yin and Yang, Five Elements, Li, Qi and "Preserving the Heavenly Principles and Eliminating Human Desire" in Neo Confucianism also deeply influenced the medical scientists in the Song dynasty. On the basis of the thoughts of Neo Confucianism, medical professionals deeply studied and developed medical specialties such as etiology, pathology and physiology, and infiltrated into many fields of TCM in China, which had an extremely important impact on the development of TCM. With the continuous influence of Neo Confucianism, China's traditional medical ethics cultural system has also been gradually improved. The main representatives of medical ethics in the Northern and Southern Song dynasties, such as Qian Yi, Pang Anshi, Tang Shenwei, Chen Wuze, Shen Kuo, have made important contributions to the development of medical ethics and the implementation of medical techniques.

5.1.2 Main Contents of Medical Ethics Culture

The vigorous development of medicine and the innovation of Neo Confucianism in the Northern and Southern Song dynasties were the important background for the development of medical ethics culture at that time. The Confucianism dominated by Neo Confucianism further enriched China's traditional medical ethics culture. In the Northern and Southern Song dynasties, medical experts consciously used Confucianism to guide themselves to practice medicine to save people. The emergence of "Confucian medical practitioners" marked that Confucian ethics began to affect all aspects of medical ethics. The medical ethics culture in this period was still based on "benevolence", "essence" and "sincerity". Contributions made by TCM practitioners in the Northern and Southern Song dynasties to the development of medical ethics culture were mainly reflected in the following aspects.

1. Diligent study and excellent medical skills

For all science and technology, only by continual study, and spending time on diligent study and continuous practice can we truly master its essence, so as to promote the progress and development of science and technology, as is the case with medicine. As a TCM practitioner, he must be diligent and eager to learn, read medical books, study diligently and assiduously, understand the medical skills, thoughts and works of his ancestors, and explore the causes and root causes of various diseases. All the famous TCM practitioners in the Northern and Southern Song dynasties were excellent TCM practitioners with noble medical ethics, and their superb medical skills were all derived from their tireless pursuit of medicine. According to the *History of the Song Dynasty*, medical education institutions such as the "Imperial Medical Bureau" were specially set up for medical education in the Northern and Southern Song dynasties, and medical experts were specially invited to teach classical medical books such as *Plain Conversation* and *Classic on Medical Problems*, so that medical students could learn the ancient ways diligently and improve their medical skills on this basis. Chen Wuze, a famous medical ethicist in the Southern Song dynasty, put forward that "how can a TCM practitioner understand the changes of Yin and Yang and decree without reading *Spiritual Pivot* and *Plain Conversation*? How can a TCM practitioner know the sacred craftsmanship and the righteousness without reading *Spiritual Pivot* and *Plain Conversation*... If a TCM practitioner doesn't read extensively, how can he know that pulse points are empty and strange diseases and different syndromes." It can be seen from this that Chen Wuze also advocates that TCM practitioners should learn the ancient medical knowledge and read medical books. One who understood all aspects of medicine can be called a TCM practitioner. He even proposed that even if TCM practitioners read all the medical books, it was far from enough. They should also be familiar with the works of hundreds of classics and history, cultivate their own morality, and strive to be a Confucian TCM practitioner who was dedicated to the people.

The famous medical practitioners in the Northern and Southern Song dynasties, whether Qian Yi, Pang Anshi, or Chen Wuze and other famous TCM practitioners, learned from their childhood about ancient medical prescriptions and read widely. They were aware that only by standing on the shoulders of giants can they see farther. Medical science is broad and profound, and they need to learn from the wisdom of their predecessors and hone their own medical skills.

2. Benevolence, value righteousness over benefits

All science and technology can only be widely promoted if they serve human beings, especially in medicine. Only those who serve as TCM practitioners with benevolence, can they truly be called "benevolent TCM practitioners". The medical ethics culture in the Northern and Southern Song dynasties was deeply influenced by "Neo Confucianism", among which the Confucian "benevolence" thought, which was founded by Confucius and Mencius, was the core connotation of the medical ethics culture, and this period also promoted the emergence of "Confucian medical practitioners". TCM practitioners must have a heart of benevolence and compassion, practice mutual survival, mutual assistance and mutual love between people, respect patients and treat patients kindly, and not just for the sake of benefits. There were many medical practitioners who practiced benevolence without seeking fame and wealth in the Northern and Southern Song dynasties. Liu Fang, a medical expert in the Northern Song dynasty, wrote in *A New Book of Pediatrics* that "as a TCM practitioner, benevolence and selfishness are indispensable". *The Medical Engineering Theory* in volume I of the famous book of the Southern Song dynasty, *The General Micro Treatise on Children's Health*, once recorded that "anyone who is a TCM practitioner must first command himself rather than other. Those who correct themselves can do their best to treat patients by their medical shills; Those who correct material can use medicine to deal with the disease... Don't exaggerate the illness at will, or describe the disease that is easy to cure as difficult. If a patient comes to a TCM practitioner for treatment, whether he or she is rich or poor, the TCM practitioner will treat equally... As long as he is a TCM practitioner, no matter how far away someone asks, he must go to save others." In addition, Tang Shenwei, a TCM practitioner from Shu area in the Northern Song dynasty, said, "Whether noble or ordinary, if someone needs help, he will go there, even if it rains or snows, and even if there is no diagnosis fee, it can be obtained." Pang Anshi, a famous TCM practitioner in the Northern Song dynasty, said, "He regarded money as garbage and regarded patients as mothers".

The medical ethics culture in the Northern and Southern Song dynasties was centered around the core of "benevolence". The TCM practitioners not only embodied the noble medical ethics with benevolence in the practice to help the world, but also advocated the idea of "benevolence" when compiling medical books. At the same time, many TCM practitioners in the Northern and Southern Song dynasties treated the patients equally, regardless of the rich and the poor. They don't pursue interests and treat patients as close relatives. They were modest and respectful to peers without pursuing of fame and wealth.

3. Take responsibilities and overcome difficulties

Due to the influence of politics, economy, science and technology, and cultural environment, medicine in the Northern and Southern Song dynasties was prosperous and developed, and medical disciplines were gradually subdivided into various small subjects during this period. Under this background, the TCM discipline in China has gradually enriched and improved. However, when faced with some difficulties such as patients, diseases and disciplines which were difficult to be treated, the TCM practitioners in the Northern and Southern Song dynasties made great efforts to save the life, bravely took the responsibility for the development of medical cause, overcome difficulties and finally became medical masters with exquisite medical skills, noble medical ethics and profound academic knowledge. As an ancient saying goes, "I would rather treat ten men than one woman; I would rather treat ten women than one child." It can be seen from this that TCM practitioners' treatment of women and children is a difficult point in medicine, but Qian Yi, a famous TCM practitioner in the Northern Song dynasty, without fearing the difficulties of pediatrics, made in-depth research in pediatrics. It took him more than 40 years to overcome the difficulties of pediatrics, and he finally became the "saint of pediatrics" and the "ancestor of pediatrics". Chen Ziming, an old man in the Southern Song dynasty, deeply understood that the condition of childbirth was complex, changeable and with great risks. In addition, there were few experiences that predecessors could learn from. However, he dared to face this condition, bravely shouldered heavy responsibilities, and finally compiled the first monograph on obstetrics and gynecology in the history of China, *The Complete Works of Women's Good Prescriptions*, which had a far-reaching impact.

In addition, some local TCM practitioners, such as Tang Shenwei, felt deeply sorry when they saw the medical experience and books of the ancients were lost. Therefore, he gave up serving as an official but sought prescriptions for the treatment of diseases. He collected, sorted out and summarized the herbal medicines and famous prescriptions of the past dynasties and finally completed the 32 volumes of *Complete Effective Prescriptions for Women's Diseases*. He bravely shoulder the responsibility of the development of TCM and overcame the difficulties of medicine. This is a profound reflection of being responsible to the public.

4. Pragmatic and devoted to research

Medical technology can not tolerate any mistake. Once mistakes are made, they may endanger people's lives. Therefore, TCM practitioners should be careful, realistic and pragmatic. The TCM practitioner must carefully inquire about the root cause of the disease during diagnosis and treatment. Be careful when using the medicine, and do not misuse the medicine and dosage. Qian Yi, a TCM practitioner in the Northern Song dynasty, learned the prescriptions of Bawei Pill in the *Synopsis of Golden Chamber* by Zhang Zhongjing, a medical saint in China. However, due to the flexible use of drugs and prudence in treating children, he prepared the pill of Liuwei Dihuang, which has been prepared by TCM practitioners of different generations and is still used today. The medical ethics culture in the Northern and Southern Song dynasties had the connotation of seeking truth and pragmatism. Song Ci, the "father of forensic medicine" in the Southern Song dynasty, required himself and other autopsy examiners not to be perfunctory and go through the motions, and be serious, responsible and realistic, which fully reflected his high respect for the profession of forensic medicine. In addition, Song Ci dares to challenge the secular world in order to find the truth. He once proposed that anyone who tests women should not feel shame and women should be carried to a bright and stable place for testing. Many TCM practitioners in the Northern and Southern Song dynasties devoted themselves to research, and even completed medical masterpieces with lifelong efforts, such as three volumes of the *Key to the Therapeutics of children's Disease* written by Qian Yi, six volumes of the *General Treatise on Febrile Diseases* written by Pang Anshi, thirty-two volumes of the *Preparation of the Classic Classified Materia Medica for Emergency* written by Tang Shenwei, eighteen volumes of the *Sanyin Ji Yi Bingzheng Fang Lun* written by Chen Wuze, five volumes of the *Record of Redressing Mishandled Cases* written by Song Ci and the *Complete Collection of Prescriptions for Women* written by Chen Ziming, twenty-four volumes of the *Complete Effective Prescriptions for Women's Diseases* and the three volumes of *Essentials of External Medicine*, have a profound impact on the development of the medical industry.

5.1.3　Main Characteristics of Medical Ethics Culture

The development of medical ethics culture is closely related to the development of medicine, and is also deeply influenced by the background of the whole era and the mainstream ideology of society. The medical ethics culture in the Northern and Southern Song dynasties not only inherited the virtues of TCM practitioners before the Song dynasty, but also made critical development on its basis. The medical ethics culture in this period mainly has the following characteristics.

1. Inheritance

Medical ethics, as the due professional ethics of TCM practitioners, has been inherited and carried forward by later generations in the process of its formation, development and improvement. The medical ethics in the Northern and Southern Song dynasties inherited the fine tradition of medical ethics formed by TCM practitioners before the Song dynasty. It still practiced the most core virtues, such as benevolence, helping the patients, valuing justice over profit, devoting to research, and the sincerity of a great physician. TCM practitioners in the Northern and Southern Song dynasties helped the patients, and they were either influenced by the ancestral family, or taught by the teacher, or guided by the official medical education, or from their own research. The official medical education in the Northern Song dynasty explicitly required that medical students must learn the basic knowledge of the Four Books and Five Classics in order to cultivate basic humanistic quality. In addition, with the progress of printing technology in the Northern Song dynasty, a large number of medical books were printed. In the books, there was not only the sharing of medical experience of predecessors, but also many medical stories that made TCM practitioners deeply influenced by medical ethics. For example, Sun Simiao, who was called the King of Medicine in the Tang dynasty, wrote in *The Thousand Golden Prescription*, "As a TCM practitioner, when you are treating your patient, you must calm down and resolve, have no desire, show mercy firstly, and devote to help patients... TCM practitioners must be knowledgeable, diligent and indefatigable, and not hearsay... As a TCM practitioner, we can't make fun of, laugh loudly, talk about people, show off others." Under the influence of the medical education system at that time and the medical ethics of famous TCM practitioners such as Hua Tuo, Bianque, Zhang Zhongjing and Sun Simiao, the TCM practitioners of the Song dynasty further developed the traditional medical ethics of China.

2. Characteristics of the times

The inheritance and development of TCM practitioners were greatly influenced by the times. Under the influence of politics, economy, science and technology, and social trend of thought, the medical ethics culture in the Northern and Southern Song dynasties had obvious characteristics of the times. First, with the development of medical education in the Song dynasty, the moral education of TCM practitioners also became particularly prominent. The offical require the TCM practitioners to learn, practice and promote medical ethics specially. Second, with the development of the Song dynasty's Confucianism and the growing popularity of Confucian scholars learning medical skills, it was a common phenomenon that scholars know some medical knowledge. The emergence of "Confucian medical practitioners" emphasizes the importance of medical ethics. Therefore, TCM practitioners under the influence of Confucianism paid more attention to health and morality, motivation for TCM practitioners, medical value, etc. The characteristics of the Northern and Southern Song dynasties were also reflected in the increase of words on medical ethics, which were gradually published and circulated. Medical ethics were becoming increasingly rich, such as the truth-seeking morality advocated by legal TCM practitioners. Medical ethics were practiced in real life by TCM practitioners, and many medical professionals adhered to the essence of medical ethics and practice benevolence.

3. Criticalness

To some extent, the medical ethics culture in the Northern and Southern Song dynasties reflected criticalness, which was mainly reflected in the conflict between medical needs and reality. On the one hand, with the development of medical education, medical technology and government institutions in the Song dynasty, many medical ethics cultures before the Song dynasty were challenged. The most typical was that with the gradual emergence of forensic medicine, forensic ethics conflicted with the "Neo Confucianism" culture in some aspects. For example, Song Ci, a famous forensic scientist in the Southern Song dynasty, in order to seek truth in handling cases, some practices during autopsy conflicted with the culture at that time. For example, in the second volume of the *Record of Redressing Mishandled Cases, Women*, it was recorded that "anyone who tests a woman should not shy away from her", which was in conflict with such doctrines as "men and women are not related to each other", "seeing, listening, speaking, moving, being rude and not doing anything", "don't take reckless actions and thought". But for the practical needs of testing, he criticized the ethics at that time. On the other hand, with the emergence of "Confucian medical practitioners", the TCM practitioners who contradicted them were criticized as "quack TCM practitioners". Those TCM practitioners were criticized for could not adhere to the medical ethics and skills of "benevolence and sincerity", and those TCM practitioners were criticized for only focused on seeking benefits, but have poor medical skills and hurt people's lives.

5.2 Representative Medical Practitioners and Their Medical Ethics

5.2.1 Qian Yi

1. Brief biography

Qian Yi, whose style name was Zhongyang, was born in Qiantang, Zhejiang Province. His grandfather moved north, so he was born in Fuzhou of Dongping in the Song dynasty (now Fucheng, Shandong Province). He was a famous pediatrician in the Song dynasty and the first famous pediatrician in Chinese medical history. When Qian Yi was three years old, his father traveled away and never returned home. His mother died long ago. He was adopted by his aunt and her husband, a TCM practitioner with the surname of Lü, and Qian Yi was regarded as a foster son. Therefore, he studied medicine with his uncle. In his medical career, his most outstanding achievement was devoting himself to the study of pediatric medicine. He has been awarded the Hanlin Chancellor for curing the disease. He saved people, summarized experience, and wrote books for transmission. He once wrote five volumes of *Treatise on Febrile Diseases*, one hundred pieces of *Treatise on Infants and Children*, eight volumes of the *Qian's Prescriptions for Children*, and three volumes of *Prescriptions for Children's Medicine*. But now there is only the *Prescriptions for Children's Medicine*, and others have been lost. *The Prescriptions of Pediatric Medicine Syndrome* written by Qian Yi has been valued by TCM in all dynasties. It was not only the earliest complete pediatrics monograph in China, but also the earliest pediatrics monograph in the world. He was also honored as the "Originator of Pediatrics" and "Saint of Pediatrics" by later generations.

2. Medical ethics

(1) Overcoming difficulties in pediatrics.

Qian Yi had specialized in pediatrics for more than 40 years and had made great achievements in pediatric treatment. But before that time, children's treatment was recognized as a tricky one by TCM practitioners. As an ancient saying goes, "I would rather treat ten men than one woman; I would rather treat ten women than one child", which can fully show the views of medical practitioners on the treatment of children.

In ancient times, TCM practitioners called pediatrics a "dumb department". There were four main reasons of the difficulty of children treatment. First, children haven't fully grown up and their moods were changeable, leading to more mixed situations, which made it more difficult to see and treat patients; Second, most children can't express themselves in accurate words, and can't communicate with TCM practitioners, which makes it more difficult for them to consult; Third, the pulse condition of children is weak, and they often cry at the hospital, which makes it more difficult to stabilize the pulse condition, increasing the difficulty of pulse diagnosis; Fourth, children are young, their bodies are not yet mature, their internal organs are particularly weak, and it is difficult to stabilize the cold and heat in their bodies. Therefore, doctors should be extremely cautious when using drugs. If they are not careful, the diagnosis and treatment will become more complex, even endanger the lives of children.

Qian Yi was deeply touched by the difficulty of children's treatment. He once said, "It is difficult to get information about the pulse, and the evidence cannot be taken out of words. It is especially difficult for infants and children." However, Qian Yi, as a TCM practitioner, still spent more than 40 years in his life, regardless of difficulties, devoting himself to research, summarizing experience and overcoming difficulties, finally made a breakthrough in pediatric treatment and achieved results, which also laid the foundation for the development of pediatric medicine in China.

(2) The wonderful use of yellow soil to cure the prince.

Qian Yi was originally a rural TCM practitioner, but was awarded the title of Assistant Director of the Imperial Academy of Medicine in the Northern Song dynasty for his skillful use of "yellow soil soup". Zhao Xu, a beloved prince of Emperor Shenzong of the Song dynasty, suddenly fell ill. After many TCM practitioners' treatment, Zhao Xu still did not improve. His illness became more serious with convulsions. The prince's body became weaker and his life was in danger. At this time, the Grand Princess recommended Qian Yi, the "highly skilled TCM practitioner" of Fuzhou, to the Emperor Song Shenzong. Qian Yi went to the palace to cure the prince. When Qian Yi saw the prince, he gave him a prescription of "yellow soil soup". Emperor Shenzong was puzzled, but he finally agreed to use the medicine to cure the prince. After the prince Zhao Xu took the "yellow soil soup", his condition gradually improved and he finally recovered. The Emperor Shenzong praised Qian Yi and asked him why yellow soil can also cure the prince. Qian Yi replied that "he is suffering from a disease of water, and the soil can fight against the water, so he can recover". In addition, he also said that all Imperial Physicians had basically cured the prince's disease before, and only on this basis can he make the prince recover. After hearing this, the Emperor Shenzong praised Qian Yi for his excellent medical skills, being modest and not greedy, and made him the Assistant Director of the Imperial Academy of Medicine.

The wonderful use of yellow soil to cure the prince was a famous medical case in Qian Yi's life. This case highlighted his superb medical skills of tailoring medicine to the situation, knowing the nature of medicine, being good at using medicinal materials, and using medicines skillfully. It reflected his noble medical ethics of not being proud of his achievements, understanding humility, and affirming the achievements of predecessors.

(3) Making prescriptions innovative and flexible.

"Liuwei Dihuang Pill" is a medicine that is still well-known today. Its original name is Dihuang Yuan (pill), which was first seen in Qian Yi's *Prescription for Children's Medicine*. Qian Yi was granted the title of Assistant Director of the Imperial Academy of Medicine by the Emperor Shenzong. He was envied by many imperial TCM practitioners, so they often took Qian Yi's medicine to "consult him". One day, Qian Yi and his disciple Yan Xiaozhong were treating a patient. A TCM practitioner came to Qian Yi with a prescription to "consult him". He slightly mocked the geology and asked him to follow the prescription of the Bawei Pill in the *Synopsis of Golden Chamber* written by Zhang Zhongjing, in which he seemed to forget the two herbs of cinnamon and aconite. [①]Qian Yi was not angry. He said with a smile that the Bawei Pill written by Zhang Zhongjing was for adults, and this prescription was for children. Children have enough Yang, so they can avoid these two kinds of fiery medicines. So he made the Liuwei Dihuang Pill to prevent the children from getting too excessive fire and bleeding after taking it. After listening to this, the TCM practitioner praised Qian Yi for his flexibility in medication and his ability to learn and use flexibly, and expressed his admiration. After the event, Yan Xiaozhong recorded it and compiled it into the *Prescription for Children's Medicine*.

---

① Yan Xiaozhong was a famous disciple of Qian Yi. He collected and sorted out Qian Yi's medical theories, medical cases, prescriptions, etc., and finally compiled them into three volumes of *Formulas for Paediatrics*.

Qian Yi did not stick to the classics of predecessors, used them flexibly on the basis of good learning, and dared to innovate and develop drugs and used them appropriately in combination with the actual situation of patients. This was the respect of Qian Yi as a TCM practitioner for patients, and was also the result of his devotion to research. Qian Yi was not afraid of or angry at others' "consult him" and was enthusiastic to explain, which was a quality of being modest and generous.

(4) Diligence made him a master.

Qian Yi became a famous master in the history of ancient Chinese medicine due to his diligence in study through his life. Qian Yi was adopted by his aunt when he was three years old and regarded as her adopted son. His uncle was a local TCM practitioner. However, his uncle always valued justice over profit. He asked patients who cannot pay for the medicine not to worry, and often taught Qian Yi to focus on curing diseases and saving people, not just on reward. Qian Yi also often followed his uncle to secretly learn how to cure and save people. He became his uncle's assistant in medicine at young age. At the age of seventeen or eighteen, he was able to cure some mild diseases independently. At the same time, Qian Yi also carefully studied medical works such as *Yellow Emperor's Canon of Medicine*, *Treatise on Febrile Diseases*, and *Shennong's Herbal Classic*. He studied those books carefully and repeatedly, which was very enlightening. He was proficient in internal medicine, surgery, gynecology and other departments, especially pediatrics. In the process of treating patients with his uncle, Qian Yi felt that children's diseases were difficult to cure and there were few monographs on treatment. He also knew that it was important to cure children, so he continued to explore, study and travel around the country on the road of treating children. Until Qian Yi was famous and became the Assistant Director of the Imperial Academy of Medicine, he read extensively, summarized and pondered, wrote books and handed them down from generation to generation, and finally became a great pediatrician.

As a TCM practitioner, Qian Yi was constantly learning in his life. Furthermore, he had shown the broadness and benevolence of China's traditional medical ethics in his life. His noble medical ethics were worth learning, inheriting and developing for future generations.

5.2.2　Pang Anshi

1. Brief biography

Pang Anshi, whose courtesy name was Anchang, was from Chuozhou of Chuoshui (now Heshui, Hubei Province) of Maqiao. He was a famous medical scientist in the Northern Song dynasty and was praised as the "Medical King of the Northern Song dynasty". His father Pang Qing was also a TCM practitioner. He was intelligent and eager to learn since childhood, and had the talent of never forgetting after reading. When he was less than 20 years old, he knew well the *Pulse Classic* and had his own new ideas sometimes, which surprised his father. Later, because of his deafness, Pang Anshi became more and more involved in learning and studying such famous medical works as the *Spiritual Pivot*, the *Taisu*, and *Canon of Acupuncture and Moxibustion*. Pang Anshi practiced medicine all his life. He was skilled in medicine, devoted himself to research, and valued justice over profit. He left many medical stories and wrote books such as the *Classic of Questioning*, the *Zhudui Ji*, and the *Supplemented Materia Medica*, but they were basically lost. There are now six volumes of the *General Treatise on Febrile Diseases*, which is an influential work in the history of Chinese medicine to study *Treatise on Febrile Diseases* written by Zhang Zhongjing. It was a classic of TCM.

2. Medical ethics

(1) Searching for water source and digging wells to cure the plague.

It is said that one year of drought caused plagues in many places. Pang Anshi worked out a good recipe to control the plague and produced good effects in many places, but it did not work for the Yangjiapu in Guoxiang, Shuicheng. He went to investigate the reason, and finally found that the water for Yangjiapu villagers to drink and other purpose was not separated, all from the muddy water of the pond, which led to many diseases among the villagers. Therefore the conventional treatment for plague was not effective. He thought it was necessary to dig wells to acquire drinking water. So Pang Anshi went up the mountain with his disciple Yang Ke to search for clean water source. At the edge of a small tree at the foot of a hillside, he saw that the grass there was thick when the weather was so dry, so he asserted that there must have a water source there. Later, according to Pang Anshi's design,

Yangjiapu villagers dug a well there to find the water source. The water was really clear. The villagers also used the well water to boil medicine to cure the plague and make the villagers healthy. In order to thank Pang Anshi and his disciples, the villagers wanted to set up a monument "Pang Gong Jing (the well of Pang Anshi)", but they were persuaded by him and finally named it "Yang Jing (the well of Yang)". Today, the well has become a national key cultural relic.

Whether searching for the root cause of the ineffective treatment of the Yangjiapu plague or looking for clean water, it showed Pang Anshi's moral character as a TCM practitioner to investigate the root cause, explore the root cause, practice and explore, as well as his modest quality. That's exactly why Pang Anshi was deeply respected by the people.

(2) Using acupuncture to save the pregnant woman.

It is said that Pang Anshi once went to Tongcheng, Shuzhou, a woman from a civilian family happened to be giving birth, but no child was born after seven days, and many methods were not effective. One of Pang Anshi's students, Li Baiquan, was a neighbor of this family, so he invited his teacher Pang Anshi to have a look. As soon as Pang Anshi saw the woman, he said that she would not die. He asked the women's family to warm her waist and abdomen with hot water and touched her belly up and down with their hands. The woman had a slight abdominal pain, and a male baby was born while her moaning. The people were surprised and delighted, but they did not know why it was so. Pang Anshi said that in fact the baby had already left the placenta, but one hand mistakenly grasped the mother's intestinal tract, which led to the failure of smooth delivery. This could not be solved by medicine. Therefore, he stroked the position of the baby's hand across the mother's abdomen, and used acupuncture at its palm edge. The baby immediately released its grasp, so he was born, and no other method was used. The family brought the child to see that there was indeed a needle mark on the edge of the baby's right palm.

Pang Anshi's superb medical skills not only saved the pregnant woman, but also her baby. As a TCM practitioner, superb medical skills should be the foundation of his career in medicine. More importantly, it is a lifelong pursuit of TCM practitioners.

(3) Benevolence and value over profit show the good medical ethics.

Pang Anshi not only had excellent medical skills, but also had good medical ethics. According to the *Records of Pang Anshi in the History of the Song Dynasty*, "The rate of curing diseases was nine out of ten. Pang Anshi made room for the patients who came to the hospital to live in, and personally inspected the patients' medicines. He must wait for the patients to recover and then let them go home. Those patients who could not be cured must tell them the truth and stop treating them. He cured countless patients, and the patients came to thank him with money and silk, but he did not accept all of them." During his medical practice, he set up his own medical workshop, where patients who needed long-term diagnosis and treatment and long-distance treatment were kept for careful treatment. When the patients recovered, they could return home. This can be said to be the pioneer of setting up a medical workshop for inpatient treatment in China, and has had a far-reaching impact so far. In addition, he was also praised for not valuing profit. His friend Su Shi once mentioned in a recommendation letter, "Pang Anshi was knowledgeable and he was excellent in pulse and medicine. This man was elegant and not interested in profit." Pang Anshi showed great benevolence in dealing with patients at that time. According to the *Preface to Pang's Treatise on Febrile Diseases* written by Huang Tingjian, "When the patient comes to the hospital for treatment, he doesn't care about whether the patient is rich or poor. He respected the old and loved the young. He regarded money as garbage and regarded patients as mothers."

Pang Anshi had a medical practitioner's morality of caring for patients, not focusing on interests, and respecting the old and loving the young. It has of great significance to the moral education of traditional medicine in China.

5.2.3 Tang Shenwei

1. Brief biography

Tang Shenwei, whose courtesy name was Zhenyuan, was originally from Jinyang, Shuzhou (now Chongzhou, Sichuan Province). At the invitation of supreme commander of Shuzhou, Li Duanbo, he went to Chengdu to be a TCM practitioner, and later moved to Huayang, Chengdu (now Shuangliu, Chengdu). He was a famous TCM practitioner and pharmacist in the Northern Song dynasty. He made great contributions to the development of pharmacy and the collection of folk prescriptions, and created a precedent for the comparison of prescription dosage in drug learning in China. He is the ancestor of the academic field of Chinese medicine in China. Tang Shenwei was born in a family of TCM practitioners. His ancestors were all TCM practitioners. He had a strong interest in medicine since he was young. He was very intelligent and kind-hearted. In addition, under the guidance of his medical family, he studied hard and had excellent medical skills, especially in medicine and pharmacy. His work, 32 volumes of the *Classic Classified Materia Medica for Emergency*, recorded 1,558 kinds of medicines. It has been highly valued by later generations of pharmaceutical masters, including Li Shizhen, and it is a medical masterpiece. Even though Tang Shenwei is a folk TCM practitioner, he independently complete his book, which is also a legend in the history of TCM in China.

2. Medical ethics

(1) A person who makes no mistake in one hundred treatments can become a miracle TCM practitioner.

Tang Shenwei was widely praised by the people at that time for his TCM practitioners' treatment in the central Sichuan area in the Song dynasty. At that time, people praised his practice of medical treatment as "no mistake in one hundred treatments". It is said that Yuwen Bangyan, father of Yuwen Xuzhong, which was the patriotic minister and great poet in the Song dynasty, once suffered from rubella and was treated ineffectively in many ways. Later, Tang Shenwei was recommended for diagnosis and treatment. After being carefully treated by Tang Shenwei, Yuwen Bangyan soon recovered. However, Tang Shenwei knew that rebella is difficult to completely cured, so he left a letter to Yuwen Xuzhong, and indicated on the envelope that the letter should be opened on a certain date. At that time, Yuwen Bangyan really suffered from rubella again. So Yuwen Xuzhong opened the letter left by Tang Shenwei and saw three prescriptions. The first one was to cure recurrence of rubella, the second one was to cure the sore caused by rubella, and the third one was to cure the cough caused by shortness of breath. Yuwen Bangyan treated his father according to the letter left by Tang Shenwei, and his father recovered after half a month. This event was well known in Chengdu at that time, and people praised Tang Shenwei as a miracle-working TCM practitioner.

Tang Shenwei, who made no mistake in one hundred treatments, had become a miracle-working TCM practitioner because of his hard study and hard work.

(2) Treating patients with skilled medical prescriptions.

Tang Shenwei not only had excellent medical skills, but also had noble medical ethics. When he went out to treat the patients, whether noble or average, if someone needs help, he will go there, even if it rains or snows. During his practice of medicine, patients were treated equally. Rather than saying too much, Tang Shenwei only touched the topic lightly, but he had already made the other party understood his intention. Rather than catering to patients with exaggerated words or pretentious actions to win favor and support, he was simple and cautious in diagnosis and treatment. What was more different from other TCM practitioners was that he did not ask patients to give much money as a reward for medical treatment, but asked patients and their relatives and friends to provide famous prescriptions as a reward. It is said that one day, a patient inadvertently told him a folk prescription during his medical treatment. Tang Shenwei was enlightened when he heard about it, and wondered why he didn't use his advantage of practicing medicine everywhere to collect medical prescriptions. Since then, Tang Shenwei made a rule that every intellectual who went to cure disease needn't to pay, but provide him with prescriptions. This rule was very popular with the intellectuals. Therefore, once the intellectuals found a medicine name or a prescription in the history books, they will definitely collect the transcripts and inform Tang Shenwei. In addition, Tang Shenwei attended the drug fairs held regularly every year in Chengdu, during which he could obtain valuable drug materials every time. In addition to his research, he often went out to practice medicine, and collect drugs and folk prescriptions. After a long period of accumulation, he finally collected a large number of medical prescriptions, which accumulated abundant medical materials for his preparations of the *Classic Classified Materia Medica for Emergency*.

(3) Accomplishing his great works.

Tang Shenwei read medical books extensively since he was a child, but he found that the medical classics before the Song dynasty were basically hand-written records or passed down from mouth to mouth. Some medical books were either lost or were repeatedly copied with errors. It was not until the prevalence of printing in the Northern Song dynasty that some medical books were printed and circulated. Tang Shenwei, as a TCM practitioner, was extremely sad by the loss of ancient medical prescriptions. In order to make the achievements of predecessors pass on from generation to generation and benefit the future generations as much as possible, he studied, collected and sorted out ancient medicines all his life. During the period, someone once recommended him as an official but was rejected by him. Instead, he devoted himself to the study of medicinal herbs. Relied on his own strength, and after hard research and extensive collection of medical prescriptions, he finally accomplish the great herbal works the *Classified Materia Medica*, which was a masterpiece of herbal medicine before the Song dynasty. After being revised and corrected, it has been used for hundreds of years. *The Compendium of Materia Medica* written by Li Shizhen, a medical master in the Ming dynasty, was also compiled on its basis. Li Shizhen commented on Tang Shenwei, "It was his contribution that all the herbs and prescriptions have been inherited for thousands of years without being lost."

As a TCM practitioner, Tang Shenwei devoted his life to curing diseases and saving people, and his craftsmanship spirit and noble medical ethics deserve to be widely inherited and carried forward by future generations.

5.2.4   Chen Wuze

1. Brief biography

Chen Wuze, whose first name was Yan, was also called Hexi Daoren (the Taoist priest at Hexi). He was born in Hexi, Qingtian in Southern Song dynasty (now Hexi Town, Jingning, Zhejiang Province). Later, he lived in Wenzhou for a long time and married the Wu in Yongjia. He is a famous medical scientist and medical ethics expert in Southern Song dynasty, the founder of Yongjia Medical School, and one of the "22 famous TCM practitioners in Tang, Song, Jin and Yuan dynasties". Chen Wuze helped patients all his life. He excelled in medical academic and medical skills, including pulse prescriptions. In his life, he founded the "Sanyin Theory (Three-Cause Theory)", compiled 18 volumes of *Sanyin Ji Yi Bingzheng Fang Lun*, which became a monograph on the etiology of TCM, and made great contributions to the development of etiology and pathology in later generations. At the same time, "Sanyin Prescriptions" also laid a solid academic foundation for the establishment of Yongjia School of Medicine in the Southern Song dynasty.

2. Medical ethics

(1) Creating "Sanyin Theory".

Although Chen Wuze was born in Qingtian village, he was smart since childhood. He was good at medicine. It is said that he can predict the death of the incurable. He was famous for his superb medical skills and noble medical ethics. Chen Wuze studied medical books and absorbed the merits of predecessors. He summarized and sorted out the ancient medical classics like *Yellow Emperor's Canon of Medicine* and Zhang Zhongjing's *Synopsis of Golden Chamber*, and on this basis finally created the "Sanyin Theory" of etiology classification, and compiled the monograph *Sanyin Prescriptions*. Chen Wuze divided the etiology into three categories: internal, external and non-external, explained it in detail and emphasized that syndrome differentiation treatment should be carried out according to the etiology. As a comprehensive and systematic monograph on etiology and pathology in the history of Chinese medicine, *Sanyin Prescriptions* has been popular for a hundred years and has had a profound impact on Chinese medicine.

(2) Tracing the origin of "Ganmao (catch cold)".

The word "Ganmao" is still used in Chinese today, although it is not created by Chen Wuze, he had a lot to do with it. According to legend, during the Song dynasty, Guan Ge (the official library and history record department) set up a system that one staff member taking turns to stay on duty every night. However, during the shift, the atmosphere of staff members skipping duties was prevalent, and the word "stomach upset" was recorded in the duty record book, so that they could ask for leave. It is said that Chen Hu, a student of the Imperial College who was forced to be on duty, wrote "Ganfeng" in order to slip away. Chen Hu's writing of this word was rooted in *Sanyin Theory* written by Chen Wuze. That is, "feng", the first of the six external causes, plus the word "gan". It is said that until the Qing dynasty, the word "Ganfeng" had evolved. All the officials who asked for leave were called "Ganmao (cold) leave", that is to say, they needed to ask for leave because they had syndromes of catching a cold. Therefore, the word "Ganmao" came from this and had been used until today.

(3) Helping the patients with noble medical ethics.

Chen Wuze pointed out in the *Imperial Medicine Practice*, Volume II of the *Sanyin Prescriptions* that "the state employs all civil and military officials as officials to support the people. There is no one who does not learn from the ancients to gain knowledge and learn the ancient ways. Although they are different, they are essentially the same." He believed that all civil and military officials were set up to support the people, whose duty was to serve the people, and that no one could make achievements without learning the ancient classics. Chen Wuze advocated that TCM practitioners should read ancient medical books such as *Yellow Emperor's Canon of Medicine, Shennong's Herbal Classic*, master the Five Classics, Three Histories and the classics of Hundred Schools of Thought. They should also learn the medical skills and ethics of famous TCM practitioners such as Zhang Zhongjing, Hua Tuo, Sun

Simiao. He believed that those who help the people must have the excellent skills and noble morality.

Throughout his life, Chen Wuze has helped patients with his excellent medical skills and noble medical ethics. He also founded the Yongjia School of Medicine. Lu Zuchang, who has a good relationship with Chen Wuze, once commented on Chen Wuzi in the *Yijian Jiumiufang*, Mr. Chen is light on money and values people. He is devoted to learning from the past. He is rational and has a good theory. It can be seen that Chen Wuze's virtue, the excellent skills and noble morality were highly appreciated.

5.2.5 Song Ci

1. Brief biography

Song Ci, whose courtesy name was Huifu, was born in Nanhe, Xingtai, Hebei Province, and was a native of Tongyou Li, Jianyang (now Nanping, Fujian Province). He was a famous criminal justice official in the Southern Song dynasty, and also a distinguished forensic scientist in ancient China. Song Ci had a scientific spirit of seeking truth and being pragmatic, serious and prudent, and dared to challenge the secular world in his life. He compiled his experience, research, thoughts and other knowledge into a book, *Collection of Grievance Relief Stories*, which was the first forensic medicine book in ancient China and the world. It was famous at home and abroad and had made great contributions to the development of medicine, especially forensic medicine. The forensics community at home and abroad also generally agrees that Song Ci created "forensic toxicology", and respectfully calls Song Ci "the father of forensic medicine" and "the originator of world forensic medicine".

2. Medical ethics

(1) A criminal prosecutor with the scientific spirit of seeking truth and being pragmatic.

Due to his father's influence, Song Ci became a famous criminal prosecutor and forensic scientist in the Southern Song dynasty. Song Ci's father, Song Gong, once served as the Guanzhou governor. He was especially responsible for the management of prisons. He often engaged in some criminal cases. His work was particularly special, and he often encountered some forensic examination cases. As a result, Song Ci had been around since childhood and had interest in criminal cases. During serving as the criminal prosecutor, Song Ci always adhered to the scientific spirit of seeking truth and being pragmatic. Some officials did not test and analyze the case, which led to many unjust, false and wrong cases. He often opposed and condemned such phenomena. He mentioned in the *Collection of Grievance Relief Stories*, "In all cases, the most important thing is the death penalty. To sentence a prisoner to death, the most important thing is to find out the clues and facts of the case. However, in order to find out the clues and facts of the case, the first thing is to rely on the means of inspection and investigation. Because whether an offender is alive or dead, whether a case is judged correctly or wrongfully, and whether a grievance is upheld or forged, all depend on the conclusions drawn from inspection and investigation." This is also the reason that all criminal officials must participate in the inspection and exploration as stipulated by the law. They must be extremely careful. At the same time, Song Ci also mentioned in the *Collection of Grievance Relief Stories* that "I, Song Ci have served as a law enforcement officer for four times. I have no other skills, but I am very serious in judging cases. It is necessary to try again after hearing. I dare not be careless." It can also be seen from this that Song Ci has always been responsible and prudent in dealing with inspection, and has never been a bit negligent. He has a high level of professionalism, as well as a moral demeanor with great respect for life.

(2) Challenge the secular world to investigate the truth.

Song Ci not only had the professional spirit of seeking truth and being pragmatic, but also had the noble character of challanging the secular world and pursuing truth. During his autopsy, Song Ci strongly opposed the ethical concept and practice of covering up the private parts to avoid "delusional thinking" and "delusional action". He believed that it was extremely disrespectful to the deceased and to the facts, and would even allow some people to use this ethical concept and practice to cover up the truth of the case itself, thus leading to some wrongful convictions. Therefore, Song Ci broke away with secular concepts and emphasized and admonished that one should not cover up private parts of the body, and all the apertures of the corpse must be carefully examined to confirm whether there are knives, needles, sharp objects and other deadly objects inside. He also pointed out that when examining the bodies of women, one should not be limited by secular perspectives, but should go to a bright place for a careful examination. Song Ci's truth-seeking attitude during autopsies conflicted with secular ethics at that time. But his spirit of defying the secular and daring to find out the truth is worthy of being inherited and learned by every official and forensic TCM practitioner.

(3) Passing on and accumulating experience.

Song Ci was an official through his life, serving four times as a criminal officer. He practiced the principle of putting people's lives first throughout his life and he strongly advocating the spirit of seeking truth. He was quite aware that autopsy is particularly important in the process of judging and settling cases, and is very technical, even much more difficult than treating illnesses and injuries for living people. It requires autopsy examiners to have not only good moral character but also profound medical knowledge. To build up his medical basis, Song Ci diligently studied medical books, especially physiology, pathology, pharmacology and other related books on medicine, and applied what he had learned in the autopsy, to "making the dead speak". He also made a comprehensive summary based on the practices of his predecessors and created new test methods to make them more rational, systematic and theoretical. With his rich forensic experience and dedicated efforts, Song Ci compiled *Collection of Grievance Relief Stories*, which recorded informative test methods, techniques, and many practical and effective detoxification and first-aid methods. It became a must-have reference book for subsequent generations of crime and prison officials, and was translated into various languages such as Korean and Japanese.

5.2.6　Chen Ziming

1. Brief biography

Chen Ziming, with the courtesy name of Liangpu and "Yaoyin Old Man" (literally means "reclusive medical elder") as pseudonym in his twilight years, was a native of Linchuan, Fuzhou (now Fuzhou City, Jiangxi Province). He was a renowned medical expert in the Southern Song dynasty, particularly proficient in gynecology and surgery. He was appraised as one of the ten most famous TCM practitioners in the history of Jiangxi and an outstanding expert in gynecology and obstetrics in ancient China. Chen Ziming was born in a family of medicine, with his ancestors engaged in medicine for three generations. He studied medicine with his father since he was a child. His family had a large collection of medical books, and he was so diligent and talented in medicine that he was reputed to have mastered medical masterpieces such as *Shennong's Herbal Classic* and *Treatise on Febrile and*

Miscellaneous Diseases when he was 14 years old. He once served as a medical official at Mingdao Academy in Jiankang Prefecture (now Nanjing, Jiangsu Province). When reading medical books, Chen Ziming found that the medical information on the diagnosis and treatment of gynecological diseases before the Song dynasty was too simple and had not been studied systematically. So he accepted the challenge and gathered the medical achievements of his predecessors, sorted them out and made a summary in clinical practice, and finally completed the compilation of the first monograph on obstetrics and gynecology in China's history, *Complete Effective Prescriptions for Women's Diseases*. In addition, he also wrote three volumes of medical books such as *Complete Collection of Effective Medicinal Prescriptions* and *Essence of Surgery*. Among these, *Complete Effective Prescriptions for Women's Diseases* and *Essence of Surgery* are preserved to the present day.

2. Medical ethics

(1) Studying diligently to cure strange diseases.

Born in a family of TCM practitioners, Chen Ziming gained a lot of knowledge and experience in medicine. In Volume 15 "No. 13 Prescription for Irritability and Sadness in Pregnancy" of *Complete Effective Prescriptions for Women's Diseases*, there is an anecdote about Chen Ziming in his youth. The legend goes that Chen Ziming had a fellow villager named Cheng Huqing, whose wife Cheng Huangshi was four or five months pregnant, but was suddenly plagued by a strange illness. Cheng Huangshi was sad and tearful during the daytime. A number of TCM practitioners and wizards were invited to treat her, but all failed. Seeing his wife plagued by a strange disease every day, Cheng Huqing was anxious and at a loss. Chen Ziming, then 14 years old, was studying medicine at home, and as soon as he learned of Cheng Huangshi's strange illness from his father, who was a TCM practitioner, he had his own idea, and asked someone to tell Cheng Huqing, "I remember that my ancestor once said that this illness is called irritability and sadness, and it will be cured with jujube soup." So Cheng Huqing consulted ancient books and canons and was very happy to see that there really was such a thing, so he applied for the right medicine, and Cheng Huangshi was cured after taking the medicine.

Chen Ziming was able to use ancient prescriptions to cure diseases that cannot be cured by other TCM practitioners when only 14 years old, which shows that he was diligent and studious since childhood and had his own thoughts and ideas. This anecdote shows that the young Chen Ziming had already paid attention to and studied gynecological diseases.

(2) Commitment to research in gynecology.

During his life, Chen Ziming had interacted a lot with TCM practitioners and patients, but he was extremely dissatisfied with various social ills that existed in the medical field at that time, such as witch TCM practitioners and quack TCM practitioners, and he was especially disturbed by the fact that gynecology was not taken seriously by TCM practitioners. Chen Ziming knew that women's diseases were extremely complicated, especially the hardship of childbirth. From time to time, maternal patients ended up losing their lives due to the unavailability of treatment, and even though some survived, they still suffered from gynecological diseases that were difficult to cure. Chen Ziming read ancient books and found that there were few records of women's diseases and that much of the knowledge and experience of his predecessors had not been systematically summarized and studied, so he assumed the task of studying gynecological diseases and compiled a book. As such, Chen Ziming read medical books extensively and collected the strengths of others, summarizing and sorting out the writings of his predecessors and integrating them with the famous prescriptions taught by his own family, finally compiled *Complete Effective Prescriptions for Women's Diseases*, a monograph with considerable influence on later generations of obstetrics and gynecology.

As stated in *Complete Effective Prescriptions for Women's Diseases*, the technique of medicine is complex, especially for women. Gynecology and obstetrics are the most risky and complicated ones, but Chen Ziming was brave enough to assume the great mission despite the difficulties.

(3) Positive thinking reveals medical ethics.

Chen Ziming was not only well-known for his excellent medical skills, but also for his medical ethics. In *Complete Effective Prescriptions for Women's Diseases*, Chen Ziming wrote that according to the ancients, there is no hard-to-treat disease in the world, but only TCM practitioners who are not good at treating it; and there is no medicine that cannot be replaced, but only TCM practitioners who are not good at using the medicine flexibly. From this, we can see that he was brave enough to treat hard-to-treat diseases and moreover, he had the medical skill and courage to use medicine flexibly. Legend has it that Chen Ziming hated quacks who only valued money and profit, especially some TCM practitioners who changed the name of their prescriptions and claimed that they were secret prescriptions handed down from his ancestors, in order to collect money and show off. Chen Ziming had noble medical ethics and treated his patients rich or poor, equally and would not even take any money from those who were really in need, and compiled his family's secret prescriptions into a book for the benefit of the world.

As a TCM practitioner, Chen Ziming was so enthusiastic, conscientious, and selfless, demonstrating his noble medical ethics.

5.3　Evaluation of Medical Practitioners and Their Medical Ethics

During the Northern and Southern Song dynasties, the social environment was fairly prosperous and stable, the economy, science and technology and culture developed rapidly, and the rulers attached great importance to medicine under the strategy of ruling the country by emphasizing literature rather than martial arts, which led to a significant improvement in the level of medical skills and ethics of the TCM practitioners, and highly recognition of medical TCM practitioners and their ethics by the people of the time.

The prosperous and stable economy provided a social setting for people and TCM practitioners to focus on health and research; the development of science and technology provided a large amount of medical resources and books for TCM practitioners; the high importance attached by the government provided good education on medical skills and medical ethics for TCM practitioners; the rise of Neo-Confucianism provided a standardized code of conduct for TCM practitioners. During the Northern and Southern Song dynasties, medical practitioners were more sophisticated in medical skills than in previous generations, and their medical ethics were also generally improved. Qin Guan, a scholar in the Imperial Academy of the Northern Song dynasty, remarked in his *Letter to the TCM Practitioner Zou Fang* that "all works are made by the saints, only TCM practitioners have books to write. TCM practitioners can bring people back from illness with common medical materials". In *Biography of Pang Anshi of History of the Song Dynasty*, Tuo Tuo of the Yuan dynasty evaluated famous TCM practitioner Pang Anshi as such, "Patients came to consult one after another, and he vacated his house to let the patients live. He personally took care of the decoction and made sure that the patients were cured before leaving. If he really can't cure some diseases, he would tell the patients honestly and stop providing them with treatment". Huang Tingjian also wrote in the *Preface for Mr. Pang's Treatise on Febrile Diseases* that "when patients came to the door, no matter rich or poor, Pang Anshi would provide them with a place to stay, so that they could live comfortably regardless of the cold or heat, and also provide them with very good food. He respected the old and loved the young. He did not care about money and treated his patients with patience like a loving mother". Lu Zuchang, a TCM practitioner of the Yongjia Medical School during the Southern Song dynasty, appraised TCM practitioner Chen Wuze as such, "He didn't care about money, only about human life. He worked hard to learn ancient medical techniques and wrote medical books. He was as serious as the great TCM practitioner Bianque when he took the pulse. He was as earnest as the great TCM practitioner Hua Tuo when he administered medicine to his patients". Fan Zhongyan also wrote that "if I can't be a good minister, I'll be a good TCM practitioner".

Back then, people called TCM practitioners who violated the code of medical ethics "quacks". As it was recorded in *History of the Economy—History of the Song Dynasty*, "Order the imperial physician to choose a TCM practitioner who is good at taking pulses, and have the magistrate provide medicine to patients based on the patients' conditions, so that the poor will not be mistreated by quacks." Lin Bo, a renowned hermit poet during the Northern Song dynasty, denounced and criticized quacks in his *Recording of Reflections*, "A person without virtue cannot be a TCM practitioner. A TCM practitioner's duty involves life and death, while the purpose of a quack is to earn money. The prescriptions prescribed by quacks may not be appropriate, and if the patient takes the medicine and fortunately does not die, the quack will demand a high price, and the patient will willingly satisfy his desire. If the patient dies after taking the medicine, the quack will argue that it is caused by improper diet and has nothing to do with the medicine. What's wrong with the dead? There are no more miracle-working TCM practitioners in this world who can save lives like Bianque and Hua Tuo. It is better to keep health properly than to give your life to a quack. Alas, it's really sad."

Generally speaking, in the Northern and Southern Song dynasty, people mainly praised the medical skills and ethics of TCM practitioners, but strongly condemned some profit-oriented TCM practitioners who violated the medical ethics and were bad at medical skills. This indicated that people paid more attention to medical ethics and skills of TCM practitioners.

5.4 Medical Education

Medical education in the Northern and Southern Song dynasty was very prosperous in the history of traditional medical education in China. During this time, the status of medicine and TCM practitioners was increasingly improved, and even surpassed that of the Tang dynasty. Meanwhile, the implementation of medical policies also highlighted the thought of benevolence. The cultivation of TCM practitioners in the Northern and Southern Song dynasty not only played a significant role for the development of the dynasty, but also significantly enlightened later generations' education in medical skills and ethics.

5.4.1 Medical Education in the Northern and Southern Song dynasty

The cultivation of TCM practitioners in the Northern and Southern Song dynasty was deeply influenced by politics, economy, society, and science and technology. Apart from the inheritance of masters and apprentices, ancestral traditions, and self-study to be a TCM practitioner, medical education was particularly prominent compared with previous dynasties. The Imperial Medical Bureaus in the Sui and Tang dynasties were the earliest medical schools sponsored by the government in the world. Based on the medical education in the Sui and Tang dynasties, the Northern and Southern Song dynasty continued to reform and improve it.

(1) Medical education institutions were independent and teaching by disciplines was more reasonable.

In the Sui and Tang dynasties, the Imperial Medical Bureau was not only responsible for the management of medical affairs of the imperial court, but also for medical education. However, in the Song dynasty, the medical management and education were clearly divided. Thus, the Hanlin Hospital and the Imperial Medical Bureau were specially set up to be responsible for medical management and medical education respectively. Of course, the establishment of the Imperial Medical Bureau, a medical education institution, also experienced a long-term development process.

In the early days of the Northern and Southern Song dynasty, the Imperial Medical Bureau was set up by imitating the bureaus in the Tang dynasty. Nevertheless, it lacked the function of medical education and a specific TCM practitioner training system. Therefore, the TCM practitioners in these bureaus were all selected from the public. In 992, the Imperial Medical Bureau was renamed Imperial Medical Academy, but medical education was still not carried out. Until the Qingli period governed by Song Renzong, Fan Zhongyan presided over the reform of national policies. The reconstructed Imperial Medical Academy aimed to select a group of medical officers with excellent medical skills, who were affiliated to Taichang Temple. Additionally, the academy recruited students and medical professionals through lectures at the Imperial Medical Academy. And the academy selected Sun Yonghe, Zhao Conggu and other imperial TCM practitioners from Hanlin Hospital as medical faculties, so as to teach the medical foundations. These medical foundations include *Yellow Emperor's Canon of Medicine—Plain Conversation* and *The Classic of Difficult Issues*. At first, the Imperial Medical Academy had no restrictions on the number of medical students, and there was no special examination system and didn't gain official recognition. However, medical education had begun to scale up at that time. Until the reform implemented by Wang Anshi, the Imperial Medical Academy formally established the official rank, and separated from the Taichang Temple. Consequently, it became an independent, formal medical education management institution.

Medical education in the Northern and Southern Song dynasty was implemented according to disciplines. In the Jiayou period, medical education was divided into nine subjects: adult's pulse (internal medicine), wind diseases, infantile pulse (pediatrics), obstetrics, ophthalmology, sores, mouth, Jinyu-shujin and Jinlian-wound. The discipline of medical education was further subdivided into thirteen subjects: adult's pulse, wind diseases, infantile pulse, acupuncture, moxibustion, mouth, throat, ophthalmology, ear, sores, wound, metal-inflicted wound and shujin. However, after the systems were changed in Yuanfeng period, the Imperial Medical Academy was subordinate to the Taichang Rites Department. And Jinlian-wound in the medical education was changed into acupuncture and moxibustion. But other subjects were the same in content compared with previous subjects. Nine subjects were still retained. Thus, this classification was more reasonable than before. Since then, the subject classification of medical education has basically remained unchanged until the late Northern and Southern Song dynasty.

(2) Establishing an entrance examination system and implementing the "Sanshe" promotion method.

In the early days of the establishment of the Imperial Medical Academy in the Northern Song dynasty, there were no entrance examinations or quota restrictions. However, with the continuous expansion of the Imperial Medical Academy, the ability of medical trainees gradually showed differences. And the medical education system was gradually formed. Therefore, an entrance examination system was set up. Apart from some public basic subjects such as *Yellow Emperor's Canon of Medicine—Plain Conversation, The Classic of Difficult Issues,* and *Zhubing Yuanhou Lun, Shennong's Herbal Classic* was also a compulsory subject. At the same time, specialty examinations would be conducted according to different subjects, which was expected to improve the overall level of medical students through the entrance examination. When the entrance examination was initially set up, the enrollment quota was 120. However, it was recorded that there were already 161 learners at that time. Therefore, 41 candidates were eliminated as alternates through the entrance examination. The number of alternates was not limited, and anyone who met the conditions could sign up. If there were guarantees from officials, alternates could be admitted to study medicine. These alternates could be selected into formal trainees through standardized selection when formal trainees were absent or eliminated. In 1060, there were 9 subjects in medical education. And it was stipulated that anyone who went to the Imperial Medical Academy to study medicine must be at least 15 years old. Firstly, students should register with the Taichang Temple. And then they should be guaranteed by destiny officers, envoys, medical officers in Hanlin Hospital and other officers in the medical school. Meanwhile, three students should provide guarantee for each other and supervise themselves. In this way, they could take the entrance examination after studying medicine in Imperial Medical Academy for one year. When students were qualified and the academy had quotas, they would officially become medical students in the Imperial Medical Academy. Once students became formal medical students in the Imperial Medical Academy, they could obtain the salary from the imperial court.

During the reign of Song Huizong, the Imperial Medical Academy was still responsible for the medical education and medical management. But the Central Medicine ("Imperial Medicine") and Local Medicine ("County Medicine") were further established to train medical students. The Imperial Medicine School established in the central government was subordinate to the Imperial College, which was consistent with the regulations of the Taixue, Wuxue and Law School. So far, medical education reached the highest status. Like the Taixue, Wuxue and Law School, Imperial Medicine School adopted the "Sanshe" method, increasing the number of students to 300, and teaching them in three different places. The entrance examination system of Imperial Medical College and Imperial Medicine Bureau was basically the same, but there were differences in the source of students. Imperial Medical College was the real national selection for medical students. The "Sanshe" promotion method founded by Wang Anshi was first applied to the education in Taixue, Wuxue and Law School, and then to the Medical Education.

The 300 medical students who passed the entrance examination were dividied into 40 superior students, 60 middle students and 200 external students according to their scores. Students would take quarterly "temporary tests" and annual "official tests". And the scope of each test would be publicly informed. At the end of each year, students would be classified into superior students, middle students and external students according to their scores in all "temporary test" and moral performance. Also, only the superior students, 30 middle students and 120 external students could be assessed. Finally, only students who were superior and first-class in the "official tests" could be directly granted the official position. Those who were assessed to first-class and middle-class, or both middle-class could participate in the three-year imperial examination. Those who were first-class and inferior-class, or middle-class and inferior-class, or both inferior-class would be rewarded as "Neishesheng". And the rest would be reduced their classes or leave college. The implementation of the entrance examination system and the "Sanshe" promotion method greatly improved the training quality of medical students in the Northern and Southern Song dynasty. Additionally, it enhanced the status of TCM practitioners and medical education, which is of great significance to the development of TCM.

(3) Developing assessment systems, strengthening local medical education.

Whether it was the Imperial Medical Bureau, Imperial Medicine Academy or County Medicine Academy, students all needed to take many examinations and assessments in their daily study after passing the entrance examination as to determine their promotion and elimination. The daily examination in the Imperial Medical Bureau was also related to subsidies. The higher the score, the more subsidies it got. The subsidies were also divided into upper, middle and lower levels. Only one-third of the total students received subsidies. Others were only free of board and lodging, and the last students would be eliminated. In addition, formal students also needed to go to designated places to treat civilians on a regular basis. And their treatment effect was also related to subsidies. After three years of study, eligible students could participate in the selection of medical officers in the Imperial Medical Bureau. If someone succeeded, he or she would officially become medical officers in the Hanlin Hospital. The Imperial Medicine Academy and County Medicine Academy implemented the "Sanshe" promotion method for assessment after students passing the entrance examination in most cases. In general, the Northern and Southern Song dynasty not only paid attention to medical education, but also constantly explored and improved the medical examination system, which was very vital to the medical education in the central and local governments.

The preliminary establishment of the medical examination system in the Northern and Southern Song dynasty was mainly reflected in the previous stages. For example, during the Jiayou period, Taichang Temple mentioned that "if someone was familiar with other medicine classics, but didn't understand *The Compendium of Materia Medica*, we would not recruit them". This reflected the preliminary norms of medical examination and the assessment focused on the clinical application of drugs. In addition, a clinical assessment system was also gradually established. Medical students were required to go to the city to treat civilians on a regular basis. And they should take turns to treat students in Taixue, Wuxue and Law school and soldiers. Their treatment effect and medical ethics would be considered in the assessment. If medical students made many mistakes, they would be punished, and even leave School in severe cases. Besides, the examination system in school continuously improved. The "make-up test" was a medical enrollment examination. And the "temporary test" was conducted three times a quarter hosted by senior officials. And the "official test" was divided into two times hosted by the officials appointed by the emperors. The recruitment and assessment system for TCM practitioners and medicine officers gradually improved due to the following reasons: setting up the recruitment and assessment system of TCM practitioners and medicine officers, establishing and developing of other test systems by "Sanshe" promotion method.

In the Northern and Southern Song dynasty, the independent medical education institutions, the rational teaching by subjects, the improving examination and assessment system, and the strong central and local medical education accumulated experience to a certain extent. And these also enhanced the status of medicine and TCM practitioners, promoting the development of traditional medical education and TCM in China. The training and assessment of TCM practitioners not only reflected in medical skills, but also in the cultivation of medical ethics. For example, the assessment included the "virtues" performance. Additionally, the learning subjects include Confucian classics such as the *Book of Songs*, the *Book of History*, the *Book of Rites*, the *Book of Changes*, the *Book of Spring and Autumn Annals*. These contents greatly promoted the formation of traditional medical ethics culture in the Northern and Southern Song dynasty and were of great importance to the cultivation of medical ethics for TCM practitioners these days.

5.4.2 Contemporary Enlightenment of Medical Ethics Culture in the Northern and Southern Song dynasty

The medical ethics elaborated by medical professionals in the Northern and Southern Song dynasty was an important part of the traditional medical ethics culture in China. They have certain enlightenment to the medical ethics education for medical workers and students these days.

(1) Strengthening medical ethics, developing correct outlooks on life, value and world.

Medical education in the Northern and Southern Song dynasty paid particular attention to personal ethics of TCM practitioners. As recorded in the volume one *Xiao'er Weisheng Zongwei Lunfang of Medical Professionals Theory*, "All TCM practitioners must have right personal ethics first, and then require other people and things to be moral". For instance, official medical education required medical students to learn Confucian culture and be familiar with hundreds of scriptures and history. Also, it emphasized that TCM practitioners must firstly have good ethics. Only in this way, they could experience and address the patients' sufferings. Today, we still know that the responsibility of TCM practitioners is related to people's lives. Thus, TCM practitioners must be careful and upright in curing diseases, and never use medical skills to harm people. Therefore, all medical workers and students should strengthen their own ethics, establish a correct outlook on the world, life and values. Also, they should practice the requirements of socialist core values. On this basis, they should correct their motivation to engage in medical work, have a healthy and positive understanding of their responsibilities, strengthen their beliefs for medical careers, and strive unremittingly for them.

(2) Studying hard to boost medical skills.

With the emergence of "Confucian medical practitioners" in the Southern and Northern Song dynasty, people often used "good TCM practitioners" and "quack TCM practitioners" to evaluate TCM practitioners. Those with exquisite medical skills and noble medical ethics were good TCM practitioners, while those with poor medical skills or violating medical ethics were quack TCM practitioners. Quack TCM practitioners not only prevent patients from getting good treatment, but also endanger their lives. As medicine is an indispensable science for human survival, medical workers and students should not only have correct outlook on the world, life and values, and good personal ethics, but also have exquisite medical skills, so as to truly save people's lives. With the continuous elaboration of medical categories, medical subjects continuedly are researched and applied to clinical practice. Furthermore, medical workers and students must study hard, observe carefully and learn until they are old. Also, they should improve their medical skills on the basis of consolidating the theoretical basis and strengthening clinical practice. For medical students, it is more important to strengthen humanistic quality when receiving medical education. At the same time, they should assiduously study medical knowledge in theories to consolidate medical foundations. Also, medical students should find their own direction in the medical field and study diligently, laying a solid theoretical foundation for each discipline. And medical students should learn more, observe more, practice more and summarize more during probation, internship and companionship, so as to lay a solid foundation to be a TCM practitioner in the future. For medical workers, it is more important to adhere to study in daily life and lifelong learning, strengthen communication and exchange between TCM practitioners, and diligently participate in training and clinical practice, so as to improve medical skills.

(3) Be sincere and kind to serve patients.

Throughout the Northern and Southern Song dynasty, all medical masters were skilled and noble, such as Qian Yi, Pang Anshi, Tang Shenwei, Song Ci and Chen Ziming. They were benevolent and had exquisite skills. And they treated patients equally regardless of their wealth and poverty. Furthermore, they didn't pursue the supremacy of interests, but valued ethics instead of interests. Additionally, they didn't pursue promotion but were modest and cautious. Meanwhile, they didn't care whether the weather was windy, frosty, rainy or snowy, and would go out to treat patients. Such sincere medical ethics are still worth inheriting and carrying forward today. With the increasing development of medical and health services, the TCM practitioner-patient relationships become particularly sensitive. A harmonious TCM practitioner-patient relationship is not only conducive to developing the medical and health services, but also building a harmonious society. As contemporary medical workers and students, we should also serve patients sincerely while providing medical treatment to patients. Similarly, no matter the patient's family is rich or poor, the patients should be treated with the same respect and treatment. It is wrong to give a special preferential treatment because of the patient's wealth. It is not allowed to charge red envelopes in order to obtain benefits, let alone prescribe unnecessary examination items and amount of drugs for patients. If there are drugs that have the same efficacy and are cheaper, priority should be given to them. The TCM practitioner doesn't degrade other TCM practitioners for his own fame and wealth, but respects and communicates with each other. In addition, the TCM practitioner should strengthen communication and exchange with patients with strong humanistic care.

(4) Be brave in shouldering responsibilities and willing to dedicate.

The responsibility of medical practitioners lies in saving lives. When encountering first aid and difficulties, medical practitioners should dare to take responsibilities and be willing to sacrifice. During the Northern Song dynasty, the plague was rampant. Pang Anshi, a famous TCM practitioner, undertook the responsibility of a TCM practitioner and entered the plague area to seek the treatment method. At the same time, he practiced physically and finally cured the local plague. As a result, Pang Anshi became well-known for thousands of years. Medical workers and students in modern times should do their utmost to treat patients. When facing the epidemic and infectious diseases, they should bravely undertake the mission of medical workers and take the initiative to fight against the epidemic. In 2020, the outbreak of COVID-19 pandemic swept the world. Countless medical workers are willing to make contributions and are not afraid of sacrifice. They are at the forefront in fighting against the epidemic. Their medical skills and sincere heart bring hope for patients. Such professional dedication is worthy of admiration and learning by every medical worker, medical student and the public.

(5) Devoting to scientific research to develop medicine.

The medical science is profound. Hence, only with TCM practitioners of all dynasties working tirelessly and devoting themselves to research, we can have a glimpse of it today. In the Northern and Southern Song dynasty, medical subjects were constantly subdivided. At that time, TCM practitioners devoted themselves to research in various medical subjects. For instance, Qian Yi specialized in pediatrics, Pang Anshi specialized in typhoid fever, Tang Shenwei specialized in Chinese materia medica, Song Ci specialized in forensic medicine, Chen Wuze specialized in "Sanyin Theory", and Chen Ziming specialized in gynecology and surgery. All laid a foundation for later development of medicine. With the development of science and technology, many medical difficulties have been overcome at present. Nevertheless, there are still plenty of medical problems that are not addressed. As a consequence, medical workers and students are required to study hard, deeply research and pursue truth. Also, medical workers and students should be good at finding problems, dare to put forth questions and be willing to research problems, contributing to the development of medical and health care for human beings.

Chapter Summary

The medical ethics culture in the Northern and Southern Song dynasty was deeply influenced by the politics, economy, society and technology at that time. It closely focused on the main line of "benevolence", "essence" and "sincerity". Also, it featured inheritance, criticality and epoch. Admittedly, some TCM practitioners inherited medical ethics, such as Qian Yi, Pang Anshi, Tang Shenwei, Chen Wuze, Song Ci and Chen Ziming. This inheritance further enriches and develops medical ethics in traditional Chinese culture.

At the same time, the medical ethics culture in the Northern and Southern Song dynasty was very vital to strengthen medical ethics cultivation for contemporary medical workers and students. To begin with, it is conducive to cultivating qualified medical workers. A qualified medical worker should not only have exquisite medical skills and solid medical foundations in theories, but also have noble medical ethics. Secondly, it is beneficial to inherit and carry forward traditional Chinese culture and help the construction of socialist spiritual civilization. Thirdly, it is conducive to promoting the healthy development of today's TCM practitioner-patient relationship. Fourthly, it can promote the development of medical technology.

Application in Contemporary Times

1. Coordinated development in medical ethics culture and health care

This chapter describes the development of TCM and characteristics of medical ethics culture in the Northern and Southern Song dynasty. Affected by social ideological trends, a new social ideological trend-Neo-Confucianism emerged. This philosophy integrated some views of Confucianism, Taoism, Buddhism and metaphysics in Wei and Jin dynasties. And then "Confucian medicine" occurred. TCM practitioners belonging to the "Confucian medicine" had a solid cultural foundation. They were good at professional research, read loads of books, and even completed medical research and medical works with their own lifelong experience.

The professional ability requirements for medical workers are very strict today. In order to master consolidated medical technologies, medical workers need to continuously learn scientific and cultural knowledge and skills. Additionally, they also should have the spirit of exploration and research. In the new epidemic era, in order to fight against the ever-changing epidemic, medical students and workers should continuously improve their scientific and cultural knowledge and professional skills. At the same time, they should pursue truth, forge ahead and serve the country scientifically. All are to be a socialist medical worker with ideals, beliefs and responsibilities.

2. Be a "warm" medical worker

The "Confucian medicine" studied in this chapter greatly demonstrates the "benevolence" of medical workers, further enriching the theoretical basis for the development of medical ethics culture. In the Northern and Southern Song dynasty, many TCM practitioners treated patients like close relatives, often with a heart of benevolence and sympathy. In modern society, a "benevolent" heart is equally important. A warm word can quietly open the frozen heart. And a warm eye can rekindle the spark of hope for the desperate. And a warm doctor can warm the hearts of countless patients.

Being a "warm" doctor is the interpretation of "doctors with benevolent hearts" in this era. Real TCM practitioner-patient communication is not necessarily verbal communication, but sometimes spiritual communication. Someone said, "The farthest distance in the world is not between life and death, but when the patient stands in front of the doctor, the doctor only sees the disease, not the person." Being a good doctor should be a warm doctor who can think from the perspective of the patients.

6

Medical Ethics Culture in the Jin and Yuan Dynasties

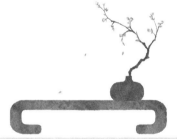

During the Jin and Yuan dynasties, ethnic and class contradictions were extremely prominent. At the same time, there were frequent wars, chaos and epidemic diseases. In the face of the contradiction between new diseases and old customs, coupled with the health needs of the rulers, the policies implemented by the rulers in medicine community were inclusive and tolerant at that time. Therefore, TCM practitioners and celebrities such as Liu Wansu, Zhang Congzheng, Li Gao and Zhu Zhenheng in the Jin and Yuan dynasty appeared one after another, creating a new situation for the medical development in China. Medical ethics culture in the Jin and Yuan dynasty not only inherited the traditional morality of helping the world and saving people, but also included cared for the people's sufferings and be enthusiastic about treatment and indifferent to fame and wealth.

6.1 Overview of Medical Ethics

6.1.1 Social Background of Medical Ethics

1. Political background

The Jin and Yuan dynasties in Chinese history were another period when ethnic minorities governed the whole country. Although it broke the rigid political situation, the rulers paid less attention to medicine than they did in the Northern Song dynasty. The rulers of the Jin and Yuan dynasties only cared about cementing their political status and had no time for the supervision and guidance of medical science. However, under this special political background, medical science of the Jin and Yuan dynasties achieved all-round development, and TCM ushered in the new "Thriving Medicine" era. On the one hand, inadequate supervision and lack of guidance from the state level gave it ample room for development. On the other hand, war, forced labor and starvation led to the spread of epidemics. This prompted a slew of innovative TCM practitioners to carry out in-depth, systematic, comprehensive and specialized research into the cause, mechanism and syndrome differentiation and treatment of diseases such as epidemics, internal injuries, and consumptive diseases. The complex historical background in the Jin and Yuan dynasties spawned large numbers of TCM practitioners. Based on their own clinical practice, these TCM practitioners elucidated *Yellow Emperor's Canon of Medicine* from different angles and different dimensions, giving rise to distinctive schools of medicine.

What's more, the ethnic policies introduced by the Jin and Yuan dynasties ruined the career of Confucian scholars. The Jurchen rulers of the Jin dynasty put a limit on the number of Han officials in important positions when appointing officials. Han officials appointed for office often could not get their hands on real power. The rulers of the Yuan dynasty adopted a policy of ethnic division. People were treated differently depending on their social rankings when it came to the selection and appointment of officials, the granting of legal status, the introduction of imperial examinations quotas, and other rights and obligations. Besides, some Han Confucian scholars felt ashamed to serve the ethnic minority regime and they voluntarily gave up on pursuing a career in the government. As a result, the ethnic policies of the rulers of the Jin and Yuan dynasties subverted Han Confucian scholars' traditional value orientation that "He who excels in learning can make an official". Those among them who thought proactively adhered to the idea of "official or TCM practitioner". They stopped pursuing a career in the government and switched to medicine. A saying of that time adequately described this phenomenon: the perfect man, if not seen in the imperial court, must have withdrawn to the medical profession. For example, Zhang Yuansu, the founder of the Yishui school of thought, devoted himself to medicine after his failure to pursue a career in the government due to his violation of the "temple taboo" during imperial examinations. Under such complex political circumstances, a large number of Confucian scholars switched to the medical profession and contributed enormously to the development of medicine. Most of them were erudite Confucian scholars with a knowledge structure different from that of those who "inherited family traditions". They were quick-thinking and innovative, and had a more comprehensive and profound understanding of diseases, which promoted the development of medical theory.

2. Economic background

During the Jin and Yuan dynasties, ethnic and class contradictions were manifest. Continuous wars and widespread epidemics inflicted heavy pain on people. During this period, the vast northern and central China were reduced to the battlegrounds of competing regimes. Politically, the rulers of the Jin dynasty suppressed the rebellion of other ethnic groups. Economically, they pushed for backward slavery and brutally exploited the working people. This ruined the economy. After Kublai of the Yuan dynasty came to power, the political situation was ostensibly stable. However, power struggle made the government corrupted and people impoverished, and prevalent infectious diseases plunged people into sickness and misery.

To help people in dire straits and protect the health of the ruling class, innovative TCM practitioners emerged in the inclusive medical sector, though the society and economy of the Jin and Yuan dynasties were in terrible conditions. They studied medical theories, explored causes of diseases, and sought new ways of saving the world. Their efforts were positively viewed by people.

3. Cultural background

During the Jin and Yuan dynasties, ethnic minorities occupied the Central Plains. This had a strong impact on traditional culture and society of the Central Plains. People even began to doubt the orthodox political philosophy which had long been regarded as eternal truth. The rise of various schools of medicine indirectly served as a reflection of the cultural diversity in the Jin and Yuan dynasties.

On the one hand, Confucian scholars' free and heated debate on academic issues contributed enormously to the rise of schools of medicine in the Jin and Yuan dynasties. "Confucianism diversified in the Song dynasty, and medicine diversified in the Jin and Yuan dynasties". This not only indicates that there were a diversity of schools of medicine in the Jin and Yuan dynasties, but also suggests that Confucian TCM practitioners played a dominant role in the development of medicine during that time. Many TCM practitioners of the Jin and Yuan dynasties, such as Zhang Yuansu, Liu Wansu, Wang Haogu, Zhu Zhenheng, Cheng Wuji, Dai Qizong, etc., were famous Confucian TCM practitioners who first practiced Confucianism and then medicine. Confucian scholars' inclination towards free academic debate necessarily made its entry into the medical profession. On the other hand, cultural exchanges across regions and in multiple fields broadened the academic perspective of the medical community of the Jin and Yuan dynasties. Territory expansion spanning Asia and Europe during the Jin and Yuan dynasties facilitated the communication between Asian and European peoples and the exchange between Chinese and Western cultures. As a result, Western and Central Asian medicine streamed into the Central Plains. In the mid-13th century, Europeans and Arabs came to China to practice medicine. They introduced Western and Arabian therapies and drugs to China, further extending the influence of Western medicine on Chinese medical culture. Moreover, war was rampant during the Jin and Yuan dynasties. People including TCM practitioners were left homeless. They had no choice but to travel around to treat people. This way of practicing medicine promoted cultural fusion in various fields as well as domestic medical exchanges.

6.1.2 Main Contents of Medical Ethics Culture

During the Jin and Yuan dynasties, ethnic and class contradictions were prominent, wars were incessant, and many powerful infectious diseases spread from place to place. Existing practices were no longer able to cope with new diseases. Liu Wansu, Zhang Yuansu, Zhang Congzheng, Li Gao, and Zhu Zhenheng emerged. They carried out research into the mechanism of diseases and sought new ways of saving people. As a result, medicine prospered. TCM practitioners in the Jin and Yuan dynasties established their own theories and were innovative in one way or another, yet the medical ethics they upheld had many similarities.

1. Studious and scholarly

Various schools of thought emerged during the Jin and Yuan dynasties, and the academic atmosphere was harmonious and inclusive. The medical community flourished despite the incessant, raging wars. Most of the medical practitioners in the Jin and Yuan dynasties were diligent and scholarly. They made new discoveries and breakthroughs in pathogenesis and preclinical medication.

The founder of Hejian School Liu Wansu was smart and keen on learning medicine when he was just a child. He began to learn *Plain Conversation* at the age of 25 and at the same time practiced medicine. This persevering scholarly endeavor continued for 35 years. He was diligent and knowledgeable. Li Gao was born in a wealthy family, which paid a lot for him to learn medicine under Zhang Yuansu in Yizhou. Li was a dedicated medical scholar. To recapitulate his decades-long practical experience in medicine and correct the mistakes made by quack medical practitioners, he studied the differences between "internal and external injuries" for 16 years. To pass his expertise on to later generations, he wrote *Differentiation between Internal and External Injuries* at the age of 68. By the time he finished *Theory of the Spleen and the Stomach*, he was already 70 years old. Li Gao was arguably a life-time medical practitioner. Zhu Zhenheng was smart and had great memory when he was just a child. At the age of 30, his mother suffered from spleen pain but the medical practitioners the family consulted were at a loss for what to do.

So he decided to learn medicine and carefully read many medical classics. Years of study paid off. At the age of 40, he specialized in medicine, and thoroughly studied *Prescriptions of the Bureau of Taiping People's Welfare Pharmacy*. He manually copied the book, and studied it day and night. Later, he decided to travel around and study under a mentor after finding that ancient prescriptions cannot cure today's diseases.

2. Helpful and indifferent to fame and fortune

Frequent wars and contagious diseases during the Jin and Yuan dynasties left people in dire conditions. Medical practitioners of the Jin and Yuan dynasties were well aware of the suffering of people. Most of them had noble virtues—helpful and indifferent to fame and fortune. These TCM practitioners did not succumb to authority nor seek fame or profit respected and loveed by people.

Liu Wansu was extraordinarily broad-minded. He despised fame and fortune, and declined the invitations to assume office in the government three times. He only wanted to practice medicine, so people called him the "noble man". Zhang Congzheng cured many scholar-officials, but the majority of his patients were common working people. He was sympathetic to the working people's plight, had no fear of power, and treated patients equally. Li Gao lived in the Southern Song dynasty. At that time, social and ethnic contradictions were glaring, and wars, turmoil, hunger and diseases caused people great pain and suffering. He was very sympathetic to the diseased people, treating them carefully and posting copies of the effective prescriptions he had personally tried on vital roads so sick people could take medicine according to prescription. Zhu Zhenheng was well versed in medicine. People came to him for treatment from near and far or requested him to pay a home visit every day. He always responded to patient's requests and visited them even if it snowed or the road was muddy. He never charged poor patients who couldn't afford drugs, and would carry medicine to treat people who were in distress.

3. Valuing education and the spread of medical science

TCM practitioners of the Jin and Yuan dynasties were diligent and scholarly. They valued education and the spread of their medical achievements, contributing enormously to the development of Chinese medicine.

Zhang Yuansu, who specialized in research into the pathogenesis of Zang-Fu diseases, was the founder of this particular field of medicine. His treatment of spleen and stomach diseases was passed on among the disciples of the Yishui School, and his students Li Dongyuan and Wang Haogu grew to be famous TCM practitioners. His article *Prescription of Drugs for Deficiency of Zang-Fu Specimens Due to Cold and Heat* was included in *Compendium of Materia Medica* by Li Shizhen, an indication of his great academic influence in the medical field. Li Gao traveled around in his twilight years to look for students with potential so that his expertise could be handed down to benefit future generations. His promotion of medicine to the benefit of people was worthy of great praise.

4. Dare to innovate

Chinese medicine prioritized the development of drugs and the collection of prescriptions after the Tang and Song dynasties. TCM practitioners and patients developed an inclination of making up prescriptions according to symptoms without concern for medical principles. TCM practitioners of the Jin and Yuan dynasties did in-depth studies of medical classics. They preserved the very best of traditional medicine and discarded what they considered to be dross. They interpreted their predecessors' medical theories and clinical experiences based on their own practice, showing an inclination of prizing established practices and innovation.

Zhang Yuansu studied ancient medical theories but did not follow them rigidly. He found that traditional methods failed to cure existing diseases. Therefore, he flexibly drew on the experience of predecessors and brought together his decades-long clinical experiences, founding a systematic syndrome differentiation system for curing the deficiencies of Zang-Fu organs with a focus on the pathogenesis. Under the influence of Zhang Yuansu's innovative thinking that "ancient prescriptions don't apply to new diseases", Li Gao analyzed the various causes of diseases. He criticized pedantic quack TCM practitioners' misuse of prescriptions and laid down his own medication principles. He not only made sure to "differentiate between endogenous and exogenous diseases" and treat the illness holistically, but also gathered clinical records. This attitude towards science which valued objective reality and opposed falsehood was very commendable. Zhu Zhenheng was the founder of the Yangyin School, one of the four major schools of medicine of the Jin and Yuan dynasties. Yangyin School was the most recent one in the four major schools. The most prominent feature of Zhu Zhenheng's medical ethics is that he did not stick to existing academic views. He acknowledged the achievements of his predecessors and affirmed the strengths of other scholars. Therefore, he did not take a negative attitude towards all other schools. He aired his own unique views and boldly applied neo-Confucianism viewpoints to medicine. All this reflects his innovative spirit and flexible use of ancient prescriptions.

5. Upright and noble

TCM practitioners of the Jin and Yuan dynasties experienced frequent wars and rampant epidemics, but they were decent and noble people beloved by others.

Liu Wansu was a studious and scholarly medical practitioner who helped those in distress and aided those in peril. He devoted his life to serving people, who held him in high esteem. Zhang Congzheng sought to benefit people with medical treatment. He emphasized virtue and honored his profession, treating all his patients equally regardless of their social status, nationality or mental ability. In his time, TCM practitioners who failed to cure patients with traditional methods would not be held accountable, but those who tried to do so with new methods faced risk. As a virtuous scientist, he treated patients with new methods, not fearing resentment if he failed nor envied if he succeeded. Li Gao was loyal, honest, sincere and serious. He was cautious when making friends, never joking with others. He emphasized the importance of medical ethics, believing that morality should be internalized and understood through practical efforts before being implemented. He strove to preserve his moral integrity. This act earned him respect and love.

6.1.3   Characteristics of Medical Ethics Culture

1. Bold innovation based on practice

Chinese medicine prioritized the development of drugs and the collection of prescriptions after the Tang and Song dynasties. TCM practitioners and patients developed an inclination of making up prescriptions according to symptoms without concern for medical principles. The preparation for curing dry dampness with aroma and tepidity, as documented in *Prescriptions* by the Song dynasty Imperial Medical Service, was frequently used by TCM practitioners and patients of that time. However, this preparation did not work with febrile diseases. The fact was that many of the diseases that were prevalent during the Jin and Yuan dynasties were potent infectious diseases (with symptoms similar to those of plague). Medical theories of that time could not cure actual illnesses. TCM practitioners of the Jin and Yuan dynasties often worked towards new theories and methods of saving people based on their predecessors' achievements. For example, Liu Wansu thought that cold medicine should be applied to diseases, which were actually fever caused by internal heat. Zhang Yuansu also held that diseases were caused by internal heat, but he advocated warm tonification. The various schools of medicine that emerged during the Jin and Yuan dynasties were an indication that all schools of thought boldly introduced innovations based on reality.

2. Emphasis on practice and well-founded argument

Medicine of the Jin and Yuan dynasties was empirical medicine. The method used was mainly observation, and clinical verification was the main means of experimentation. TCM practitioners of this period attached great importance to clinical observation. They gathered medical cases, based their theory on facts, and advanced arguments based on their predecessors' theoretical achievements. They respected facts, valued practice, and supported their arguments with solid evidence. In addition, TCM practitioners of the Jin and Yuan dynasties respected science and accepted truth. They neither prioritized the past over the present, nor vice versa. They respected established practices but did not follow them rigidly. They combined what they learned from medical classics with their own experiences to innovate their predecessors' findings.

3. Seeking common points while reserving difference

Diverse theories of medicine rose in the Jin and Yuan dynasties. The four schools of thought had their own theories, insights, academic views, and even contending arguments. However, the rise of various schools of thought did not come at the expense of collaboration and mutual respect. Liu Wansu and Zhang Yuansu, for example, were respectively the founders of the Hejian and Yishui Schools. Liu Wansu thought that cold medicine should be applied to fever, while Zhang Yuansu advocated warm tonification for curing it. They had different views but broke the pernicious habit of disparaging each other as peer scholars. Initially, Liu Wansu despised Zhang Yuansu. Zhang Yuansu didn't care. He won recognition and respect from Liu Wansu for the therapeutic effect his methods produced. Liu Wansu not only admired Zhang Yuansu for his medical expertise and virtue, but also spoke highly of his medical skills. Zhang Yuansu also drew on the strengths of Liu Wansu. He prepared the "Nine-Taste Notopterygium Soup" to treat typhoid fever and the three Yangs based on

Liu Wansu's "dual processes". This shows that TCM practitioners of the Jin and Yuan dynasties contended with each other not for fame but for medical development and the welfare of people. This upright, all-embracing purpose ensured the seeking of common ground while reserving differences and the respect for each other. It is a lofty character that scientists should have in their innovative academic activities.

6.2 Representative Medical Practitioners and Their Medical Ethics

The Jin and Yuan dynasties saw the birth and growth of a multitude of TCM practitioners. Most of them were excellent medical practitioners of a lofty character. In addition to their common points such as readiness to save lives and innovate, each of them had concepts and characteristics of their own. The following is an introduction to the medical ethics of five influential TCM practitioners of the Jin and Yuan dynasties: Liu Wansu, Zhang Yuansu, Zhang Congzheng, Li Gao and Zhu Zhenheng.

6.2.1 Liu Wansu

1. Brief biography

Liu Wansu, who styled himself Shouzhen and nicknamed himself Shouzhenzi, was a native of Hejian (now Hejian, Hebei Province) living under the assumed name Scholar Proficient in Metaphysics in the Jin dynasty. People called him "Mr. Hejian" or "Liu Hejian". Liu Wansu was a great fan of medicine. He was erudite, helpful, indifferent to fame or wealth, keen on medical research and creative. He was a pioneering medical figure in the Jin and Yuan dynasties as the No. 1 TCM practitioner among the four major schools of medicine. People loved and respected him deeply.

2. Medical ethics

(1) Medical ethics on therapeutic effect.

"TCM practitioners should seek to save the world and the sick," Liu Wansu said. The key to evaluating a doctor's medical practice and ethics is the effectiveness of medical treatment—to what extent he saves the world and the sick. Saving the world is the macro-effect, whereas treating diseases is the micro-effect. Broadly speaking, his responsibility was to save the world and cure patients. It was documented that Liu Wansu did not charge his patients. He treated every patient wholeheartedly. Of the typhoid patients he treated in 30 years, four to five thousand recovered within two to five days or five to seven days. This indicates that Liu Wansu made every effort to ensure the efficacy of treatment.

(2) Helpful and indifferent to fame and fortune.

Liu Wansu began to study medicine at the age of 25. He would hold a medical book in his hands and read it avidly every day, often forgetting to sleep or eat. This perseverance continued for years. Thanks to his efforts, Liu Wansu made tremendous contributions to the classification of diseases and meteorological medicine. At the same time, Liu Wansu built close ties with his patients. In addition, Liu Wansu traveled around to treat patients. This earned him love from people. However, he declined the imperial court's invitation to serve the government. Emperor Zhangzong's daughter fell ill in 1191. Even the imperial physician could do nothing about it. Wu Rui, the magistrate of Hejian, recommended Liu Wansu to the emperor. Liu Wansu cured her with only three doses of TCM. The emperor requested Liu Wansu to serve the imperial court three times but in vain. He only wanted to practice medicine for the working people. This earned him the title "Noble Man". Liu Wansu was well respected by the people for his hard work and dedication to medicine. After his death, people built Liu Shouzhen Tomb, a stone tablet and Liuye Temple in his hometown. The temple housed a statue of Liu Wansu. Liu was one of the top ten famous TCM practitioners documented in the Temple of the King of Medicine in the west of Hejian and east of Beijing. This is an indication that Liu Wansu enjoyed a nationwide reputation.

(3) Propensity to Humanitarianism.

Liu Wansu developed the theory of "five elements' motion and six kinds of natural factors", stressing the importance of motion and natural factors. On the one hand, he acknowledged that "five elements' motion and six kinds of natural factors" objectively depended on the four seasons, noting that climate change in nature was closely related to the occurrence and development of human diseases. On the other hand, he emphasized the subjective initiative of human beings in adapting to nature, believing that human beings were able to control their lives. Those who lost their lives were responsible for the loss, those who survived were the rescuer of their own lives, and those who were considered morally unacceptable or couldn't live long should blame themselves. This reflected Liu Wansu's way of keeping in good health, which emphasized the key role of man himself in self-cultivation and illustrated that people could control their own lives. Liu Wansu attributed the departure, retention and continuation of life to man himself. And he believed that people in general, including TCM practitioners and patients, could control their own destiny. This represents a new development in medical humanitarianism and embodies Liu's humanistic spirit which respected human dignity and human values.

(4) Proposition that TCM practitioners should have extensive knowledge.

Liu Wansu was smart and studious in his childhood. He loved reading medical books. He began to study *Plain Conversation* at the age of 25 and at the same time practiced medicine. He traveled all over northern China to treat patients. He was diligent and thoughtful, with profound medical knowledge. He maintained that TCM practitioners should have extensive knowledge. According to him, a qualified medical practitioner should be proficient in astronomy and geography, understand the changes in Yin and Yang. Liu Wansu studied the *Internal Canon of Medicine* day and night for 35 years. His hard work, diligence and immense learning made him a role model for others.

6.2.2　Zhang Yuansu

1. Brief biography

Zhang Yuansu, with the courtesy name Jiegu, was a native of Yizhou (now Yixian County, Hebei Province) of the Jin dynasty. He started his medical learning with the cold and heat and the deficiency and excess of Zang-Fu organs to study the occurrence and development of diseases. As the founder of the Yishui School, he established a relatively complete academic system centered on the Zang-Fu disease detection theory. Zhang Yuansu's academic thinking was inherited and developed by his disciples and later-generation TCM practitioners. In the Yuan dynasty, his school of medical thought became the rival of the Hejian School. The two schools competed for influence and in doing so, promoted each other, leading to the prosperity of medicine throughout the Jin and Yuan dynasties.

2. Medical ethics

(1) Academic and creative.

Zhang Yuansu studied ancient medical theories modestly, but he did not stick to ancient prescriptions. He said, "Motion and natural factors of the past differ from those of the present. Ancient prescriptions naturally are not applicable to today's diseases." According to him, illness changed with time, climate, and the patient's constitution; old prescriptions no longer suited today's diseases. Under the guidance of this approach to syndrome differentiation and treatment, he flexibly drew on the experiences of previous generations, and made new breakthroughs based on his decades-long clinical experiences. His treatment of spleen and stomach diseases was inherited by the disciples of the Yishui School, among whom Li Dongyuan and Wang Haogu were famous TCM practitioners in the history of Chinese medicine. His article *Prescription of Drugs for Deficiency of Zang-Fu Specimens Due to Cold and Heat*, which explored the efficacy and clinical application of drugs, was later included in Li Shizhen's *Compendium of Materia Medica*—an indication of his great influence.

(2) Open-minded and inclusive.

Zhang Yuansu had little fame at the beginning of his medical career. The fact that he helped Liu Wansu treat patients was the evidence that he was inclusive of other schools of medical thought. When the renowned TCM practitioner Liu Wansu suffered from typhoid and didn't eat anything for eight consecutive days, Zhang Yuansu paid him a visit upon hearing the news. Liu Wansu was scornful of Zhang Yuansu. He faced the wall and didn't utter a single word when Zhang entered the house. Zhang Yuansu was not upset. He felt the pulse of Liu and told him what his pulse suggested. When he asked if Liu had taken some kind of drug, Liu nodded his head. Zhang Yuansu told Liu that the drug he had taken was cold and that it would only make matters worse. Liu Wansu began to admire Zhang Yuansu at that moment. He took the medicine that Zhang prescribed for him and soon recovered. Zhang Yuansu rose in fame from then on. He almost rivaled Liu Wansu. Later, he established his own school of medicine—the Yishui School. Zhang Yuansu did not hold celebrities in awe, and he would embarrass people when needed. After he voluntarily treated and saved his peer TCM practitioner Liu Wansu, he frankly pointed out his mistakes—another indication that he was open-minded and inclusive of different academic views. He advocated mutual respect and mutual learning; he proposed to make the best of the both worlds and oppose provincialism. So he was humble and discreet in his interactions with his peers. Liu Wansu and Zhang Yuansu belonged to two different schools of thought, but Zhang did not try to alienate Liu, nor did he totally reject Liu's treatment methods. The profound attainments and inclusiveness that he displayed while treating Liu for typhoid earned him recognition and respect from Liu Wansu. Since then, he became immensely popular.

6.2.3　Zhang Congzheng

1. Brief biography

Zhang Congzheng, with the courtesy name Zihe, lived under the assumed name of Dairen. He was a native of Kaocheng, Suizhou (now Lankao County, Henan Province). He began to study medicine at the age of 19 and treated people at the age of 20. He wrote the masterpiece *Confucians' Duties to Their Parents* after he reached 60, leaving behind precious medical heritages. He is one of the four most influential TCM practitioners of the Jin and Yuan dynasties. Zhang Congzheng was an innovative practitioner of the Hejian School.

2. Medical ethics

(1) Confucianism-oriented medical ethics.

Confucians' Duties to Their Parents was Zhang Congzheng's masterpiece. He believed that one must first understand Confucianism to master medical principles. The dutiful son should not fail to understand medicine, and Confucianism should serve as the guiding thought for medical ethics. According to him, Confucian thinking of the pre-Qin period advocated "filial piety as the foundation of virtue". People learned medicine to serve their family, so filial piety was the foundation of medical ethics.

Zhang Congzheng also ardently advocated the Confucian idea of "benevolence." He believed that treating disease and administering drug were actually the process of delivering benevolence. The introduction of benevolence into medical practice reflected Zhang Congzheng's idea that medicine and Confucianism shared the same goal. He saw the medical profession as a cause of benevolence, devoted himself to his work, and emphasized in-depth discussion of treatment methods. He treated all his patients equally regardless of their social status, nationality or mental ability. He respected his peers and the sick, not deceiving himself nor others. Benevolence was the theoretical foundation of medical ethics, and the idea of benevolence was the foundation of the ethical thinking of Chinese TCM practitioners. "Saving people with benevolence" and "medicine is benevolence" are the embodiment of the concept of "benevolence" in medicine. Zhang Conzheng regarded medicine as an important means of realizing his ideal of "benevolence". Raising medicine to the height of benevolence and filial piety was his new understanding of Confucian medicine.

(2) Principled and responsible.

Zhang Congzheng did not discriminate against those who were considered sinners by the government in medical treatment. Zhang Congzheng cured many scholar-officials, but the majority of his patients were common working people. He sympathized with the suffering of the working people. When Zhang Congzheng passed through the old town of Guxi, he saw a man who had been wrongfully flogged. The man was suffering from sores, and inflammation went deep into his flesh. He clenched his jaws. All the treatments had been proven ineffective, and his family were preparing for his death. Zhang Congzheng immediately treated him. He saved the dying man using the method of vomiting and perspiration.

He said, "Motion and natural factors of the past differ from those of the present. Ancient prescriptions do not apply to today's diseases." Zhang Congzheng boldly used new methods to treat diseases that couldn't be cured with traditional methods. He said, "All the diseases that I treated were very severe. The patients were in grave danger or dying, but I managed to save them. I fear no resentment if they die. And I fear no envy if they survive." This shows that Zhang was principled and responsible. He didn't fear resentment nor envy when using new methods to cure illness. He was a lenient TCM practitioner.

(3) Appropriate love for patients and flexible in approach.

Under the feudal hierarchical system of that time, TCM practitioners had a lower status than prominent officials and wealthy merchants. Some patients, taking advantage of their social status and wealth, ordered TCM practitioners to prescribe them everything they wanted, such as expensive medicine and restoratives. Many TCM practitioners, in order to please the powerful and suit their needs, often prescribed them restoratives regardless of the state of their illness. Zhang Congzheng mocked those powerful people who put themselves at the mercy of quacks once they got sick. He called on TCM practitioners to delve into medicine, believing that TCM practitioners should have lofty ideals and feel ashamed of not stepping up their studies.

(4) Opposing superstition and fatalism with behavioral therapy.

The weather is not predictable, and every dog has its day. War, plagues, and hunger constantly posed danger to man. As a result, fatalism became widespread. Zhang Congzheng did not believe ghosts were the cause of illness. He said, "It is a fallacy to say that ghosts caused illness. Prayer does not cure illness, only treatment can. Superstition would only aggravate the condition." In his view, it is ridiculous that people should attribute illness to ghosts. He once cured an extremely upset person by showing deliberate contempt for witchcraft. His method diverted the patient's attention. A patient who had wept copiously felt a heart attack. In just a month, the patient felt as if there were a clog in his heart causing unbearable pain. Zhang Congzheng imitated a witch, and used funny language to mock her. This made the patient laugh uncontrollably. In just a day or two, the patient felt ok again.

(5) Trust in technology preceding trust in the TCM practitioner.

Zhang said that conservatism and arrogance will betray the trust of patients. Innovation should conform to science and there should be a limit to it. TCM practitioners should not only believe what patients say, but also make sure to analyze the disease. He outlined eight situations in which vomiting is prohibited: ① Unreasonably emotional patients; ② Patients disagreeing with the TCM practitioner; ③ Failure to properly understand medicine; ④ Failure to distinguish between pathogenic factors and symptoms; ⑤ Nonsensical talk on the part of the patient; ⑥ Critical conditions; ⑦ Yang depletion and blood deficiency as a result of vomiting; ⑧ Hematemesis, hemoptysis, metrorrhagia and other types of blood loss. The eight situations in which vomiting is prohibited reflect not only Zhang Congzheng's trust in patients, but also his responsible attitude that TCM practitioners must suit the remedy to the case.

6.2.4　Li Gao

1. Brief biography

Li Gao, who styled himself Mingzi, was a native of Dongyuan, Zhending (now Zhengding County, Hebei Province). He was called "elderly man of Dongyuan" in his twilight years. Li Gao learned medicine from Zhang Yuansu. He put forward the viewpoint of "internal injury to the spleen and stomach causes all kinds of diseases" based on his long-term clinical experiences, establishing a unique theory of spleen and stomach internal injury. He was one of the four famous scholars in the history of Chinese medicine in the Jin and Yuan dynasties and the founder of "Spleen and Stomach Theory" in TCM. He emphasized the important role of the spleen and stomach in the human body. The spleen and stomach were considered earth among the five elements. His teachings were also categorized as the "school of invigorating the earth".

2. Medical ethics

(1) Opposing fabrication and valuing objectivity.

Li Gao was born in a wealthy family. His diseased mother sought medical care everywhere but couldn't know the cause. She died as a result of the misuse of drugs. Li Gao was very regretful that he did not know medicine. Li Gao strongly felt that medicine mattered a lot to life. So he paid a visit to Zhang Yuansu in Yizhou in order to learn medicine from him. This marked the start of his medical career. TCM practitioners should study medicine out of love, he thought, and the purpose of studying medicine is to treat diseases and save people, not to seek fame or wealth. Under the influence of Zhang Yuansu's thinking that "ancient prescriptions don't apply to new diseases", Li Gao analyzed the various causes of diseases. He criticized pedantic quack TCM practitioners' misuse of prescriptions and laid down his own medication principles. He not only made sure to differentiate between endogenous and exogenous diseases and treat the illness holistically, but also gathered clinical records. To sum up his decades-long practical experience in medical treatment and correct the medication mistakes of quacks, Li Gao explained the theory of "differentiation between internal and external injuries" in 16 years. He completed the book *Differentiation between Internal and External Injuries* at the age of 68. This attitude towards science which valued objective reality and opposed falsehood was very commendable.

(2) Dignified and serious.

Li Gao was loyal, honest, sincere and serious. He was cautious when making friends, never joking with others. He never visited the downtown area or leisure spots. Some of his peers were jealous. They arranged prostitutes to test Li Gao under the cover of banquet. Some prostitutes even dragged his clothes, which Li Gao denounced. He burned the clothes when back at home. At that time, messengers came and left serving as a bridge of communication between the Southern Song dynasty and the Jin dynasty. At a banquet held by the local squire for receiving the Jin messenger, an officer heard that Li Gao was young and upright. He secretly arranged a prostitute to encourage him to drink. Li Gao could not decline that. He tried to cover his embarrassment but couldn't put up with it. He threw up and left the banquet. Li Gao lived under a feudal hierarchical system, but he was proud and unwilling to flatter the "scholar-officials." However, he was loyal, friendly and generous towards ordinary people. He emphasized the importance of medical ethics, believing that morality should be internalized and understood through practical efforts before being implemented. He strove to preserve his moral integrity. This act earned him respect and love.

(3) Caring, valuing medical ethics education and promoting the spread of medical knowledge.

Li Gao lived in the Southern Song dynasty. At that time, social and ethnic contradictions were glaring, and wars, turmoil, hunger and diseases caused people great pain and suffering. He was very sympathetic to the diseased people, treating them carefully and posting copies of the effective prescriptions he had personally tried in public spaces and on vital roads so sick people could take medicine according to prescription. Li Gao traveled around the country in his twilight years to look for students with potential so that his expertise could be handed down to benefit future generations. One day, his friend Zhou Duyun told him, "Luo Tianyi from Liantai County is honest and simple. He regrets that he himself alone couldn't master medicine. He wants to continue his studies. He could be a good student if you want to teach medicine." In his conversation with Luo Tianyi, Li Gao asked, "What's your purpose of learning medicine, to make a fortune or to inherit and promote medicine?" "I want to inherit and promote it," said Luo. Li Gao happily admitted him as a student. Luo Tianyi was from a poor family. To make him focus on studies without worries about the fees, Li Gao offered him food and accommodation, and 20 taels of silver to settle down. Before Li Gao's death, he collated the books he wrote and put them on the desk by category. He told Luo Tianyi, "Keep these books. They are not for me or you; they are for the future generations. Take good care of them. Protect them and pass them on to our children." It was commendable that Li Gao valued medical ethics education and selflessly imparted medical knowledge to benefit later generations.

6.2.5 Zhu Zhenheng

1. Brief biography

Zhu Zhenheng, with the courtesy name Yanxiu, was a native of Yiwu, Wuzhou (now Yiwu City, Zhejiang Province). He lived along the Danxi River, so people called him "elderly man of Danxi" or "Mr. Danxi." He was educated by Liu Wansu's disciple Luo Zhiti, and was a famous eclectic TCM practitioner. Zhu Zhenheng believed that "excess Yang suggests deficiency in Yin." He stressed the importance of Yang and Yin in the human body. He was the founder of the "School of Enriching Yin." He sympathized with the suffering of patients and was enthusiastic in treating them. He was not fearful of hardship and didn't charge his patients, which made him highly respected by the people.

2. Medical ethics

(1) Eclectic towards schools of medicine.

Zhu Zhenheng was the founder of the School of Nourishing Yin, the lastest founded school of the four major schools of medicine during the Jin and Yuan dynasties. The most prominent feature of Zhu Zhenheng's medical ethics is that he did not stick to existing academic views. In his view, Zhang Zhongjing's theory focused on external contraction while Li Gao's theory focused on internal injury. They should learn from each other. He adopted an eclectic attitude towards Liu Wansu's and Zhang Yuansu's theories, which formed the basis of his school of medical thought. He thought the method of purging fire adopted by Liu Wansu and Zhang Yuansu was superior to that of their predecessors when the patient didn't show signs of indication. Li Gao's theory of the etiology of improper diet and overstrain was also superior to that of his predecessors. However, the living and eating conditions of residents in the northwest and the southeast were different. The Buzhong Yiqi Decoction was not applicable to all cases. Zhu Zhenheng acknowledged the achievements of his predecessors and affirmed the strengths of other scholars. Therefore, he did not take a negative attitude towards all other schools. This shows how open-minded he was.

(2) Removing worries, controlling desires and encouraging late marriage.

Zhang Zhenheng believed that Yin was difficult to cultivate, and if it was unduly consumed, deficiency of Yin would result. Therefore, he opposed indulgence, and advocated that men and women couldn't get married until they are 30 and 20 respectively. He put forward the theory of pure heart and few desires, and pointed out that cultivating the mind and resisting the temptation of material desires were the key to this goal. According to Zhang Zhenheng, if a person could devote himself to his career, he would not have superfluous desires. He divided desires into two categories: appetite and lust, and pointed out that curbing appetite and lust could lead to asceticism. Zhu Zhenheng admitted that these two desires are normal human needs, but people should curb them if they wished to pursue a "successful career". According to him, "excessive lust can cause deficiency of Yin and Yang", and "uncontrolled human lust can ruin health". Asceticism is conducive to fitness—the ethical basis of the school of nourishing Yin.

(3) Studious and modest.

Zhu Zhenheng lost his father when he was young and lived with his mother. He was "eager to learn since childhood, and had an extraordinary memory". At the age of 30, his mother fell ill, but the medical practitioners whom the family consulted were at a loss for what to do. So he decided to learn medicine and carefully read many medical classics. Years later, Zhu Zhenheng made up the prescription he wrote out and cured his mother. At the age of 40, Zhu Zhenheng specialized in medicine. Prescriptions authored by Chen Shiwen and Pei Zongyuan was popular at that time. He did an in-depth study of it and made a copy of it. Later, he found that "ancient prescriptions cannot cure today's diseases". Then he bought all the things he needed and went on a tour to seek a mentor. He traveled all over the country, but could not find an ideal mentor. Finally he returned to Wuling (now Hangzhou, Zhejiang Province). In Wuling, he learned that Luo Zhiti was well versed in medicine. So he made ten visits but failed to see Luo. Zhu Zhenheng was sincere and serious. He stood in front of the door of Luo Zhiti's residence despite rain or wind every day for three months. His sincerity moved Luo Zhiti, who finally was willing to see him. By then, Luo Zhiti was too old to treat patients himself. He asked his disciples to feel the pulse and watch the complexion of the patient. Then, he wrote out prescriptions according to what his disciples said about the patient. The teacher was professional and the student was diligent. In less than two years, Luo Zhiti imparted all that he knew to Zhu Zhenheng, whose medical skills developed very quickly. Zhu returned to his hometown to practice medicine after his study under Luo. Back home, all the TCM practitioners were very surprised at first. They didn't know what special skills he had acquired away from home. When they found his prescriptions unorthodox, they dismissed him as neither fish nor fowl. Zhu Zhenheng did not argue. He would convince them with action. He cured his teacher Xu Qian of rheumatic arthralgia which had persisted for more than ten years using "deviant" methods. This made the people who mocked him quiet. His fame soared in just a few years. Patients and students came to him seeking treatment or knowledge.

Zhu Zhenheng remained humble after becoming famous. He would consult specialists when he felt unsure about a disease. As a well-known TCM practitioner, Zhu Zhenheng sincerely consulted TCM practitioners younger than himself. This studious spirit was really commendable. It was not allowed to prescribe medicine casually, otherwise people would get killed. This reflects his high medical ethics and responsible attitude towards patients.

(4) Eclectic, innovative and emphasizing sexual morality.

Zhu Zhenheng established the theory of nourishing Yin by drawing on the strengths of the Hejian School and the Yishui School. He creatively applied Neo-Confucianism to medicine, believing that "excess vitality means deficiency of blood." In addition, Zhu Zhenheng believed that if sexual desires were unrestrained, Yin would be exhausted, and Yang would have nowhere to go. He called on people to exercise restraint in lust and vigorously promote sexual morality. Zhu Zhenheng was good at integrating the achievements of various schools of thought and was innovative. Therefore, his profound medical attainments opened the way for later generations of physicians to treat deficiency of Yin and fever. Although he began to study medicine at an old age, he wrote quite a lot. In addition to his own unique opinions and insights into medical theory, he advocated syndrome differentiation and treatment. He made good use of the drugs for nourishing Yin and reducing heat, as well as those for warming Yang and invigorating qi. Zhu Zhenheng was well known for his method of "nourishing Yin and reducing heat" and "removing phlegm depression." He had many famous disciples, who played an important role in Chinese medicine.

(5) Helpful, resilient, open-minded and sincere.

Zhu Zhenheng was well versed in medicine. People came to him for treatment from near and far or requested him to pay a home visit every day. He always responded to patient's requests and visited them even if it snowed or the road was muddy. One day, a patient visited him when Zhu Zhenheng had just returned home from work. His entourage told the patient that the master was overworked. When Zhu Zhenheng learned this, he said to his entourage, "The patient is suffering from misery. How can I refuse to save him and lie back in my seat?" In addition, he would treat patients free of charge if the patient couldn't afford the treatment. He would carry medicine to treat people who were in distress. The journey might seem long, but Zhu Zhenheng would feel no fatigue. He didn't care about himself. He treated people sincerely, worked tirelessly, and led a humble, frugal life. At the age of seventy, he was still energetic. To remember him, the local people built Danxi Tomb in the town of Chi'an, and engraved "Epitaph of Mr. Danxi" by Song Lian on the tombstone. The Danxi Temple built beside the tomb housed the statue of Zhu Danxi.

6.3　Medical Education

Medical education in China was in its heyday during the Jin and Yuan dynasties. Medicine enjoyed a high social status, and the implementation of medical policy was listed as a category of benevolent governance. The state set up medical education institutions on a large scale and took a series of measures to develop medical science. As a result, practicing medicine became an effective way for aspiring people in pursuit of government positions, and the title "Confucian medical practitioner" has emerged. During this period, although ethnic groups ruled the state, they prized Han culture and emphasized cultural harmony. This greatly boosted overall national development. Medical technology developed rapidly in this period. Famous medical practitioners emerged in large numbers, and various schools of medicine emerged. TCM practitioners were skilled and unique in terms of working methodology. As a result, the medical sector achieved great academic development, and medical education ushered in a new wave of reform and displayed unprecedented characteristics. This, coupled with the flourishing of printing, enabled the preservation and circulation of numerous medical works, contributing enormously to the development of medical education and the preparation of TCM practitioners.

6.3.1　Education of TCM Practitioners

1. Education of TCM practitioners in the Jin dynasty

The education system of the Jin dynasty was modeled on the imperial examination system of the Song dynasties so as to recruit talent. The education of TCM practitioners was mainly modeled on that of the Northern Song dynasty. Medical education institutions at both the central and local levels adopted the "Sanshe" promotion method to select TCM practitioners of truly high medical standards. Medical education institutions adopted a subdivided educational model, with one professor per subject, a limited number of students in each prefecture and county, a test every three years and a 10-course test. This guaranteed the quality of medical students.

2. Education of TCM practitioners in the Yuan dynasty

Thanks to the cultural fusion, medical technology of the Yuan dynasty prospered, producing a huge number of talents. At the same time, TCM practitioners' education experienced a new wave of reform and displayed completely new characteristics.

(1) Extensive establishment of local medical schools—"Imperial Medicine".

The biggest feature of medical education in the Yuan dynasty was that there were no central medical education institutions. All medical education institutions were locally established, and medical schools are collectively called "Imperial Medicine."

In 1261, the government officially ordered the establishment of medical education institutions in various localities to improve the education of TCM practitioners. In order to implement the national decree of promoting medical education and prevent the local government from ignoring the policy, the state also took a series of effective measures: the imperial court appointed the Deputy Superintendent of the Imperial Hospital as its inspector, the local supreme governor was ordered to directly manage school-running, the local medical administrators were given a certain salary, and school buildings were built. By imitating Confucian education, the Yuan dynasty set up "Imperial Medicine" in Dadu, Shangdu and various local places. Staffing was also modeled entirely on Confucian education, with one medical professor and one educational officer in each administrative region. According to statistics, over 200 medical teachers worked nationwide at that time.

(2) Specialized medical education management positions in local regions—Medical Education Administration.

Considering that the Imperial Hospital was busy, to strengthen the supervision and management of medical education quality in various places and select high-quality medical teachers, the Yuan dynasty set up Medical Education Administration in various places and Administrative Region Medical Education Administration in the Imperial Hospital to take charge of the overall situation. This shows that the management of medical education in the Yuan dynasty was comprehensive and that a medical education management system from the local to the central, level was set up. It was close to the medical education management mechanism in today's society.

The Medical Education Administration managed medical education institutions across the country and also served as a government body for selecting medical teachers. The Medical Education Administration was headed by the administrator. Because the Yuan dynasty didn't unify the north and the south at the same time, the medical education management system of the north was completed when the south was unified. In addition, the south was distant from the central government, so the setting of Medical Education Administration in the whole country was different between the north and the south. In the north, Medical Education Administration was established in all the administrative regions, and Medical Education Bureau was established in the prefectures and counties. In the south, Medical Education Administration was established in the provinces, Medical Education Bureau was set up in the administrative regions, and Collusion-free Regulator was set up in the prefectures and counties.

(3) Special educational institution— the Three Emperors Temple.

During the Yuan dynasty, the rulers prized Han culture, especially Confucianism. Confucius Shrine was seen wherever there was a school. For various reasons, the Yuan dynasty located medical education at the Three Emperors Temple.

Medical professionals generally believed that the founders of Chinese medicine were Yellow Emperor, Fu Xi and Shennong, or the "Three Emperors". Correspondingly, medical education was provided at the Three Emperors Temple. However, this practice caused widespread dissatisfaction. Medicine did not enjoy the same high status in all dynasties. Despite the opposition, the policy of locating medical education at the Three Emperors Temple continued into the Ming dynasty.

(4) The official medical examination—Medical Imperial Examinations.

Although imperial examinations were opposed by many Mongolian nobles in the Yuan dynasty, the first imperial examinations were held in 1315. Medical imperial examinations were not implemented this time for various reasons. In 1316, the state issued a decree formally establishing a medical examination system. It was the first official medical examination in the true sense of the word.

The specific content of the medical imperial examination system was very detailed. It was very similar to that of the imperial examination system of that time. The examination was held once every three years, with two examinations each time. The Provincial Examination preceded the Metropolitan Examination. Those who took the exam were recommended TCM practitioners, and those who were not recommended couldn't sign up for the test. There was no limit to the number of candidates in the Provincial Examination, after which 100 candidates were selected, and 30 candidates were selected after the Metropolitan Examination. The scope of the examination included the topics released by the Imperial Hospital over the years, and the questions covered principles of medical science, treatment methods and drug properties. 30 people were admitted finally: the candidate who took the first place would fill the imperial physician vacancy, the candidate who took the second place would fill the education administrator vacancy, and the third would get teaching positions. The medical imperial examination system didn't last long, but it ushered in a new era for the selection of medical talent and provided a frame of reference for the selection of medical personnel in later times.

6.3.2　Management of TCM Practitioners

1. Management of TCM practitioners in the Jin dynasty

The medical management organization of the Jin dynasty was the Imperial Hospital Palace Dispensary. The Imperial Hospital was the highest medical management body of the Jin dynasty. It performed both management and education functions. The number of personnel in each section was different, and Collusion-free Regulator was established. There were also medical institutions in counties and other local places called "Hospital". Generally, the hospital had one physician and eight medical workers. In the Jin dynasty, medical personnel were highly valued, and they were ranked four grade, which surpassed that of the Northern Song dynasty.

2. Management of TCM practitioners in the Yuan dynasty

(1) Specialized medical administration—the Imperial Hospital.

The Imperial Hospital was the highest medical management organization in the state during the Yuan dynasty. It was founded in 1260. Local medical education, medical officers and medical practitioners were under its control. Before that, there were also medical institutions in the court. The basic system followed the example of the previous dynasties and gave equal consideration to management and education. The Imperial Hospital of the Yuan dynasty performed only management functions and did not perform educational functions.

During this time, the official position of the Imperial Hospital was second level. It was in charge of all medical and pharmaceutical matters, as well as all its branch medical institutions, including pharmaceutical management institutions such as Medical Education Administration, Official Medical Education Administration, Guanghui Department and Huimin Pharmacy Bureau. In 1283, the Imperial Hospital changed its name to medical superintendent, and the post was downgraded to the fourth grade. This was the lowest post in the Yuan-dynasty Imperial Hospital, but higher than all the medical posts of previous dynasties. In 1285, medical superintendent was renamed the Imperial Hospital and the old system was restored, with a third-level position, four tidian, and two medical envoys, deputies and judges, each of whom was granted a silver seal. In 1288, the Imperial Hospital was detached from Xuanhuiyuan, becoming an independent body again.

In 1301, the Imperial Hospital carried out a large-scale reform again. Its rank was promoted to second level, higher than the six ministries. The post of hospital deputy was set up as the chief of the Imperial Hospital. The number of hospital deputies increased from 2 up to 12. Hospital deputies were diverse, including both Hans and Mongolians. Most of them were second-level officials, and the lowest post was not lower than third level. The number of other personnel in the Imperial Hospital increased from 16 to 46. The degree of importance attached to medicine by the Yuandynasty regime shows that the integration of different cultures gave rise to a free management style.

(2) Classified medical education examination system.

① Examinations for medical teachers.

In the Yuan dynasty, medical teachers were constantly tested to ensure their quality. The specific procedure is divided into three steps: First, there must be a peer-to-peer recommendation. The person needed to have a higher reputation among the peers and be skilled in the medical profession. He must provide his treatment cases. Second, the selected person should register at the local Medical Education Administration and take an examination there. Third, TCM practitioners who have passed the examination in the Medical Education Administration were recommended to the Imperial Hospital (or medical superintendent), where they were appointed after passing another examination.

The examination was conducted once a year. The specific subjects to be tested in the examination were principles of medical science and clinical treatment. The Department for Administration and Integrity responsible for supervising local administrative officials would oversee the examination of medical teachers in order to prevent cheating. The strict examination system for medical teachers ensured the quality of medical education.

② Management and examination of official TCM practitioners.

Official TCM practitioners were under the unified management of the Imperial Hospital, and the specific management organization was the Official Medical Education Administration. The Official Medical Education Administration was different from the Medical Education Administration. In the north, it was only set up in Dadu, Baoding, Daning and 14 other administrative regions. The specific number of officials varied. In the south, it was set up in Henan, Zhejiang, Jiangxi, Hubei, Hunan, and Shaanxi provinces. Medical Education Bureau was set up in the administrative regions under the provinces, and Collusion-free Regulator was established in counties and prefectures. The staffing was customized according to the grade of the region.

In the early days of the Yuan dynasty, war continued and medical personnel were in short supply. So the official TCM practitioner system was formulated. After the war was over, the official policies towards TCM practitioners were maintained and the number of official TCM practitioners was stabilized through mandatory professional inheritance and medical knowledge training for the children of official TCM practitioners. At the same time, the central authorities took some necessary measures to maintain the level of medical care provided by medical practitioners in the course of inheritance.

Since the emergence of medical practitioners, only medical officers or teachers had been selected through examinations, and no local medical practitioners had been assessed in any form. Medical practitioners were a special profession, and their work was directly related to people's lives. In the past, the government only punished some unscrupulous medical practitioners who caused the death of their patients through negligence or fraud. There was no preventive measures to regulate the overall situation. When Emperor Renzong acceded to the throne, he formally decreed that local medical practitioners must take the qualification examination before they could practice medicine. The above measures, together with the official TCM practitioners management policy in the Yuan dynasty, could enable the court to effectively grasp whether official TCM practitioners passed the examination or not, as well as the level of their proficiency. The contents of the examination were determined by the Imperial Hospital. Official TCM practitioners were required to study and take the examination regularly, and the results of the examination were documented. This system of compulsory medical examination ensured the medical standards of medical practitioners. It was an important part of the history of Chinese medicine and the first medical examination for medical practitioners equivalent to the modern medical examination system.

TCM practitioners' ability to treat diseases generally was not passed on to people other than their disciples and family members. In addition, the Yuan dynasty prohibited TCM practitioners from changing careers. This ensured that medical skills were passed on from generation to generation, but reduced academic exchanges between TCM practitioners, hindering the development of medicine to a certain extent. In view of this, the Yuan dynasty, in addition to the examination of medical practitioners, would organize the medical practitioners who participated in the study. They would have discussions and learn from each other's experiences. In addition, the Yuan dynasty also organized medical clients to perform voluntary consultations and assessments, and submitted the reports of the cases they diagnosed to the local medical teachers for unified calibration, evaluation, and documentation. The outstanding ones would be named medical teachers or other medical officers. In short, the Yuan dynasty's policies aimed at medical practitioners to a large extent ensured the standard of medical care in the private sector, and at the same time prepared talent for national needs.

③ Examinations for medical students.

In the Yuan dynasty, medical education institutions were all located in local areas, making medical education examinations closer to the ordinary people. The candidates were mainly children of medical practitioners and those who volunteered to study medicine. The state imposed a mandatory requirement on every medical household to send a member of their household to participate medical examinations, while other people were free to sign up. 13 subjects would be tested in the examinations, of which 10 were Broad Internal Medicine, Narrow Internal Medicine,

Wind Diseases, Obstetrics and Women's Miscellaneous Diseases, Ophthalmology, Pharynx and Larynx, Bonesetting, Scratch Fever, Acupuncture, and Prayer-based Treatment. The other three subjects were optional. The contents of the examination for the above 10 subjects were different, and the Imperial Hospital later laid down the specific scope of the examination, which set the scope of the questions. Students took an exam once a year. During the year-long study, there would be an assignment every month, which would be handed in at the end of the year and revised as part of the assessment results.

The examination system for medical students in the Yuan dynasty was complete and strict, but there was no clear stipulation on the length of study for students, nor definite direction. According to regulations, medical students who had just studied for a few years couldn't take the post of medical teacher, and the first phase, "peer recommendation", could not proceed. Therefore, students with a medical background usually went home to inherit the family business, and those without a medical background would start their own businesses locally. The medical education of the Yuan dynasty not only produced talent, but also repaid society with the results of medical education. A medical atmosphere spread to every corner of society.

Chapter Summary

1. The rise of various schools of medical thought wrote a new chapter for the development of medicine in China

Schools of medical thought are a long-term phenomenon in China. After the 12th century, the schools of thought began to air differing views. According to *Synopsis of the General Catalogue of Complete Library in the Four Branches of Literature*, "Confucianism diversified in the Song dynasty and medicine diversified in the Jin and Yuan dynasties." In terms of the geography and lineage of the founder, two schools had emerged: "Hejian School" represented by Liu Wansu, and "Yishui School" represented by Zhang Yuansu. In terms of academic point of view and its influence on later generations, four schools had emerged: Liu Wansu's School of Cold Medicine, Zhang Congzheng's Cathartic School, Li Gao's School of Invigorating the Spleen and Zhu Zhenheng's School of Nourishing Yin. The four schools of thought in the Jin and Yuan dynasties represented a new page in the development of medicine in China.

2. The legacy of medical ethics culture is a valuable asset for the development of medicine in China

In addition to inheriting the traditional virtue of saving lives, the medical ethics culture in the Jin and Yuan dynasties highlighted the morality of caring for people's sufferings, being enthusiastic about treatment, being indifferent to fame and fortune, and having a decent style, the innovative spirit of being diligent and studious, respecting the ancient but not being bogged down in the ancient, and boldly exploring, as well as the scientific attitude of loving the medical profession, attaching importance to education, popularizing medicine, and being brave in practice.

3. The education and training of TCM practitioners is the Core force of the continuation and development of Chinese medicine

The medical culture and technology in the Jin and Yuan dynasties were well inherited and developed, and famous TCM practitioners emerged in an endless stream. All of them had outstanding medical skills and styles, which greatly boosted the development of medicine. Medical education also witnessed a new wave of reform and new features that have never been seen before. In addition, the development of printing in this era enabled the preservation and circulation of numerous medical works, which contributed to the development of medical education and the production of TCM practitioners.

Application in Contemporary Times

1. Medical practitioners should put virtue first

This chapter describes some Jin and Yuandynasty TCM practitioners' path to study and their excellent quality that "put ethics first". In their course of study, they were hardworking and scholarly and attached great importance to the development and inheritance of medical ethics education. Filial piety is the foundation of virtue. Both Li Gao and Zhu Zhenheng studied medicine because of their mother's illness in order to perform filial piety. Li Gao looked for students with great potential to spread medical skills and benefit future generations. As society developed and time marched on, the demands on the comprehensive training and comprehensive quality of medical students became increasingly high, and the concept of medical education, which put moral education first, became more necessary and urgent.

Virtue is the capital of talent. Virtue is the foundation of man and his growth, and it is also the primary task of education. Medical education should put morality first, adhere to the fundamental task of "fostering character and civic virtue," combine moral education with the entire process of education and teaching, and promote the comprehensive development of contemporary medical students through ideological education.

2. TCM practitioners and patients should value medical ethics and build harmonious relationships

This chapter describes the friendship and harmonious relationship between TCM practitioners and patients in the Jin and Yuan dynasties and provides a frame of reference for building new TCM practitioner-patient relations. Liu Wansu was extraordinarily broad-minded. He despised fame and fortune, and declined the invitations to assume office in the government three time. He only wanted to practice medicine, so people called him the "noble man". Zhu Zhenheng was sincere and tireless. He lived in a humble place and advocated frugality and economy. To remember him, the local people built Danxi Tomb in the town of Chi'an, and engraved "Epitaph of Mr. Danxi" by Song Lian on the tombstone. The Danxi Temple built beside the tomb housed the statue of Zhu Danxi. TCM practitioners of the Jin and Yuan dynasties moved their patients with noble medical ethics and they also showed the virtues that should be possessed to establish a harmonious medical practitioner-patient relationship for future generations.

TCM practitioners must be virtuous. A TCM practitioner is measured by his benevolence and skills. Benevolence precedes skills. Contemporary TCM practitioners and patients should take pride in their ethics. While improving medical services for patients, practitioners should enhance the sense of well-being and acquisition of medical practitioners and build harmonious medical-patient relationships so as to comprehensively promote the orderly and healthy development of China's medical and health undertakings.

7

Medical Ethics Culture
in the Ming Dynasty

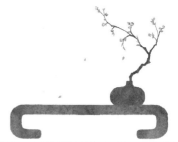

In 1368, Zhu Yuanzhang established the Ming dynasty. The centralization of power deepened. Zhu Yuanzhang adopted a policy of tax cut, promoted the development of productive forces, greatly increased the population, quickly recovered and developed the economy, made frequent exchanges with foreign countries, and made great achievements in science and technology, all of which provided favorable social conditions for the development of medicine. The invention of human pox vaccination and advances in infectious diseases have opened a new era in ancient Chinese medicine. Tremendous progress was made in drug research, and Compendium of Materia Medica was a bright pearl in China's pharmaceutical history. Medical disciplines of the Ming dynasty further developed on the basis of the Yuan dynasty, forming a more complete theoretical system. The number of medical works spiked. According to Grand Dictionary of Chinese Medical Works, 362 medical works were written before the Yuan dynasty, and 981 medical works were authored in the Ming dynasty, exceeding the sum of those produced in previous times. The development of medicine in the Ming dynasty showed the characteristics of comprehensive applied science. It formed as a result of long-term experience and specialization. It was strongly influenced by traditional culture and way of thinking. By promoting classical Chinese medicine theories, summarizing new clinical experience, and innovating, the Ming dynasty established a unique theoretical system of medicine.

7.1 Overview of Medical Ethics

7.1.1 Social Background of the Ming dynasty's Medical Ethics Culture

1. Strengthening of political centralism

After the establishment of a political power to unify the whole country, Zhu Yuanzhang tried his best to strengthen the centralized system in view of the lesson of the demise of the Yuan dynasty. First, the prime minister system was abolished, the bureaucratic establishment was adjusted, and monarchy centralization and power centralization were strengthened unprecedentedly. In 1380, the prime minister system, which had been practiced for more than 1,600 years since the Qin and Han dynasties, was abolished. The six departments of officials, households, rituals, soldiers, penalties and workers were directly responsible to the emperor. The power of the prime minister and monarch power were combined into one. The Ming emperor monopolized the power. The Ming dynasty reformed the old system of the Yuan dynasty, abolished the province system, divided local authorities into three, and set up respectively the Administrative Commissioner's Office, the Command Commissioner's Office, and the Penalty and Investigation Commissioner's Office. The three powers were not affiliated to each other but restricted each other. Local governments were directly accountable to the central government. Second, enfore strict social management. Strict spy politics was practiced in the Ming dynasty. The main spy agencies included Royal Guards, Dong Chang and Xi Chang. Their main duties were to monitor political forces, such as government officials, social dignitaries, scholars, and so on. They had the right to report the results of such surveillance directly to the emperor and were authorized to put people under arrest and proceed secret interrogation. The Ming dynasty garrison system, which was created by imitating the military system of the Northern Wei, Sui and Tang dynasties and of the Yuan dynasty, was the most important part of the military system of the Ming dynasty. It was a self-sufficient military reclamation type. The sergeants under the garrison system were hereditary, proving a stable source of troops for the regime. The Ming dynasty further tightened and standardized the Yuandynasty system of classifying family registration, established the yellow registers system, and divided registered families into civilian, military, and medical according to occupation. Once a family was registered, it couldn't be changed and it would be hereditary. The Lijia system was intended to control the grass-roots people. A certain number of households formed Li, and a certain number of households formed Jia, to each of which a chief was assigned. Third, enforce cultural autocracy. In 1370, Zhu Yuanzhang adopted Liu Ji's suggestion. He set up the imperial examination system, selected scholars according to stereotyped writing limited to the content of Four Books and Five Classics. Zhu Xi said that stereotyped writing on behalf of sages confined intellectuals' thoughts within the scope of Neo-Confucianism. Stereotyped academic atmosphere restricted the freedom of thought, pushing a group of intellectuals into the field of medicine. This was objectively beneficial to raising the cultural literacy and research attainment of medical personnel.

2. Economic recovery and the emergence of capitalism

In the early days of the Ming dynasty, in view of the economic depression brought about by war, the Ming dynasty adopted a series of measures to stimulate the economy, such as promoting the use of land in the fields, encouraging the reclamation of land, and encouraging the recovery of land. The development of water conservancy projects and the reduction of taxes stimulated the vigorous development of the agricultural sector. Starting from the middle of the Ming dynasty, Grand Secretary Zhang Juzheng pushed through the single-whip-tax reform, under which land tax, compulsory laboring and other miscellaneous levies at the county and prefecture level were combined into one. Tax was collectively collected by size. This greatly simplified the collection procedures and made it difficult for local officials to cheat. This method freed peasants without land from the burden of labor, and peasants with land could spend more time cultivating their land, playing a certain role in agricultural development. Agricultural production of the Ming dynasty exceeded that of previous times. The scale of the production of textiles, porcelain, iron and other handicrafts was greater and involved more advanced technology. At the same time, by changing compulsory laboring into the payment of silver, farmers gained greater personal freedom and found it easier to leave the land. This provided more labor sources for the urban handicraft industry. Landless businessmen were exempted from tax. This had a positive impact on the development of business. In the middle and later periods of the Ming dynasty, capitalism emerged, employment was common, and the handicraft industry developed further. Industrial centers began to take hold. A typical example was the silk-weaving factory south of the Changjiang River. The development of the commodity economy facilitated the movement and concentration of the population. This not only stimulated the further development of health services, but also accelerated the occurrence and spread of diseases, as is the case with the introduction of syphilis. The development of transportation broadened the range of activities of TCM practitioners, increased opportunities for contacts and learning from each other's academic perspectives, and created favorable conditions for medical development.

Economic prosperity brought about a stable political situation and created good conditions for the development of medical science. For example, in Jiangsu and Zhejiang where the economy was well-developed, a large number of famous medical practitioners emerged. According to *A Practical Dictionary of Chinese Medicine*, 72% of TCM practitioners in the Ming dynasty who had verifiable residence lived in Jiangsu, Zhejiang and Anhui. In the south of Jiangsu, there were fewer than 100 TCM practitioners before the Yuan dynasty. In the Ming dynasty, the number increased to 489.

3. New developments in thought and culture

In order to consolidate the position of feudal autocratic rule, the Ming dynasty implemented an autocratic policy on ideology and culture, and respected Confucianism. Zhu Yuanzhang, the great emperor of the Ming dynasty, appointed *Imperial Mandate* as the standard for students. Candidates in the imperial examinations were tested on the principle of feudal moral conduct. In the early Ming dynasty, Confucianism developed further and Neo-Confucianism occupied a dominant position. The masters of Confucianism, such as Song Lian and Fang Xiaoru, all honored Cheng and Zhu. Zhu Yuanzhang set Zhu Xi's *Notes on the Four Books* as the standard of the imperial examination, and Zhu Di headed the compilation of books such as *The Complete Book on Neo-Confucianism* which preached Cheng and Zhu's Neo-Confucianism. In the middle and later stages of the Ming dynasty, Wang Shouren's criticism of Cheng and Zhu's Neo-Confucianism gradually gave rise to the predominance of Lu Wang's studies.

The social function of medicine was close to Confucians' humanistic pragmatism and governance ideas. Under the influence of the idea of "official or medical practitioner", a large number of Confucian scholars joined the medical field. In addition, the Confucian idea of filial piety and fraternal duty treated medicine as a means of practicing filial piety. He who doesn't know medicine would fail to perform filial piety. Entrusting diseased parents to quacks was considered as an act not in accordance with filial. Medicine is easy to connect and Confucianism and medicine are connected. A large number of scholars with profound Confucian accomplishments practiced medicine, thus improving the social status of medicine and the cultural literacy of medical staff and greatly improving the theoretical and clinical research of TCM. Classic works of TCM were collated and annotated, and the exchange and dissemination of medical knowledge was promoted. In the Ming dynasty, a large number of Confucian TCM practitioners such as Li Shizhen, Wang Kentang, Li Zhongzi, Wang Ji and Zhang Jingyue emerged. During the late Ming period, materialist thinkers such as Li Zhi, Wang Fuchi and others stressed practical experience and applied learning to application. This had a positive impact on medical science, and open-minded medical practitioners such as Chen Shigong, Chen Sicheng, and Shen Gongchen emerged.

4. Innovation in science and technology

Economic prosperity and political stability promoted the development of science and technology. In the Ming dynasty, some achievements were made in science and technology, such as astronomy, calendar, mathematics, architecture and water conservancy, and some outstanding scientists such as Xu Guangqi and Song Yingxing appeared, as well as scientific and technological works such as *The Complete Book on Agricultural Administration and Exploitation of the Works of Nature*. Disciplines permeated each other. The development of science and technology in the Ming dynasty had a major impact on medicine in terms of theoretical viewpoint, method, technology and data.

The printing of the Ming dynasty was updated from the Yuan dynasty. At the end of the 15th century, copper movable type printing became popular. In the Wanli period, chromatic printing appeared. Advancements in printing made the publication industry of the Ming dynasty unprecedentedly prosperous, creating conditions for the publication of medical works and the popularization of medical knowledge. Take surgery as an example. There were only 40 surgical monographs before the Ming dynasty. In the Ming dynasty, the number increased to 50. They were beautifully printed and many have survived to this day. Agricultural technology provided conditions for the acclimatization and planting of herbs, promoted the development of herbal medicine. The development of pharmacology enriched agricultural knowledge. *The Complete Book on Agricultural Administration* contained all the contents of Zhu Di's *Herbal for Relief of Famines*. Scientific and technological progress rapidly penetrated into the medical field. Iron and steel works with an annual output of 400 tons appeared, and steel quality also improved. This created favorable conditions for the production of surgical instruments. According to *Orthodox Manual of External Medicine*, the forging needles made with gag bit in the past were not sharp. After they were made with steel, the quality of the forging needles was greatly improved. As a result, surgery outcomes were taken to the next level.

5. Frequent exchanges between China and foreign countries

The advanced shipbuilding industry provided a good foundation for navigation, and trade facilitated the introduction of overseas drugs and the discovery of new drugs. The Ming dynasty had frequent exchanges with foreign countries, and more than 120 countries and regions had trade and diplomatic relations with the Ming dynasty. Between 1405 and 1433, the Ming dynasty ordered Zheng He to sail to the West for seven times. More than 180 medical officers and TCM practitioners accompanied each trip, as well as excellent pharmacists to identify the medicinal materials that were traded between countries. In its contacts with many countries, the Ming dynasty expanded the sources of Chinese medicinal materials, especially precious medicinal materials, such as olibanum, myrrh, sangusis draconis, hematoxylon, rhinoceros horn, ivory, sulfur, lilacs and aloe vera.

After the middle of the Ming dynasty, western missionaries came to China one after another, bringing medical knowledge. In cooperation with Chinese intellectuals, Matteo Ricci from Italy translated many works on Western science and technology. Neurology was described in *Science from the West*, which introduced western neurology and psychology to China. The Italian missionary Alfonse Vagoni's book *Physical Meteorology* dealt with the theory of four elements from Greece and some anatomical physiology. Italian missionary Sabatino de Ursis wrote about digestive physiology in his *Hydraulic Machinery of the West*. In 1621, the Swiss missionary Johann Schreck arrived in Macao to practice medicine. He then went to Beijing to write *Chongzhen Calendar*. In his late years, he tried to introduce Western anatomy to China. The books he translated and reviewed included *Overview of the Human Body* and *The Human Body with Illustrations*.

6. Other factors

The Ming government and emperors attached importance to medicine and had always personally organized and participated in the writing of medical works. Zhu Yuanzhang's fifth son, Zhu Nan, compiled works such as *Herbal for Relief of Famines, Health Keeping Notes, Miniature Prescriptions, Prescriptions for Universal Relief*, etc. He made tremendous contributions to the development of China's pharmaceutical industry. Formulated by him personally, *Prescriptions for Universal Relief*, compiled with the help of Teng Shuo and Liu Chun, was the largest monograph on Chinese prescriptions in the history of ancient Chinese medicine. It was considered as a detailed masterpiece. The book not only discussed various diseases in detail, but also provided corresponding prescriptions and treatments. Emperor Yongle of the Ming dynasty organized the compilation of *The Yongle Canon*, which covered medical classics. Voluminous medical documents, including *Prescriptions for Universal Relief and The Yongle Canon: Medicine*, were exhaustive. They preserved a large number of medical documents written before the Ming dynasty, providing valuable research materials for future generations.

The prevalence of infectious diseases was an important factor in moving medicine forward. According to *History of the Ming Dynasty* and *Analects of the Ming Dynasty*, at least 30 cases of large-scale infectious diseases occurred in the Ming dynasty, and the number of deaths was estimated at 178,898. The epidemic caused TCM practitioners to carry out relevant medical research, thus promoting the development of medicine. After he ascended the throng, Zhu Yuanzhang formulated a series of measures to strengthen local medical education and meet the need to fight the epidemic. The rise of the School of Warm Diseases was the inevitable result of the experience and academic accumulation of medical practitioners in the Ming dynasty in fighting epidemic diseases.

7.1.2　Medical Ethics Culture of the Ming dynasty

The Ming dynasty provided relatively favorable conditions for the development of medicine for the centralized system, the recovery and development of the economy, the flourishing of scientific and technological thinking, the innovation of science and technology, and frequent exchanges between China and the world. A large number of medical works emerged in the Ming dynasty, forming a systematic and perfect theoretical system of Chinese medicine. The Ming dynasty produced more works about medical ethics than previous times.

The Ming dynasty was an important period for the development of medical ethics in China, and many excellent literatures on medical ethics appeared. Chen Shigong put forward "five precepts and ten commandments" in *Orthodox Manual of External Medicine*. In 1978, the *Encyclopedia of Bioethics* published by the New York Press in the United States and classified it as a classical medical literature. Li Ting set clear requirements for the study and morality of TCM practitioners in *Requirements for TCM Practitioners*. Li Zhongzi divided the common feelings of people into those of patients, those of others, and those of TCM practitioners, and put forward the principle of "humanitarianism" to adjust the relationship between TCM practitioners and patients. Miao Xiyong expounded on the medical ethics of TCM practitioners through the "five principles in medicine" in *Shennong's Herbal Classics*. *Medical Treatment of Yesterday and Today* the chapters of "quacks", In order to compile *Compendium of Materia Medica*, Li Shizhen traveled around the country for medical advice from people, demonstrating that he was earnest in learning and combined theory with practice. Xu Chunfu founded the first non-governmental medical academic organization in China, the "All-in-one Medical Association," and made 22 specific demands on TCM practitioners' professional qualities, ways of treating students, ideological and moral qualities, and attitude toward patients. In the practice of medical ethics, the Ming dynasty TCM practitioners advocated four consultations and eight programs of identification, and further standardized and systematized the medical record format.

7.1.3 Main Contents of Ming Dynasty Medical Ethics

1. Benevolence of TCM practitioners

The medical practitioner must serve society in a benevolent way. The Ming dynasty TCM practitioners believed that medicine was a benevolence technique, and any person who encountered a patient should find ways to treat the patient as best as possible. All people have been learning Confucianism from their youth, and the Confucian idea of "benevolence" permeated their medical career as a TCM practitioner. According to Wan Quan, "The TCM practitioner should be a man of good will and a man of love regardless of the circumstances." In the event of a call for help, whether you are a relative or not, TCM practitioners must do their best to treat the patient. Xu Chunfu cited from *Activated Complex Theory* that "a TCM practitioner cannot be trusted if he is not a benevolent man, nor can he be trusted if he is not a wise man." The primary virtue of a good TCM practitioner is to be benevolent. The Ming dynasty TCM practitioners believed that TCM practitioners should treat people equally if they are "benevolent" and should do their best to treat people, whether they were poor or rich. Gong Tingxian wrote in *Recovery of Diseases* that "TCM practitioners of today's world are often ignorant of this. They discriminate between the rich and the poor in treatment. However, this is not benevolence and

TCM practitioners are responsible for saving life. Those who are my colleagues should try to save people regardless of their status."

2. Medical literacy of TCM practitioners

To fully discharge their duties, TCM practitioners must have excellent medical skills and be able to effectively and efficiently deal with the disease of patients. Incompetence would harm patients and put them at great risk. The Ming dynasty TCM practitioners thoroughly explored the medical literacy of TCM practitioners, and the TCM practitioners one after another stressed the harm caused by imprecision in medicine. Xu Chunfu believed that "medicine is harmful if it is not precise." The Ming dynasty TCM practitioners put forward their own opinions on what goals TCM practitioners should reach and how to upgrade their medical skills. Zhang Jiebin thought that accuracy was key to medical treatment. "If the cause cannot be determined, we should wait and watch. Once we get to know it, we can use a one or two-ingredient prescription to get rid of it. If the disease is persistent, we can apply more ingredients in our prescriptions. However, all the other ingredients that we add to the prescription serve to bring out the efficacy of the previous one or two ingredients. Those who treat diseases with one core ingredient is arguably a master." The Ming dynasty TCM practitioners insisted that there was no distinction between Confucianism and medicine. Gong Tingxian pointed out in *Ten Commandments for Medical Practitioners* that "One who has a kind heart and is disciplined can perform his duties outstandingly. He must also be proficient in Confucianism and well aware of what is right and what is wrong." According to Chen Shigong, "Confucianism precedes medical skills." Gong Xin proposed that medical practitioners should "read a large number of books and be proficient in medicine, and have a good understanding of Yin and Yang etc." Li Ting pointed out that TCM practitioners should strictly and prudently diagnose diseases, and should treat patients well and ask them when the symptoms appeared. "He should examine the patient carefully and determine what is the cause. If the symptoms are serious and the cause is clear, it is not necessary to consult and feel the pulse. Otherwise, the symptoms must be carefully examined. First, we should look at the local symptoms and then observe the overall conditions." Most of the Ming dynasty TCM practitioners emphasized the importance of diagnosis and treatment based on an overall analysis of the illness and the patient's condition. The eight principles for disease identification matured in the

Ming dynasty. In *Compendium of Medicine*, Lou Ying stated that "patients must first be treated in a way that is thorough. We should look at the blood, the complexion, the body, and the inner parts of the body and treat the deficiency. We should make sure there is no excess or deficiency of Yin and Yang and the organs are in good conditions. The methods we take should suit the patient." In *TCM practitioners' Line Marker—Typhoid Fever*, Fang Yu said, "Though future generations may cope with diseases in different ways, the key areas that we should watch carefully are always external symptoms, internal symptoms, deficiency, excess, Yin, Yang, cold, and heat."

In order to enhance the practical guidance of medical treatment for patients and to enhance the continuity and effectiveness of treatment, the medical practitioners of the Ming dynasty further standardized and systematized the medical record format. In *Medical Practitioner*, Han Mao proposed the six step method of watching, smelling, asking, feeling the pulse, thinking, and treating. Wu Kun's *Language of Pulse* further summed up the format of the medical record. He called it "pulse case" and wrote it in seven steps: First, time, place of origin, and name; Second, observation and diagnosis through auscultation and olfaction; Third, the patient's bitterness, the cause and the time of the disease; Fourth, the onset of the disease, the treatment measures and the efficacy of the treatment; Fifth, the status of the disease, whether the disease is more severe during the day or night, whether the patient feels cold or heat; Sixth, the name of the disease and the diagnosis; Seventh, the prescription and the purpose of the medication. The TCM practitioner should sign the medical record to show he is the responsible person. Han's "six concurrent methods" and Wu's supplement played a fundamental role in standardizing the medical record format and had a major impact on the development of medicine.

3. The doctor's view on righteousness and interests

The Ming dynasty TCM practitioners opposed using medicine as a means of seeking profit. They deplored the practice of extorting money from medicine and stressed that the relief of the world was a matter of prestige. In Sun Zhihong's *Concise Medical Use*, he wrote an article "Notes for Medical Practitioners", which required TCM practitioners to despise wealth and profit, refrain from overcharging patients, and treat all equally. Miao Xiyong said that TCM practitioners should learn constantly to improve their skills. Good pay is not what they should seek, though they may have achieved a lot. Wang Kengtang was generous about his medical achievements. He wrote and published his medical experience to the public. He provided a way for others to learn and save themselves. According to him, "The doctor's sole aim is to cure patients, not to make profit."

4. The moral integrity of TCM practitioners

In order to do a good job in medical work, TCM practitioners must enhance their moral integrity and cultivate their own inner self so as to standardize their behavior. TCM practitioners in the Ming dynasty analyzed the ways to cultivate morality from many aspects. First, don't deceive people. Li Ting believed that the most important thing for medical practitioners is not to deceive people. Second, be humble regarding learning. Miao Xiyong stated in *Shennong's Herbal Classics* that the medical practitioner must be humble when it comes to learning medicine. Third, seek truth and be pragmatic. Wu Youxing witnessed the terrible consequences of epidemic disease, and the treatment of typhoid by TCM practitioners was not effective. Feeling that ancient methods didn't apply to present disease, he wrote the first monograph on acute infectious diseases in the history of China's medical development, *The Theory of Plague*, making indelible contributions to the development of the School of Warm Diseases and the study of infectious diseases. Fourth, in-depth practice. In order to write *Compendium of Materia Medica*, Li Shizhen conducted in-depth research and study on the basis of extensive reading of the literature and materials. Miao Xiyong interpreted the functions documented in *Shennong's Herbal Classics* and *Supplementary Records of Famous* Physicians, emphasizing clinical utility and focusing on the production, taste, five elements, channel tropism and curative effect of drugs. Fifth, respect peers. Gong Tingxian once said, "There are people in our profession who boast their own strengths and amplify the weaknesses of others. They would scare the patient and attribute the illness to previous TCM practitioners. How can he be useful if other TCM practitioners have failed? Nobody is perfect. We cannot blame previous TCM practitioners. People belonging to the same profession should respect each other. Even if there is a difference, they should protect each other." He seriously criticized TCM practitioners who vilified peers in front of patients and stressed that TCM practitioners should protect each other's reputation.

5. Harmonious practitioner-patient relationships

Due to the development of the commodity economy and the emergence of the nascent capitalist system, there had been much discussion among the Ming dynasty's TCM practitioners on the relationship between TCM practitioners and patients. Gong Xin and Gong Tingxian prized the study of medical ethics and comprehensively expounded the relationship between TCM practitioners and patients and the norms of medical behavior. In *Guide to Ancient and Modern Medicine*, Gong Xin put forth clear requirements for TCM practitioners, referring to the mistakes that patients often make. "Patients of today are stingy; They would wait for the body to heal; They don't take the trouble to find a skillful medical practitioner. They seek treatment everywhere without concern for their real conditions. They pray to ghosts in the hope of getting their help. They are not cautious. When good TCM practitioners come to their aid, the illness is already incurable. They don't understand that delay can cost their lives. They often say it is their fate. Such patients should correct their wrongs!" Gong Xianting proposed "Ten Commandments for Medical Practitioners" and "Ten Commandments for Patients" in order to standardize the behavior of both sides in building a harmonious relationship between TCM practitioners and patients. Li Zhongzi put forward the principle of "impersonal" in adjusting the relationship between TCM practitioners and patients.

7.1.4   Characteristics of Medical Ethics in the Ming Dynasty

1. Influence of Neo-Confucianism

Neo-Confucianism occupied an absolute dominant position in the culture of the Ming dynasty and was highly respected by the rulers. Zhu Xi's theoretical foundation is the word "logic," emphasizing that "logic" exists in all things, and that "logic" requires "investigation and research of things." Thus, "study the nature of things" became "knowledge and logic acquired from studying things". Zhu Xi believed that there were endless truths in all things in the world. Once we understand the truth, we will know all things in the world, have a broad mind, and be fearless. The scope of the investigation and research of things includes reading, doing things, and studying natural things. Understanding the cause is key to learning, which takes reading in a gradual way. Zhu Xi's concept of "studying the nature of things" had a positive effect on the study of medicine. As the core idea of Confucianism, "benevolence" has been further practiced in the Ming dynasty medicine. The Ming dynasty medical practitioners believe that "TCM practitioners represent benevolence, and what they do is a matter of benevolence." It is clear that the Ming dynasty TCM practitioners adopted the concept of "benevolence" as a golden standard. The concepts of Yin and Yang and Tai Chi, which were explored by Neo-Confucianism of the Song and Ming dynasties, have also been introduced into the medical system, and have promoted the improvement of the basic theories of Chinese medicine practitioners in the Ming dynasty. For example, Sun Yikui's "Theory of Life Gate Motion", Zhao Xianke's "Theory of Life Gate Hyperactivity", Zhang Jingyue's "Theory of Life Gate Fire and Water". "Both men and women contain the essence of life that gives birth to offspring. It resides in the kidney, which looks like a fruit. Between the two petals is the base of the fruit that represents life, also called motion or essence". In *Thoughts on Medical Principles: the Life Gate*, Sun Yikui pointed out that Primordial Qi is Tai Chi itself. He considered the movement between the kidneys to be the Primordial Qi of man and pointed out that it was the gate of vitality. Neo-Confucianism played a guiding, penetrating, and catalytic role in the medical science of the Ming dynasty, and was an important cultural background for medical development.

However, Confucianism's respect for ancient scriptures hindered the innovation and development of Chinese medicine. Confucianism emphasizes that "the body must be well protected for it's a gift from parents." Surgery, which lacks an anatomical foundation, is unable to make progress. This seriously constrained the development of China's surgical studies.

2. Harsh criticism of quacks

The Ming dynasty TCM practitioners detested and relentlessly exposed the behavior of quacks. In *Reminders to Good Medical Practitioners* and *Reminders to Quack Medical Practitioners*, Gong Xin commented on the requirements that TCM practitioners should meet in terms of ethics, knowledge, and technology, and criticized the behavior of quacks. "Quacks tend to play tawdry tricks. They do not read or write. They are deceitful. Quacks often come to visit patients without being asked to. However, their skills prove useless for lack of knowledge and evidence. They do not question the patient. They treat the patient vaguely. They do not care about the cause of the disease. They do not distinguish between facts and falsehood.

They are reckless. When illness deteriorates, they vanish. Their only purpose is to make money. They do not care about life or death. It is shameful to have such quacks." Xu Chunfu revealed that quacks unskilled in the medical profession "harm patients and themselves," pointing out that a person with poor medical skills and unproven medical skills should be called a quack. He cited the five major crimes of quacks and severely condemned them. Pei Yizhong said, "The quack kills a man without leaving a trace. So people tend to approach him. He is like a tyrant who is quick but incompetent." He stressed the dangers of quacks.

3. Civilian medicine promoted the development of medical ethics

Xu Chunfu founded the first non-governmental medical academic organization in China, the "All-in-one Medical Association," which had 46 imperial physicians and famous TCM practitioners. The famous typhoid expert Ba Yingkui, the pediatrician Zi Bingzhong, the teacher of Xu Chunfu, Wang Huan, and his students Xu Liangzuo, Li Yingjie, and Wang Tengjiao were all members of the association.

Xu Chunfu emphasized that TCM practitioners should be kind. The purpose of the Medical Association was to conduct academic research, promote the study of *Yellow Emperor's Canon of Medicine* and the study of the four major medical theories, exchange medical experience and knowledge, enhance medical skills, attach importance to TCM practitioners' cultivation of medical ethics. The assoliation require members to "refrain from the evil of favoritism and profit" and "misconduct," treat each other sincerely, unite each other, and help each other when in distress. The Medical Association had a sound organizational form and purpose. It had clear requirements for the medical ethics, skills and obligations of its members. These included good faith, rationality, research, review, authentication, perseverance, force, teaching, pulse feeling, prescription, good intentions, kindness, selflessness, self-respect, respect for nature, medicine, anti-corruption, sympathy with the poor, self-sufficiency, knowledge, medical maxims, and avoiding mishap. The content, methods, attitudes and ideological quality, moral quality, and methods of dealing with the world that should be possessed by the medical profession were dealt with in detail.

The association gathered together many TCM practitioners and scholars to give lectures, conduct academic exchanges, and delve into medical science. It was innovative and promoted academic exchanges and practices in Beijing and the whole country. It regulated medical ethics, improved medical technology and promoted the development of Chinese medicine. The charter contained an in-depth and pertinent statement on the ethics of TCM practitioners. It held that TCM practitioners should first of all have a caring spirit and refrain from fame and profit. As regards medical treatment, they should strive to be prudent and to distinguish between the different ways, value medical ethics, and lash at acts that violated medical ethics. It proposed a comprehensive standard for practicing medicine and implementing medical ethics.

7.2 Representative Medical Practitioners and Their Medical Ethics

7.2.1 Chen Shigong

1. Brief biography

Chen Shigong, with the courtesy name Yuren and the assumed name of Ruoxu, was a native of Nantong, Jiangsu. He was a famous surgeon of the Ming dynasty, with extensive practical experience and theoretical knowledge in the field of surgical medicine since he was young. He wrote *Orthodox Manual of External Medicine* in 12 volumes and 157 chapters on the causes, diagnosis, clinical symptoms and characteristics of various surgical conditions. The treatment methods for various diseases, the indications for surgery, contraindications, the composition of pharmaceutical preparations, etc. were all discussed in detail. A number of medical cases were analyzed thoroughly. The analysis in *Orthodox Manual of External Medicine* was "the most detailed and refined of all". It reflected the important achievements of Chinese surgery before the Ming dynasty. Chen Shigong never asked for thanks in his practice of medicine, and was trusted by patients. He attached great importance to the medical ethics of TCM practitioners. In *Orthodox Manual of External Medicine*, he put forward the "five precepts and ten commandments."

2. Medical ethics

Chen Shigong's *Five Precepts for Medical Practitioners* called on TCM practitioners to be approachable. Whether the patients are adults or children, the poor or the rich, they should be treated in the same way. In the course of medical practice, medicine practitioners should respect the privacy of patients, especially female patients. Medical practitioners should remain in their posts, couldn't go out and play, and should serve the patient carefully in person. They should stick to classic prescriptions, and should not make any arbitrary fabrications.

The Ten Commandments for Medical Practitioners emphasized the professional and moral obligations of TCM practitioners. Medical practitioners should first understand classical works, study them thoroughly, and use them flexibly. They should follow rational methods when making drugs. They must be humble and tolerant toward others, not insult or slander others. They must conform to natural law and take personal interests lightly to avoid disasters. They should not compete for vain. They should live a frugal life. They must not charge the poor, monks, clerks. They should not waste money. All kinds of medical equipment should be prepared in advance, and medical books should be collected and studied. They should abide by the law.

Chen Shigong's "five precepts and ten commandments" embody rich traditional medical ethics. Its core contents include: Medical practitioners should be indifferent to fame and have a lofty pursuit. Patients' privacy should be strictly observed. Medical practitioners must be attentive and responsible. Studying and passing on Chen Shigong's traditional thinking on medical ethics is of great practical significance for promoting and strengthening medical ethics.

3. Historical evaluation

Chen Shigong attached importance to the study of the basic theories of Chinese medicine and surgery, and advocated both internal and external treatment. He successfully created and used drainage, boiling, nasal polyp removal, amputation, scabysmal fistula needles and hemorrhoids, making outstanding contributions to the development of the surgical sciences. At the same time, Chen Shigong had noble medical ethics. He attached great importance to the building of medical ethics. He placed strict demands on TCM practitioners, and formulated a comprehensive system of medical ethics, such as treating the rich and the poor equally according to the "five precepts and ten commandments". He did not charge the poor for treatment, and donated money and gifts to them. Chen Shigong built five bridges for the benefit of the local people, according to *Records of Tongzhou*.

7.2.2 Gong Tingxian

1. Brief biography

Gong Tingxian, with the courtesy name Zicai and the assumed name of Man in the Yunlin Mountain, was a native of Jinxi, Jiangxi. He was born in a medical family. He learned from the strengths of many and was well versed in medical theory. He was adept in internal medicine, surgery, gynecology, and especially pediatrics. He was known as the "No.1 scholar in medicine", and was one of the top ten famous TCM practitioners in Jiangxi's history. His books included eight-volume *Jishi Quanshu*, four-volume *Apricot Prescriptions*, eight-volume *Recovery of Diseases*, six-volume *Book of Eye Surgery*, four-volume *Yunlin Medicine*, four-volume *Forbidden Prescriptions in the Prefecture* of Lu, six-volume *Introduction to Medicine*, ten-volume *Shoushi Baoyuan*, three-volume *Children's Massage*, four-volume *Medical Yardsticks*, eight-volume *Jingshi Quanshu*, three-volume *Exanthema Variolosum* and thirteen-volume *Measure of Herbal Medicine Properties*. Among them, Children's Massage was the first pediatric massage monograph in China's medical history. Gong Tingxian practiced medicine for many years. He once said, "A good medical practitioner trying to save the world should display both skills and virtue." He wrote profusely throughout his lifetime, and made positive contributions to the development of the Ming dynasty's medical business.

2. Medical ethics

Gong Tingxian attached *The Ten Commandments for Medical Practitioners and The Ten Commandments for Patients* to the end of *Recovery of Diseases* to specifically discuss medical ethics and medical sociology, analyze normal and abnormal medical-patient relationships, and set specific requirements and ethical norms for both TCM practitioners and patients. These were creative contributions to traditional medical ethics and research on medical ethics.

To ensure normal medical practitioner-patient relationships, *The Ten Commandments for Medical Practitioners* requires medical practitioners to be benevolent, proficient in Confucianism, skillful in feeling the pulse, conscious of the cause of diseases, understand motion and natural factors, know meridians and collaterals, cognitive of drug properties, know how to prepare medicine, and be indifferent to fame. On the whole, TCM practitioners should first be benevolent.

Second, they should upgrade their medical knowledge and skills, and finally, they should raise their moral quality and make sure they have the right attitude and style when practicing medicine. *The Ten Commandments for Patients* requires patients to choose a good medical practitioner, be willing to take medication, accept treatment, control desires, limit anger, end wishful thoughts, go on diet, live a quiet life, stop believing in superstition, and be willing to spend money on treatment. Gong Tingxian suggested that patients should take the initiative to consult a good medical practitioner, be ready to spend money on treatment, and stop believing in superstition. They should follow the medical practitioner's advice, develop good behavior and lifestyle, and maintain a healthy state of mind.

Gong Tingxian analyzed abnormal medical practitioner-patient relationships in *Common Problems with Medical Practitioners and Patients*. First, some TCM practitioners despise the poor and favor with the rich. He said "They carefully treat rich patients but neglect poor ones. This is not what they should pursue, nor is it benevolence." Medical practitioners should regard "benevolence" as their aim. They should treat patients equally, whether they were poor or rich. Second, some patients were short-sighted. They did not understand the law of the development of disease. They sought quick results. If not, they would immediately change their TCM practitioners. This was detrimental to the treatment of diseases and would result in disharmony between TCM practitioners and patients. Third, some patients did not respect TCM practitioners. They judged people by their appearance, unilaterally denied the hard work of TCM practitioners, and were unwilling to pay TCM practitioners for their work. Fourth, some patients tried to find fault with TCM practitioners. They did not tell TCM practitioners about their conditions in detail and prevented TCM practitioners from conducting comprehensive examinations. In particular, some women put a curtain between them and TCM practitioners when the latter felt their pulse. Fifth, some TCM practitioners denigrated their peers and boasted their strengths and dismissed the weaknesses of others in front of the patient. Gong Tingxian stressed that TCM practitioners should safeguard their reputation as a whole and protect their professional image.

3. Historical evaluation

Gong Tingxian, who studied medicine from his father and inherited the family business, was good at summing up practical medical experience and was quick to learn from others. He preserved traditions but did not follow them rigidly. Gong Tingxian comprehensively expounded on the relationship between patients and TCM practitioners and the norms of TCM practitioner behavior, condemned the bad behavior of both patients and patients, analyzed and examined both patients and patients on the same level, and advocated the new concept of equality between TCM practitioners and patients. His medical ethics were creative and enlightened the building of harmonious medical practitioner-patient relations in modern society.

7.2.3 Li Ting

1. Brief biography

Li Ting, with the courtesy name Jianzhai, was a native of Nafeng, Jiangxi. He was a famous Ming dynasty TCM practitioner, who once practiced medicine in Jiangxi and Fujian. He had a high reputation and rich clinical experience. Li Ting was one of the top 10 medical TCM practitioners in Jiangxi's history. He wrote the 9-volume *Introduction to Medicine*, a book written for beginners in Chinese medicine. It covered biographies, health keeping, motion and natural factors, etc. The book reclassified ancient works and reflected the very best of them. It was written in the form of fu (ode) and it was simple and practical and highly recommended by readers. He published *Requirements for Medical Practitioners*, which set out requirements for the learning and integrity of TCM practitioners.

2. Medical ethics

As a monograph on medical ethics, *Requirements for Medical Practitioners* set out requirements for TCM practitioners' study and medical ethics. First, TCM practitioners must be aspirational and persistent. He said that "the work of a TCM medical practitioner matters a lot to the lives of his patients. They must adopt a serious attitude toward the learning of medicine." Only those who are honest and upright, who have real learning, who are determined to excel and who do not demand pay can study and practice medicine. Second, TCM practitioners should read and be reasonable and studious. Li Ting pointed out that medical practitioners should first read and understand the principles, comprehensively master the knowledge of various medical subjects, know the basic theoretical knowledge and skills, and integrate them into one. Second, TCM practitioners should be diligent, read thoroughly and ponder, and examine the significance of what they learn. They should ask their peers when they had doubts. Third, be accountable to the patient. After the diagnosis, the TCM practitioner should tell the patients the facts about their disease. They should not draw a hurried conclusion or even scare patients. Women, in particular, should be treated with care. Fourth, TCM practitioners should be kind and treat people equally. He said, "Treating disease is TCM practitioners' duty. They should lead a frugal life and refrain from unduly charging patients. If a sick person is destitute, they should receive treatment for free. This is what the kind medical practitioner should do." Treating and rescuing patients is the essential part of TCM practitioners' duty. Fifth, TCM practitioners should not deceive patients. Li Ting analyzed a deceitful medical practitioner's "deception behavior": The medical practitioner is not proficient in medicine, but he thinks that he can become a good medical practitioner if he is familiar with just some theories; The medical practitioner does not think and don't know how to use his expertise flexibly; The medical practitioner understands medicine but he does not practice or concentrate on treatment; The medical practitioner does not fully reveal the diagnoses to patients; The medical practitioner is hasty in writing out prescriptions; The medical practitioner only cares about pay after treating patients; The medical practitioner keeps his skills to himself. Finally, "deception can lead to the demise of medicine and honesty can make it prosperous." Deception and non-deception matter to the rise and fall of medical ethics and medical skills. Only non-deception can bring about the prosperity of academic studies and highlight the principles of medicine.

3. Historical evaluation

Li Ting was a famous, well-read medical educator in the Ming dynasty. He was diligent in clinical diagnosis and treatment, often explaining medical principles in terms of Confucianism. The core of his medical ethics was "honesty" on the part of TCM practitioners, which emphasized the basic professional qualities and moral qualities necessary for TCM practitioners. He severely criticized TCM practitioners who did not read thoroughly, who did not think, who did not follow medical ethics, who only cared about pay, and who cheated patients. The viewpoint of "in-depth understanding and honesty in treating diseases and saving others" still serves as a guide for modern-day TCM practitioners to improve their medical ethics.

7.2.4 Li Shizhen

1. Brief biography

Li Shizhen, whose courtesy name is Dong Bi, was born in a TCM practitioner's family in Zhanzhou (now Zhanchun County, Hubei Province). He was a renowned Ming-dynasty medical scientist. In 1552, Li Shizhen began to author *Compendium of Materia Medica* based on *Classified Materia Medica* by Tang Shenwei of the Song dynasty. *Compendium of Materia Medica* represented the very best of Tang and Song-dynasty research into Chinese materia medica. It overcame the deficiencies of books on Chinese herbal medicine written in the Jin, Yuan and Ming dynasties, developed a unique approach while maintaining China's herbal medicine tradition, and took herbalism to the next level. According to Joseph Needham, Li Shizhen's *Compendium of Materia Medica* was the greatest scientific achievement of the Ming dynasty.

2. Medical ethics

Li Shizhen's medical ethics was embodied by his medical practice. *Compendium of Materia Medica* was an extraordinary achievement made by Li Shizhen under harsh conditions, through diligent practice and in-depth summary of previous experience. Li Shizhen dedicated his life to writing *Compendium of Materia Medica*, which bore testimony to Li Shizhen's medical ethics that valued innovation, investigation and rigor. Li Shizhen adopted an innovative academic approach. He poured creativity into his research methods, and ameliorated the ancient approach to science based on his own practical experience. He accumulated new experience in scientific research, and successfully applied observation and experiment, comparison and classification, analysis and synthesis, and critical inheritance and historical research. He abandoned the established "top, middle, bottom" three-grade taxonomy in herbalism, and established the more scientific "three-domain, sixteen-section" taxonomy. In addition, he developed a more thorough taxonomy of the main treating drugs based on Tao Hongjing's classification of the main treating drugs and founded the channel tropism taxonomy. Li Shizhen was keen on practice and investigation. On the basis of extensive reading of literature materials, he went deep into the field and personally collected specimens for research and investigation. Despite hardships, he trekked across mountains and rivers, reaching Wudang in the south and Sheishan,

Maoshan, Niushoushan and other places in the east. He visited the sites for investigation, covering Hubei, Hunan, Hebei, Henan, Jiangxi, Jiangsu and Anhui, and consulted herb farmers, woodcutters, hunters and fishermen with an open mind. Li Shizhen had always adhered to the spirit of prudent, rigorous and truthful scholarship. In order to write the *Compendium of Materia Medica*, he had successively read 277 ancient medical books and 84 herbal works, cited 440 scholars in modern and ancient classics and history at that time, and quoted works of 151 scholars as a secondary source. When studying each medicine, he always referred to works on herbal medicines of various scholars, assessed their similarities and differences, observed the test results by himself, and referred to relevant works. Through research, Li Shizhen corrected some errors in previous herbal works, criticized some wrong views and methods, and analyzed the causes of errors. For example, there were many superstitions about mercury recorded in the past dynasties. Li Shizhen criticized them deeply.

3. Historical evaluation

Compendium of Materia Medica was compiled for 27 years, and Li Shizhen had revised his manuscripts three times. It can be said that this book is the outcome of Li Shizhen's long-term persistence and assiduous study. He climbed mountains, visited TCM practitioners and collected herbs, traveled thousands of miles, and sought advice from the working people at the bottom of the society, reflecting the spirit of diligence, hardworking, modesty, and the combination of theory and practice. During the time of Li Shizhen, the pursuit of immortality was extremely popular in the society, including both the emperor and the ordinary people. However, Li Shizhen dared to break the contemporary problems, informed the people of the harm of taking the so-called immortality pills, and revised the records on mercury. Li Shizhen's scientific spirit of rigorous scholarship, adhering to the truth and daring to challenge authority is the concentrated embodiment of TCM practitioners' professional quality and professional ethics.

7.2.5　Li Zhongzi

1. Brief biography

Li Zhongzi, with the courtesy name of Shi Cai and the pseudonym of Niane, authored the *Essentials of Internal Classic* (2 volumes), *Yao Xing Jie* (6 volumes),

Essential Readings for Medical Professionals (10 volumes), *Shang Han Kuo Yao* (2 volumes), *Ben Cao Tong Xuan* (2 volumes), *Bing Ji Sha Zhuan* (2 volumes), *Zhen Jia Zheng Yan* (2 volumes), *Subtle Essays on Nourishing Life, Revised and Supplemented* (4 volumes) and *Li Zhongzi Collation of Traditional Chinese Medical Cases*. He attached great importance to the theoretical research of TCM and drew on the strengths of all scholars. He had many works, which are easy to understand, concise and practical. As an introduction to medicine, his works were widely circulated in the field of TCM in Wu, becoming a famous TCM practitioner in the south of the Yangtze River during the Ming and Qing dynasties and making great contributions to the popularization of TCM.

2. Medical ethics

Li Zhongzi believed that the diagnosis of diseases should not be separated from human feelings, and put forward the principle of "no loss of human feelings" for relieving the relationship between TCM practitioners and patients. He divided the normal feelings of people into three aspects, i.e. the feelings of patients, the feelings of others, and the feelings of TCM practitioners, and made a profound discussion. The so-called patient's feelings refer to different treatments for the same disease due to different physical fitness; Prejudice against TCM practitioners or diseases due to different personal preferences and different financial conditions; Influence on disease treatment due to excessive caution, excessive care about gains and losses, personality reasons; Unwillingness to tell TCM practitioners the actual situation of the disease, etc. The so-called feelings of others refer to that the third party, other than TCM practitioners and patients, uses its social status to interfere with the diagnosis and treatment of TCM practitioners, interfere with the selection and evaluation of TCM practitioners, and even misrepresent and comment randomly, damaging the reputation of TCM practitioners and destroying the relationship between TCM practitioners and patients. The so-called TCM practitioner's feelings refer to that under the temptation of fortune, TCM practitioners speak sweetly to deceive or please patients, defend for deception, or speak for scaremongering. Some TCM practitioners seeking quick success and instant benefits adopt arrogant or skillful methods in order to obtain positions, reputations and other benefits. These situations often eventually aggravate patients' distrust of TCM practitioners and worsen the relationship between TCM practitioners and patients. It was the disharmony among patients, others and medical practitioner that led to the final medical practitioner-patient relationship. If a patient does not know medical practitioners, he/she will like some medical practitioner only. If the medical practitioner fears to be blamed, he/she will treat the patient with medicines perfunctorily. Patients do not understand the medical practitioner and change the medical practitioner frequently, and medical practitioners are afraid of incurring risks, so they adopt superficial conservative treatment. The deterioration of medical practitioner-patient relationship eventually leads to a delay in the treatment.

3. Historical evaluation

Li Zhongzi has special works on the study of medical ethics, such as *Conformance to Human Nature* and *Theory of Being Bold and Being Wisely*. TCM practitioners should fully understand the patient's feelings and diagnose the patient's condition in detail from the aspects of the patient's physical fitness, personality characteristics, activity preferences, dietary preferences, etc. TCM practitioners should exclude the interference of the patient's family members and friends, public opinions and other feelings and focus on interrogation. This is of great significance to improve the relationship between TCM practitioners and patients from multiple aspects and enhance the medical ethics of TCM practitioners.

7.2.6　Miao Xiyong

1. Brief biography

Miao Xiyong, with the courtesy name of Zhong Chun and the pseudonym of Zhongchun, was born in Haiyu (now Changshu, Jiangsu Province). At the age of 17, he suffered from malaria and read medical books to treat himself. After recovery, he determined to become a TCM practitioner, and started to search for medical prescriptions, study medicines and extensively read various medical books. He was especially proficient in the study of herbs and completed *Annotation on Shennong's Herbal Classic*, *Extensive Notes on Medicine from Xian Xing Studio*, *Annotation on Shennong's Herbal Classic*, *Traditional Chinese Medicine Prescription Contraindications*, *Medical Cases of Zhongchun*, *Simple Recipe of Herbs*, etc. The *Extensive Notes on Medicine from Xian Xing Studio* was compiled and recorded by his disciple Ding Zhangru, which was simple in expression, well-prepared and practical. It covered internal medicine, surgery, gynecology and pediatrics, and contained many unique opinions. Among them, the three important treatment methods of hematemesis, which are especially valued by later generations, have been used in clinical practice so far.

2. Medical ethics

Miao Xiyong discussed "Five Principles for TCM Practitioners" in *Annotation on Shennong's Herbal Classic*, which reflects his medical ethics and elaborates on the medical ethics of TCM practitioners. Principle one: "As a TCM practitioner, you should be responsible for your tasks, feel commiserative, examine the prescription book in detail, seek medical advice, think deeply, and fulfill your obligations." In other words, TCM practitioners should sympathize with patients, have compassion and love, seek medical advice, and try their best to help patients. Principle two: "Anyone who is a TCM practitioner should read first. Anyone who wants to read should be literate first. Words are the beginning of writing. Illiteracy makes it impossible to understand books, and failure of understanding makes a person feel suffocating." Miao Xiyong stressed that it was essential for medical practitioners to get literate before reading and understanding Confucianism. A illiterate TCM practitioner can only be called "secular workers", who scams and delays the timing of treatment of patients. Principle three: "Anyone who is a TCM practitioner should first learn medicines." TCM practitioners should understand and recognize medicines. Different places of origin and different harvest times of drugs will lead to different efficacy, and there are inferior medicinal materials on the market. Hence, it is necessary to recognize the inferior medicinal materials. For recognition of medicinal materials, confirm the shape and quality, smell the flavor, and prepare the medicine in person. Principle four: "As a TCM practitioner, it is advisable to be open-minded, and the spiritual knowledge is void without anything inside. If you are self-opinionated, you put yourself in opposition against the real world. If you are opinionated, you will look down on others." TCM practitioners should treat others with an open mind. Excessive stubbornness will lead to opposition between yourself and the real world and contempt for others. Be open-minded and do not feel ashamed to learn from the subordinates/inferiors. Principle five: "Some TCM practitioner worries about insufficient reward instead of proficiency in medical skills. He gives up his career and pursues interests. He pretends to admire a nobleman, hoping that the praise of this nobleman will make him well-known in the world. With a lot of money acquired without efforts, it will not be rewarded in the next life. The study of medical skills is a hard-working process. Therefore, it is necessary to be diligent in seeking medical skills and using them to help patients. If your treatment has effects, let the patient pay at his/her will, and do not blame him/her for ample reward. Treat patients equally instead of being discriminatory. In this way, your high morality will be praised by all people in the world." Miao Xiyong pointed out that medical skills are not the means to gain reputation and wealth. TCM practitioners should study medical skills, try their best to treat patients instead of seeking good reward through the treatment, treat patients equally, and should not despise the poor and curry favor with the rich.

3. Historical evaluation

Miao Xiyong traveled a lot in his life and often visited teachers and friends, aiming to collect prescriptions, learn from each other and discuss medical science. He had unique insights into medical skills, such as the three important treatment methods of hematemesis. Warm tonification prevailed in the Ming dynasty. However, he distinguished himself from such an atmosphere, attaching importance to clearing heat and nourishing Yin and activating the academic atmosphere, which played a positive role in correcting deviations and preventing cheating at that time. Miao Xiyong, with noble medical ethics and indifferent to fame and wealth, often treated poor people without remuneration. He wrote the *Annotation on Shennong's Herbal Classic* and the *Extensive Notes on Medicine from Xian Xing Studio* to record his experiences in researching drugs in his lifetime, with the *Methods for Processing of TCM* attached to share the knowledge gained from his practice to the world.

7.2.7　Xu Chunfu

1. Brief biography

Xu Chunfu, with the courtesy name Ruyuan and the pseudonym Donggao, Simin or Sihe, was born in a cultured family in Qimen (now Shexian County, Anhui Province). In his early years, he worked hard for the imperial examination. Due to hard study and lack of nutrition, he was weak and diseased, so he turned to studying medical skills and learned from Wang Huan, a local TCM practitioner. He wrote *The Great Collection of Ancient and Modern Medicine* (100 volumes), *The Six Books of Introduction to Medicine* (6 volumes), *Insights into Cardiomyoscopy, Li Si Guang Yu, Collection of Pediatrics, Purgation of Acne*, etc. *The Great Collection of Ancient and Modern Medicine* is one of the top ten existing medical books in China, including the essentials of internal meridians, biographies of TCM practitioners, collection of TCM practitioners, pulse methods, yun qi, meridians and collaterals, acupuncture, herbal medicines, health preservation, clinical treatment and medical cases. It is an informative medical book, which still has high reference value for clinical application and theoretical research now. Xu Chunfu was the initiator and founder of "Yititang Benevolence Medical Association", a folk medical academic group in China. His actions have a positive effect on promoting medical development, carrying out academic exchanges and cultivating good medical ethics.

2. Medical ethics

Xu Chunfu divided TCM practitioners into six categories in the *Differences of TCM Practitioners*: "A good TCM practitioner is a tolerant and philanthropic person who knows the world, who can Distinguish the auspicious and inauspicious conditions of life, illusion and reality, good or poor conditions, determine the severity of disease, determine the dose of medicines, has an insight into deep and subtle truths and does not neglect the subtle issues. An enlightened TCM practitioner is a person who knows the essence of integrity of man and nature, disregards wealth, takes the firm stand even thousands of horses and enormous wealth are provided, observes the objective laws for everlasting existence. A hermit TCM practitioner is a person who specializes in medical skills, helps patients get rid of the diseases, stands in awe of the nature. As a saint, the hermit TCM practitioner lives at the clinic instead of an imperial court. Hence, such a TCM practitioner is called as a hermit TCM practitioner. A lucky TCM practitioner is a person who cures the patient by a fluke although he has not read any medical works and does not observe the principles of medical science. TCM practitioners can even hold lives of patients in their hands. Hence, TCM practitioners may not practice fraud. A charlatan overcharges for his work, but does not perfect his medical skills. The sixth category is the witch TCM practitioner who has no spirit of perseverance."

Xu Chunfu explained the differences between the bright TCM practitioner, the good TCM practitioner, the lucky TCM practitioner, the quack TCM practitioner and the witch TCM practitioner. Bright TCM practitioners are proficient in medical skills, good TCM practitioners are good at medical skills, lucky TCM practitioners can keep the emperor in good health, quack TCM practitioners are poor in medical skills and cannot understand the medical principles, and witch TCM practitioners only can dance and pray. He was very disgusted with quack TCM practitioners and deeply revealed the ugly phenomenon of quack TCM practitioners. Under the name of the medical family, the quack TCM practitioner plagiarizes the existing prescriptions and believes it is easy to learn medical skills although he only has a slight understanding of some pulse diagnosis skills. Xu Chunfu pointed out that the purpose of TCM practitioners is to cure diseases and save people. TCM practitioners should study carefully, instead of believing that it is easy to learn medical skills and deceive people by chance. As long as a TCM practitioner has good medical skills and noble medical ethics, he will be known by others. Even if he cannot always bring benefits to himself, justice naturally inhabits hearts of people. He blamed some TCM practitioners for using medical skills to squeeze money from patients, which is an unethical act of a snob.

3. Historical evaluation

Xu Chunfu, a Confucian TCM practitioner in Xin'an, has a good reputation and great influence. He was noted for his meticulous scholarship throughout his life, and believed that good TCM practitioners should be proficient in acupuncture and medicine and that medication should be conducted based on the specific conditions of the patients. He opposed the medical practice of "being unreasonable at first, but never changing at last", and emphasized that "prescriptions only wait for diseases, but not for diagnosis." The *Great Collection of Ancient and Modern Medicine* lists "quack TCM practitioners", "lucky TCM practitioners", "famous TCM practitioners" and others, and criticizes the violation against medical ethics. Xu Chunfu initiated Yititang Benevolence Medical Association, which was an early medical academic group, bringing together 46 imperial physicians and famous TCM practitioners from 8 provinces and autonomous regions in China. The Association put forward 22 specific requirements for the members, including medical skills of TCM practitioners, medical attitude, medical concept, medical understanding, relation between medical treatment and interest, relation between medical treatment and society, etc. It is of great practical value to the development of medical practice standards and medical ethics for TCM practitioners.

7.3 Medical Education

The Ming dynasty attached great importance to the development of medical education and established a central-to-local medical education and management system. Medical education in the Ming dynasty was characterized by attaching importance to medical education, strengthening local medical care, protecting family inheritance, allowing becoming a TCM practitioner by self-study, and encouraging medical exchanges. Medical education in the Ming dynasty consisted of official medical education and folk medical education, of which, the official medical education occupied an important position and assumed the responsibilities of medical treatment, education, and medical administration. Official medical education was the medical education resource established by the government, which was divided into two parts, i.e. the central part and the local part. The central part was the Imperial Academy of Medicine, and the local part included the People-benefit Drug Bureau and the medical education agency. Folk medical education mainly included forms of family inheritance, master-apprentice inheritance, self-study, and private school teaching. Both official medical education and folk medical education jointly promoted the development of medical education in the Ming dynasty and trained a large number of excellent TCM practitioners for the Ming dynasty.

1. Central official medical institution—Imperial Academy of Medicine

The Imperial Academy of Medicine was the highest official medical institution in the Ming dynasty. The Imperial Academy of Medicine of the Ming dynasty has two branches at Beijing and Nanjing, with the one at Beijing playing a dominant role. The Imperial Academy of Medicine had officials of the administrator, administrative assistants, imperial physician, and a medical clerk. The official allocation and ranking system included one administrator of standard rank 5, and administrative assistants of standard rank 6. There had been four imperial physicians of standard rank 8. The number of imperial physicians was increased to eighteen then... There was a medical clerk of secondary rank 9, and a commissioner and a vice commissioner in the Herbs Repository and the People-benefit Drug Bureau respectively. The Imperial Academy of Medicine mainly functioned to meet the demands of the royal family for medicine. Its another important responsibility was to assess and select national medical officers and train local medical officers and TCM practitioners.

(1) Source of TCM practitioners in the Imperial Academy of Medicine.

TCM practitioners of the Imperial Academy of Medicine were mainly selected from local TCM practitioners via examinations, while teachers were selected from the original TCM practitioners of the Imperial Academy of Medicine. In the Yuan dynasty, practitioners were divided into ten categories: officials, clerks, monks, Taoists, TCM practitioners, workers, hunters, craftsmen, Confucian scholars, and beggars. The Ming dynasty, following the example of the Yuan dynasty, formulated a more stringent inheritance system of branches and households and sons inheriting their father's industry. The TCM practitioner inheritance system in the Ming dynasty stipulated that those selected as learners of the Imperial Academy of Medicine were called TCM practitioners. TCM practitioners were generally selected from the children of original TCM practitioners. If a TCM practitioner had no direct descendants or his direct descendant was ineligible for recruitment, one of the TCM practitioner's nephews could be selected to participate in the study and examination for approval. The TCM practitioner inheritance system in the Ming dynasty stabilized medical practitioners to a certain extent and had some positive effects. However, the excessively strict household registration restrictions were not conducive to the innovative development of the medical science.

There was a TCM practitioner examination and selection system in the Ming dynasty. In 1527, Jiae, Minister of Rites; other officials addressed the issue of TCM practitioner selection. They believed that the employment of TCM practitioners was limited to descendants of original TCM practitioners only, resulting in impossibility of selecting Lu Bian and Cang Gong who were well-known among the people, making the Imperial Academy of Medicine a shelter for quack TCM practitioners. Hence, they advocated expanding from the simple inheritance system to the selective examination system. The selective examination system provided opportunities for students not from TCM practitioner families who wanted to take up jobs as TCM practitioners, and was conducive to level improvement of TCM practitioners. At the same time, local governments could recommend TCM practitioners to take the examination of the Imperial Academy of Medicine in order to widely attract medical talents. The descendants could get positions as medical officers by "donating money", thus exempting from the examination. According to the *Veritable Records of the Ming Dynasty*, "if an officer of Yin and Yang, medicine, monks or Taoists is needed, the candidates may send 200 dan of rice to the Ministry of Official Personnel Affairs for being selected without examination." "Medical officers selected via donation" increased the number of medical practitioners, but lowered the standards of TCM practitioners, resulting in uneven medical levels and hindering the development of medical undertakings in the Ming dynasty to a certain extent.

(2) TCM practitioner examination and assessment system of Imperial Academy of Medicine.

The Imperial Academy of Medicine in the Ming dynasty mainly functioned to train TCM practitioners for the Imperial Academy of Medicine. Its number of students was far less than that of Tang and Song dynasties, and the management of medical students was extremely strict. Descendants of TCM practitioners were selected to teach medical skills in the Imperial Academy of Medicine in the past. Such teaching mode was promoted again in the fifth year of Hongzhi period. Two or three teachers were selected to teach, with examinations arranged quarterly, and an administrative officer and two medical officers took the examination every three or five years. Those who thoroughly understood the medical knowledge would be recruited as TCM practitioners with food and salaries provided by the government. Those who are not familiar with the medical knowledge would be ordered to study for one year. Those not selected after two or three attempts would be dismissed. If there were many students who had passed the five-year examination, their teachers would apply to increase the quantity of promotion.

(3) Medical education courses in Imperial Academy of Medicine.

Medical education in the Imperial Academy of Medicine was divided into 13 departments: adult's pulse, infantile pulse, gynecology, ulcer, acupuncture, ophthalmology, stomatology, pharynx and larynx, massage, orthopedics, jinlian, zhuyou and typhoid. Two to three teachers worked as the trainers, and medical officers and TCM practitioners selected their specialties to study. *Plain Conversation, Shennong's Herbal Classic, The Classic of Difficult Issues* and *Pulse Technique* were compulsory courses. Familiarity with the compulsory contents and fine explanations was required for the students. Specific courses of each specialty should also be completed. Since these classic works were not easy to study, some TCM practitioners started to write readable books for medical students. For example, Li Zhongzi's *Essential Readings for Medical Professionals* was readable and simple to understand, which was helpful to guide medical students to enter the medical industry.

(4) Medical household registration administration.

The household registration management was very strict in the Ming dynasty due to the TCM practitioner inheritance system. New medical practitioners were required to register immediately, and should be regularly examined together with other medical practitioners. Besides registration at the Department of Household Registration, TCM practitioners should also file in the Ministry of Rites. The household registration records of medical practitioners may not be changed at will, and strict punishment measures were formulated for manipulation of household registration records.

2. Local official medical schools

The Ming dynasty attached great importance to the establishment and development of local medical schools and took a series of measures to promote the development of local medical education, which played a positive role in popularizing medical knowledge and training local medical talents. In terms of the local official medical schools, the government of the Ming dynasty stipulated that "a chief officer and a principal of the Medical School should be arranged for each province and prefecture; A principal of a subprefectural medical school should be arranged for each subprefecture, and a principal of a district medical school should be arranged for each county". According to the *Veritable Records of the Ming Dynasty*, all the old prefectures and counties in the Ming dynasty generally set up medical schools, and the new prefectures and counties set up medical schools as well as schools for Confucianism and Yin-yang theory. At that time, prefectures lacking medical schools were allowed to allocate TCM practitioners from nearby prefectures and counties for provision of medical services at the local place. The local medical schools mainly functioned to provide medical services at the local place, train medical personnel for the local place, prepare and publish local medical literature, and inherit the medical culture. Local medical schools were widely established throughout the country, which promoted the development of local medical education to a certain extent.

Local medical schools also had strict regulations on examinations. During the Zhengde period, Wei Xiao instructed the governments of areas under his jurisdiction that "each chief officer of the Department of Personnel should cherish life, choose those who are good at medical skills, gather TCM practitioners for training. Besides, they should take examinations as required, arrange TCM practitioners to treat patients based on their physical conditions, and reward and punish TCM practitioners based on efficacy of their treatment. Those who fail to master medical skills were prohibited from medical practice." Lü Kun, a famous thinker, called for the development of local medical schools and emphasized the professionalism and proficiency of TCM practitioners' medical skills. Beside, he encouraged TCM practitioners to get familiar with medical books. He pointed out that reading should be focused and selective rather than being proficient. Lü Kun believed that books such as *Plain Conversation*, *Spiritual Pivot* and *Ten Books of Dongyuan* were hard to understand and not suitable for most local TCM practitioners, while the *Medical Biography*, *A Collection of Elementary Medical Canon in Rhyme*, *Six Texts on Cold Damage*, *Shortcuts to Medical Prescriptions*, *Prescriptions for Poxes* and *Prescriptions of Famous TCM Practitioners* were of high practical value and were easy to understand and suitable for most local TCM practitioners.

3. Folk medical education

Folk medical education in the Ming dynasty mainly included family inheritance, master-apprentice inheritance, self-teaching and private school teaching. The TCM practitioner inheritance system of the Ming dynasty created many medical families, passed down the medical knowledge and skills from generation to generation, promoted the emergence of different academic groups, and formed a number of family TCM practitioners, such as Xin'an Medical School, Zhang's Family at Xin'an, Cheng's Family at Huaitang, and Yu's Family at Shexian County, which had far-reaching influences in the Ming and Qing dynasties. Yang Jizhou learned from several generations of experience and compiled the *Great Compendium of Acupuncture and Moxibustion*, Xue Kai and his son Xue Ji co-authored the Summary for Infant Preservation, and Yu Kua inherited his ancestral heritage and wrote *Medical Biography*. All of them are examples of family inheritance. Sun Yikui is a typical case of master-apprentice inheritance. Wang Jishi, learned after Zhu Danxi and Li Dongyuan, founded the clinical evidence idea of strengthening the foundation by cultivating Yuan. Sun Yikui also learned from Wang Ji, preferred warm tonification in prescriptions, and proposed the "Theory of Mingmen Dongqi" and created the "Zhuangyuan Tang" and "Zhuangyuan Powder" for warm tonification of kidney. There were many TCM practitioners in Danxi School, a private school. Yu Kua and Wang Lun were apprentices of Danxi School in the early Ming dynasty.

In 1568, Xu Chunfu established the early folk medical academic group of China, "Yititang Benevolence Medical Association", with members from all over the country, aiming to explore medical knowledge and improve medical skills. The medical association attached great importance to the medical ethics of TCM practitioners, and clearly stipulated the professional quality, study and research modes, moral characters and attitude towards patients of TCM practitioners. These requirements were expectations of the society for TCM practitioners at that time, and played a positive role in promoting the medical ethics of TCM practitioners.

Chapter Summary

The recovery and development of social economy, the prosperity of Neo-Confucianism, scientific and technological innovation, and frequent exchanges between China and foreign countries provided favorable conditions for the development of medicine in the Ming dynasty. The emergence of numerous TCM practitioners, the release of plentiful medical works and a large number of clinical medical practices jointly promoted the development and research of medical ethics culture in the Ming dynasty. Medical ethics and medical ethics practice were very rich at that time.

The Ming dynasty attached great importance to the development of medical education and established a medical education and management system from the central to local levels. The prosperity of folk medical education played a positive role in the development of professional quality and professional ethics of TCM practitioners. As TCM practitioners in the Ming dynasty were deeply influenced by Confucian culture and emphasized the position of "benevolence", Confucian TCM practitioners played an important role in the medical ethics culture and practice of the Ming dynasty, thus the overall quality of TCM practitioners was improved to some extent. The development and research of medical ethics culture in the Ming dynasty mainly focused on the benevolence of TCM practitioners, professional quality, view of justice and benefit, moral qualification, TCM practitioners-patient relationship, etc., and especially criticized quack TCM practitioners deeply.

Application in Contemporary Times

1. Medical ethics education should prevail in medical training

The Ming dynasty attached great importance to the development of medical education and established a medical education and management system from the central to local levels. The prosperity of folk medical education played a positive role in the development of professional quality and professional ethics of TCM practitioners. After Zhu Yuanzhang, Emperor Taizu of Ming, ascended the throne, he designated a series of measures to strengthen local medical education so as to meet the needs of fighting against the epidemic. TCM practitioners in the Ming dynasty analyzed the ways of moral qualification development for TCM practitioners from many aspects, including integrity, modesty, pursuit of truth and practicability.

Moral education prevails in training of talents in modern times. The Ministry of Education stated that the essence of medical education is elite education. For elite education, we should put moral education in the first place. For TCM practitioners, medical ethics education is an important part of moral education. Therefore, to establish a correct "view of justice and profit" as a medical worker, we must clearly understand our job responsibilities and social responsibilities and should be loyal to the country, the people and medical career.

2. Be a medical worker who "remains true to original aspiration"

TCM practitioners of the Ming dynasty discussed in this chapter opposed the use of medical skills as a means of profit-making only, and were deeply disgusted with the behavior of extorting properties using medical skills. They emphasized the medical ethics of saving patients and not for fame and fortune, sharply denounced the behaviors against medical ethics, the pursuit of fame and fortune, and lack of medical skills, and put forward a more comprehensive medical practice standard, which was of great practical value to the establishment and development of TCM practitioners' medical practice standard and medical ethics. This is the embodiment of "staying true to their original aspiration" and abiding by their duties of TCM practitioners.

It is the mission of the Party and the people of China to build socialism with Chinese characteristics and realize the great rejuvenation of the Chinese nation. Being specific to the medical staff, the mission is to provide health services for hundreds of millions of people, improve the physical fitness of the people, promote the physical and mental harmony of the people, and contribute to the health of the people. As people's TCM practitioners in the new era, we should not slack off, but take actions to integrate our medical career into the fulfilling of the great Chinese Dream.

8

Medical Ethics Culture
in the Qing Dynasty

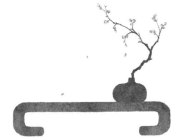

Traditional Chinese medical ethics is a reflection of ideology and culture in the medical field in a certain historical period. Being influenced by dynasty change and productivity development, traditional Chinese ideology and culture showed different characteristics in various historical periods. At the same time, along with the social progress, economic prosperity and cultural development, TCM has been continuously developed and improved to a higher level. By the Qing dynasty, traditional Chinese ideology and culture gradually entered the stage of conclusion and criticizing, while TCM continued to develop on the basis of previous dynasties and began to be impacted by western medicine. Under the influence of internal and external factors, the medical ethics culture in the Qing dynasty not only summarized the medical ethics of predecessors, but also reflected the new changes of the times.

8.1   Overview of Medical Ethics

The Qing dynasty was the last feudal dynasty in the history of China, with the reign of 268 years. The Qing dynasty was the last period of reorganization and restoration of China's feudal society. The rulers used a series of improved means to maintain their ruling. The social contradiction was relatively moderated, the politics, economy, culture and other aspects were developed to a certain extent, and an apparently stable feudal society was maintained. A large number of famous TCM practitioners emerged at that time, and many ancient classic books, which fully reflected the basic situation of medical ethics culture in the Qing dynasty, were passed down.

8.1.1   Political, Economic and Cultural Overview of the Qing dynasty

1. Politically, the centralization of absolute monarchy reached its peak

The rulers of the Qing dynasty were originally a Manchu aristocratic group in northeast China. It entered the Central Plains at the period of the late Ming dynasty bothered by political decay, social turmoil and frequent wars, defeating all opponents by force and strategies, and gaining a dominant position over the whole China.

In order to consolidate the regime, in the early Qing dynasty, the rulers absorbed the lessons from the decline of previous dynasties, and the official governance was relatively clean, upright and effective. They proposed and formulated some regime organization forms that were in line with the social development at that time on the basis of practice, pushing the centralized power system of monarchy to the peak.

Before the troops of Qing dynasty entered Shanhai Pass, the Deliberative Council of Princes and Ministers was the central authority, which was also the remnant of the clan military democracy. After entering the pass, in order to respond to the new changes in historical conditions, the rulers of the Qing dynasty made corresponding adjustments to the authority: the Grand Secretariat was reformed on the basis of the old system of the Ming dynasty. The Grand Secretariat was composed of members of both Manchu and the Han people, dominated by Manchu. There were also specific regulations on the quotas of Manchu and Han officials in central departments. In the early Qing dynasty, the Grand Secretariat was only the nominal supreme administrative body, while the Deliberative Council of Princes and Ministers was the real supreme authority. This form of Manchu aristocrat autocracy contradicted the imperial power and was not conducive to the rulers of the Qing dynasty to further seek the support of Han bureaucrats. During the reign of Yongzheng, in order to strengthen centralized ruling, the government set up the Grand Council by taking advantage of the military promotion in the northwest. The Grand Council functioned to handle military issues, gradually replacing the power of political participation of all princes in the Deliberative Council of Princes and Ministers. The ministers of the Grand Council were selected by the emperor from scholars, ministers and assistant ministers of Manchu and Han people at any time. All ministers selected into the Grand Council were favored by the emperor and could participate in the military affairs. However, the decision-making power rested with the emperor. The ministers of the Grand Council only acted as the confidential secretaries of the emperor. They only passed on the exact words of the emperor without comments or opinions. The establishment of the Grand Council marked further improvement of the centralized system of monarchy and autocracy in the Qing dynasty.

Although the Qing government adopted a series of policies of conciliation for the people of Han, the Manchu aristocrats always suppressed the people of other ethnic groups, except some upper Mongolian aristocrats, and the anti-Qing activities often occurred. The rulers of the Qing dynasty cruelly suppressed the anti-Qing activities and even killed them by mistake or indiscriminately. At the same time, literary inquisition was launched to defeat intellectuals. There were more than 80 cases of literary inquisition in the Kangxi and Qianlong dynasties, and the most influential ones were the prison of Dai Mingshi's *Corpus of Nanshan* and the prison of Lü Liuliang. In order to control the intellectuals, the rulers of the Qing dynasty organized compilation and revision of books, and deleted contents in books which were not conducive to the rule of Manchu people as well. For example, in the process of compilation and revision of the *Complete Library in Four Sections*, the personnel were ordered to examine the documents and destroy the books against the Qing dynasty and autocratic rule.

In the middle and late Qing dynasty, the ruling class became increasingly corrupt and incompetent. The resistance movement rose and fell, and the national power fell from the pinnacle. However, the government of Qing dynasty was unable to resist the invasion of the western powers, and China gradually became a semi-colonial and semi-feudal society at that time.

2. Concerns under economic prosperity

The 40 years of war in the late Ming and early Qing dynasties severely damaged the economy of both the northern and southern regions. At the early years of Kangxi period, there were arable fields, but there were no cultivators. The decay of the social economy led to a situation in which the people had no means to live, and the Qing government was lack in taxes, resulting in financial difficulties. In order to consolidate the rule, the Qing government took some measures to restore and develop production, such as stopping land enclosure, rewarding land reclaiming, launching water-conservancy projects, and reforming the taxation system.

In the early Qing dynasty, "land renaming" was implemented. That is, the land occupied by the seigniors in the Ming dynasty was returned to the original owners and was taxed the same as that of the land of farmers, thus the farmers acquiring the renamed land becoming land-holding farmers. In terms of the taxation and servitude system, the *Complete Book on Taxes and Corvée Labor* was compiled in 1646 in view of the drawbacks of the old system without quota, based on the old books of Wanli period in the Ming dynasty, with the total amount of land and taxes recorded, supplemented by the fish-scale registers (land registration book) and yellow ledgers. *The Simple Complete Book on Taxes and Corvée Labor* compiled in Kangxi period, with the mantissa of the original land taxes deleted and the integers left, solved the problem of disordered taxes and corvée labors, and unjustified financial levies. In the 51st year during the reign of Emperor Kangxi (1712), in order to stabilize the tax amount, it was announced that the tax amount in the 50th year of Kangxi period (24.62 million labors in the very year, 3.35 million taels of silver) would be used as the basis, and no tax would be added even though the population rose in the flourishing age. In Yongzheng period, the policy of "combining head tax and land tax" (also known as "unity of land and labor force"), was implemented to merge the head tax into the land tax, thus no head tax would be levied from then on. Previously, there were a variety of taxes, mainly including land tax and head tax (poll tax). After the combination of head tax and land tax, i.e. merging the head tax into the land tax, the poor and landless people were exempted from the head tax, thus relieving the personal dependence relation of farmers and the government.

As the Qing government took a series of relatively effective measures, the situation in many places gradually improved. For example, land abandoning had been severe in Huainan and Huaibei regions, while no land was abandoned or uncultivated in the middle Kangxi period. According to the *Veritable Record of Qing Dynasty*, the cultivated area in the 18th year of Shunzhi period (1661) was 5.62 million hectares, that in the 24th year of Kangxi period (1685) was 5.89 million hectares, that in the 61st year of Kangxi period (1722) was 8.51 million hectares, and that in the 3rd year of Yongzheng period (1725) was 8.9 million hectares. In terms of population, the national population was 150 million in the thirty-ninth year of Kangxi period (1700), reached 310 million in the fifty-ninth year of Qianlong period (1794), and rose to more than 400 million during the Daoguang period.

In the middle of the Qing dynasty, after the brilliant "Kangxi-Qianlong Prosperity", the economy of the Qing dynasty began to decline in Jiaqing period. In the early Qing dynasty, the self-sufficient natural economy, which combined traditional small-scale agriculture and cottage industry, occupied a dominant position in the economy. In the middle of the Qing dynasty, land annexation became increasingly serious. A large amount of cultivated land was held by the rulers of the Qing dynasty and the bureaucratic landlords, while the farmers, who accounted for the vast majority of the population, had little or no land at all. The rich had vast fields, while the poor did not have a place to stand. A vast number of farmers were trapped in the tragic situation of poverty, bankruptcy and displacement.

In terms of foreign exchanges, the Qing government continued the policy of self-imposed seclusion of the Ming dynasty and basically gave up foreign trade, with the purpose of preventing foreign personnel and cultural idea exchanges, and avoiding the threat to the rule caused by the impact on politics. However, such a closed manner aggravated the arrogance and backwardness in the Qing dynasty. Policies of self-imposed seclusion and stressing agriculture and restraining commerce continued to stifle the emergence of capitalism in the Ming and Qing dynasties. Hence, the economy of the Qing dynasty was restricted in the shackles of feudalism and it was difficult to realize modern transformation.

3. In terms of ideology and culture, textual research prevailed and thoughts were initiated

In Ming-Qing transition, Gu Yanwu, Huang Zongxi, etc. advocated that academic research should be practical and useful, denied the existence of so-called independent Neo-Confucianism outside Confucianism, opposing the malpractice of empty talk of Neo-Confucianism in the Ming and Qing dynasties, and advocating the practice of self-discipline. In terms of understanding and cognition of Confucian classics, they advocated to start from the primary school and using the method of exegesis to achieve its true meaning. Their "Thought of Pragmatism" is a reflection on the fall of the Ming dynasty. From Shunzhi period to the middle of Kangxi period, the rulers adopted the policy of leniency and conciliation to the remnants of the Ming dynasty. However, along with the regime consolidation of the Qing dynasty, the ideological constraints became increasingly severe. On the one hand, the Qing government strengthened ideological restraint by literary inquisition. On the other hand, it advocated sorting out and examining classical documents to distract the attention of the public from fighting against the Qing dynasty. In this context, the spirit of attaching importance to the study of real social issues advocated by Gu Yanwu and others was restrained, but their academic style of attaching importance to reading and opposing empty talk had a profound influence on later scholars. In this harsh reality, scholars turned to the textual research of ancient books, gradually forming a style of study that was separated from social reality and the textual research irrespective of the actual demands.

Textual research was roughly divided into two factions of Wu and Anhui in the Qianlong and Jiaqing periods. The faction Wu, represented by Hui Dong, believed in family discipline and advocated ancient precepts. In their textual research, they considered that "all ancient books are authentic, and all books of Han are good". They stuck to convention and had little impact on later generations. The faction Anhui, represented by Dai Zhen, believed that from the practical evidence, there should be an objective attitude of "speculating about opinions and viewpoints of others, and treating opinions and viewpoints of yourself objectively", and textual research should be practical, realistic, innovative, and impartial. Although the rise of textual research hindered the development of progressive thinking, it still made great contributions to the collation of Chinese classical literature.

By the Daoguang period, the situation of internal and external troubles of the Qing dynasty was increasingly apparent. In order to save the nation from the crisis, some scholar-officials tried to break the ideological and cultural atmosphere of silencing. Insightful scholars such as Gong Zizhen, Lin Zexu, and Wei Yuan, among feudal literati, perceived that empty talks and doctrines could not solve real social problems. They began to face the social reality, uncovered corruption, called for the elimination of maladies, advocated "Thought of Pragmatism", and guided people to break free from the yoke of the rationalism of Cheng and Zhu critiques.

They combined the advanced ideas of enlightenment thinkers in the early Qing dynasty with the social reality of that time and put forward some thoughts about reform and strengthening, which had a great impact on later generations. Gong Zizhen utterly detested social corruption. He believed that "the utmost shame of the country is that scholars do not know what is the shame". He also advocated political reform to strengthen the country, abolished the eight-part essay examination for selecting scholars, and insisted on "exploiting talents regardless of conventions". Lin Zexu, who was appointed as Imperial Secretary, was in charge of the ban on smoking in Guangzhou and advocated learning advanced foreign technologies. Lin Zexu also asked Wei Yuan to compile the *Illustrated Records of the Maritime Nations* and *Annals of the Four Continents*, opening up a new atmosphere of learning from the West in modern China. Wei Yuan, who advocated the spirit of seeking truth from facts and the promotion of benefits and elimination of harms believed that, "There are no methods that have been used without harms for hundreds of years, and no methods that remain infinitely unchanged. There are no methods that can bring benefits without dropping disadvantages, and no methods that are difficult but flexible."

In the late Qing dynasty, with the aggravation of imperialist aggression, Western ideology and culture were spread more widely in China, and the corruption and incompetence of the Qing government were gradually exposed. This prompted intellectuals to awaken further and gradually became a large trend for reform and renovation.

8.1.2　Main Contents of Medical Ethics Culture

During the Qing dynasty, China was in the end stage of feudal society and gradually entered into a semi-colonial and semi-feudal society. During that period, traditional Chinese medical ethics culture also entered the summary stage and was challenged by western medicine. In general, in terms of theoretical exploration and medical practice, the medical ethics culture in the Qing dynasty not only inherited the essence of its predecessors' medical ethics culture but also played a new role in keeping pace with the times.

1. *Principle and Prohibition for Medical Profession* and the thought of "sympathy for patients"

Principle and Prohibition for Medical Profession by Yu Jiayan is a prominent representative of medical ethics in the Qing dynasty. In this book, more detail about principles and norms of professional ethics that TCM practitioners should abide by are discussed. He breaks from the previous tradition of writing medical ethics in the form of maxims such as "Five Precepts" and "Ten Commandments", and takes the principles of four clinical diagnoses and eight principles of syndrome differentiation as the "principle" of the medical profession, and the prohibitions easy to be committed in clinical diagnosis and treatment as the "prohibition" of the medical profession, which is used to judge the responsibility and mistake of misdiagnosis. So the combination of the "principle" and "prohibition" is named "Principle and Prohibition for Medical Profession". This discussion that stresses medical ethics more than medical practice is called "clinical ethics" by later generations. *The Principle and Prohibition for Medical Profession* clearly put forward TCM practitioners' medical ethics and standards in diagnosing and treating patients and getting rid of the empty preaching about medical ethics, which is a significant breakthrough in ancient Chinese medical ethics.

In the *Principle and Prohibition for Medical Profession: Inquiry*, Yu Jiayan once said that "Medicine is a kind of benevolence. A good man with benevolence will be full of sympathy for others. If you are sympathetic, you will regard others as your own, and ask them their pains carefully". "Sympathy for Patients" is to have sympathy for the patient and think for the patient from their standpoint, so as to truly gain their trust. Similarly, good treatment results can in turn enhance mutual trust between TCM practitioners and patients, which furthers the construction of a harmonious TCM practitioner-patient relationship.

Under the guidance of the core value of medical ethics that must be "sympathetic" to patients, many TCM practitioners in the Qing dynasty served patients sincerely and earnestly by practicing what they advocated. So they were deeply loved by people. He Qiwei, a famous TCM practitioner during the Jiaqing period and Daoguang period, was worried about the country and the people. He once wrote the book *Effective Methods for Ending Addiction* for Lin Zexu, which effectively promoted the anti-smoking movement. He Xiaoshan, the younger brother of He Qiwei, treated patients regardless of their wealth, distance, or reward. He was only 43 years old and died of illness in the process of selfless treatment in the summer. He Hongfang, the son of He Qiwei, also nicely prepared many medicine pots and charcoal stoves in his Shoushantang medicine shop for free, so patients from afar can take medicine in time. This may be the origin of boiling medicine for the customers in the traditional medicine shop in the future. Also, He Hongfang often comforted poor patients and gave them medicine for free. The deeds above can reveal that they practiced the medical ethics of "Sympathy for Patients".

2. Criticize current problems and advocate the value of "value righteousness over benefits"

During the Ming and Qing dynasties, many new problems appeared in the process of social development, especially under the influence of the commodity economy, and the phenomenon of "greed for profit and neglect of justice" in medical activities. The issue of the relation between justice and interest had attracted extensive attention. Advocating the importance of justice over interest had become one of the focuses when people talk about medical ethics thoughts in this period. Associated with this, TCM practitioners in this period had many discussions on how to solve the issue in medical ethics. They criticized current problems, promoted good and suppressed evil, which played a positive role in redressing bad medical practices.

In the Qing dynasty, TCM practitioners were concerned about the development of medicine, so they exposed and criticized many adverse factors affecting medical development. Xu Dachun criticized that medicine should not be used as a way of earning a living. At that time, TCM practitioners did not read half a volume of prescription books, but only remember a few medicines. No matter what disease the patient get, liver cancer, esophagus cancer, stroke, tuberculosis, typhoid fever, or malaria, the TCM practitioner would only use the four diagnostic methods, look, listen, question, and feel the pulse, to determine. If the TCM practitioner wants to be an opportunist, he just needs to inquire about what is the commonly used medicine by TCM practitioners recently. If he tries it, the medicine may work by chance, which is rarely seen. If he fails for trying the medicine, he will be confused without any thoughts. If his patient die for his trying, he would only say the medicine is good, but the disease is stubborn. Xu Dachun also criticized the bad phenomenon of the TCM practitioners's favor use of tonics and strong medicine. He pointed out that the abuse of ginseng was to please patients and covered up their inability. Yu Jiayan criticized the current problems of the medical world in the *Principle and Prohibition for Medical Profession*, "TCM practitioners in this generation have a common problem, which is choosing to use dozens of non-toxic medicines for relief. The patient have been ill for two or three days and could not be cured. The TCM practitioner covers up his inability, and delays in saving people, which causes the death of the patient. This TCM practitioner even wants to live longer than others and his children and grandchildren live longer. How could that be?" Zhou Xueting criticized those TCM practitioners who were fluttered, "When he went out, his clothes were light and loose, and he spurred on the flying horse riding on the road. How spirited he is. When he felt the pulse, he concentrated his mind, closed his eyes, and sat for a long time. How elaborative he is! When he wrote his prescription, he meditated for a long time. How concentrated he is! But when we check out his prescription, there are only dandelion, white atractylodes rhizome, aconitum carmichaelii debx, and dried ginger help to keep colds away but those medicines have too strong effects, which would intensify the disease. So the prescription would be abandoned. It was a pity!" Shi Dian put forward many shortcomings of current medicine in the *Collection of First-aid Methods* and raised his own suggestions. For example, he was very resentful of the behaviors of TCM practitioners who treated their children as passers-by during the epidemic. He suggested that fellow TCM practitioners go to the village together for diagnosis and treatment. When seeing TCM practitioners who were irresponsible in diagnosing, he was deeply disgusted and advised TCM practitioners to put life first without hesitation.

Emperor Kangxi of the Qing dynasty who liked medicine and treating people's diseases also had a lot of discussions on medical ethics. He was deeply disgusted with the common problems of some quacks in society at that time. Once he pointed out that, "Nowadays, TCM practitioners are shallow in learning but self-interest and unsound in the heart. How could that TCM practitioner cure others?" He had quite an insightful statement about the medical ethics of TCM practitioners: "The TCM practitioner should put the energy of socializing into reading, researching, studying, learning medical cases, feeling the pulse, and treating people's diseases. If TCM practitioners do not care about fame, wealth or dignity, they must have some ideas about the clinical symptoms and have some understanding of using medicines. If TCM practitioners do it in this way and feel well, they can achieve a lot."

Emperor Kangxi believed that it is difficult for TCM to diagnose only by feeling the pulse, and the combination of four ways of diagnosis is a comprehensive means of diagnosis in TCM. He warned the patients, "It is quite common that some patients do not talk about their diseases honestly, and try to test whether the TCM practitioner can figure out the disease or not. Those patients think it is a tough task, but actually, they will delay their illness." This talk emphasized the significance of collecting medical history in diagnosis and criticized the wrong views and ways of patients who hide their medical history to test TCM practitioners' medical skills.

Influenced by the medical morality of "TCM practitioner is benevolence" in traditional Chinese medical ethics concepts, ancient TCM practitioners believed that the essence of medical practice was "benevolence". So it was a serious medical ethics problem to regard the medical practice as a way to make profits. Emphasizing the importance of justice over profit, the value of justice over profit, and the precedence of virtue before surgery are the main connotations of traditional Chinese medical ethics. Those are also the mainstream of medical ethics in the Qing dynasty. For example, Huang Kaijun, a TCM practitioner in the Qing dynasty, said in *Medical Notes of You Yu Zhai*, "TCM practitioners should not delay their way to save patients due to poor remuneration, not be afraid of long distances due to the heat or rain. TCM practitioners can walk rather than take a boat because boating would spend patients' money. TCM practitioners should give medicines without waiting for payment." However, with the prosperity of the commodity economy, the equivalent exchange had been recognized by people. Some TCM practitioners believed that avoiding interests may unreal the medical practitioner-patient relationship, so many TCM practitioners had also begun to advocate both righteousness and interests and legitimate interests. Yan Yuan, a TCM practitioner, also put forward the view that "a benevolent man justifies his righteousness but does not seek personal gain and he clarifies his ways but does not count his own merits".

3. Attach importance to the realistic spirit

The textology in the Qing dynasty emphasizes "seeking truth from facts" and "seeking truth from evidence". The academic tendency of TCM practitioners in the Qing dynasty is particularly affected by textology. TCM practitioners had devoted a lot of effort to textual research and annotation on classic medical works. Many TCM practitioners had proofread, identified and compiled ancient medical books by means of words, phonology, exegesis and textual research. They often used logical methods like comparison, analysis and induction in research, so they made outstanding achievements in the research of classical medical books and documents. For example, Hu Peng compiled *Yellow Emperor's Canon of Medicine—Plain Conversation Edition* based on the Song dynasty's *Yellow Emperor's Canon of Medicine* as the blueprint, and with reference to the version of Xiong Lizong in the Yuan dynasty and the version in the Ming dynasty, as well as literature before the Tang dynasty. In his book, more than 30 inexplicable words, sentences, and articles in *Plain Conversation* were extracted and interpreted through textual research and exegesis. In the late Qing dynasty, Ye Lin, a TCM practitioner, wrote the *Correct Meaning of Classic of Difficult Issues*, whose discussion is essential and detailed. It is a good version of the annotations and discourses of the *Classic of Difficult Issues*. In the Qing dynasty, the sorting and research of *Treatise on Cold Pathogenic* were also relatively comprehensive. In many TCM practitioners' works, commonly, they would have textual research on the preface, indiscernible words, compilation, different versions, etc. And their special attention is paid to the verification of compilation. Influential works concerned about *Treatise on Febrile Diseases* include *Supplementary Treatise on Zhang Zhongjing's Treatise on Febrile Diseases* by Yu Jiayan, *An Annotated Edition of Treatise on Febrile Diseases for Renewal of Patients* by Ke Qin, and *A String of Beads from Treatise on Cold Damage Diseases* by You Yi. In addition, the study and collation of the *Synopsis of Golden Chamber* are also prominent. For example, the *Heart Canon on Synopsis of Golden Chamber* compiled by Youyi is a good one among many annotated editions.

With the matter-of-fact attitude, TCM practitioners in the Qing dynasty studied and compiled ancient medical books, improving the medical documentation and leaving a rich medical legacy for future generations. However, overemphasizing the "source" and neglecting human creativity hinder the further development of the medical undertaking.

Affected by the policy of self-imposed seclusion, there was a lack of scientific and cultural exchanges between China and the West during the Qing dynasty, while the development of physical science and experimental medicine after the Renaissance brought subtle changes to the field of TCM, promoting the exploration of TCM from experience-based medicine to experimental medicine, and bringing a great impact on traditional medical ethics. Wang Qingren, a TCM practitioner during the Qing dynasty, was the first TCM practitioner in the history of Chinese medicine to accept the transformation from experience-based medicine to experimental medicine and from traditional medicine to modern medicine. He was engaged in scientific research with a matter-of-fact attitude, and had many innovative ideas in anatomy. He observed the corpses with the torn abdomen, corrected the mistakes made by the predecessors in combination with animal anatomical practices, and wrote the book *Yi Lin Gai Cuo* (*Correcting the Errors in the Forest of Medicine*) based on the predecessors' anatomical practices. Wang Qingren's medical research is the embodiment of the realistic and innovative spirits of modern experimental medicine, but it has a strong collision with the traditional moral concept of feudalism. In the face of various feudal moral thoughts, such as "Preventing damage to your body, for all of you is from your parents", "Parents give us a sound body, we should protect our body from damage", and "Medicine practice was practicing benevolence, and TCM practitioners should not rip off their patients", he had the courage to seek truth and innovate, and conduct the anatomical research with a strong sense of responsibility and self-discipline spirit of medical ethics. He went to the execution ground to examine corpses for many times. He made medical achievements in observing corpses and checking medical books.

8.1.3 Contemporary Features of Medical Ethics Culture

The objective laws, practical needs and medical ethics practices of the development of TCM are the internal impetus for the formation and development of medical ethics culture in various periods. Politics, economy and culture in the same period also play a vital role in the formation and development of medical ethics. Affected by the political system, economic development and ideological and cultural atmosphere of the Qing dynasty, the medical ethics culture in this period had obvious contemporary features.

1. Preconceived ideas hinder medical exchanges

As the trend of textual research prevailed in the medical community during the Qing dynasty, a large number of medical classics that could be passed down to the next generation were published, which spurred many academic schools, such as Dongyuan School, Danxi School, Zhezhong School, Fugu School, and Panjing School. These academic schools harbored preconceived ideas and attacked each other, and it was difficult for them to reach consensus.

The preconceived ideas among TCM practitioners were not conducive to the unity within the medical community, and greatly hindered the development of TCM and the exchanges with Western medicine. In the early Qing dynasty, the debate between the School of Epidemic Febrile Diseases and the School of Cold Medicine in TCM was mainly the academic debate. However, some TCM practitioners' debates went beyond the academic sphere, and even acted on impulse, violating the medical ethics of "respecting peers" and "drawing on each other's strengths" in traditional Chinese medical ethics. For example, Xu Dachun regarded the academic ideas of the School of Epidemic Febrile Diseases as "heresy", and said that Zhao Xianke's *Yi Guan* (*The Key Link of Medicine*) was a "demon book". So he wrote *Yi Guan Bian* to derogate Zhao's book word by word. Chen Xiuyuan followed Xu Dachun's practice and wrote *Jing Yue Xin Fang Bian* (*Comment on New Prescription for Eight Arrays*) to criticize Zhang Jingyue. The TCM practitioners of both schools were confined to their preconceived ideas and expressed their own opinions, forming different academic views. However, both sides had aggressive rhetoric against each other in order to defend their own thoughts, which affected academic seriousness and scientificalness.

With the signing of a series of unequal treaties after the Opium War, the self-imposed seclusion policy of the Qing government failed, and Western medicine was introduced, thus TCM and Western medicine formed their own preconceived ideas. Due to the different focuses and different methods of scholarly research between TCM and Western medicine, TCM practitioners of TCM and Western medicine took up positions in different camps. The introduction of Western medicine greatly impacted TCM. Due to the different understanding of the prospect of TCM, the TCM teams were following divergent trajectories, leading to more preconceived ideas within TCM and between TCM and Western medicine, as well as different ideas and opinions. The heated debates between TCM and Western medicine went beyond the academic sphere. Those who advocate that TCM should learn Western medicine or Western medicine should learn TCM were regarded as heresy. For example, some people were dissatisfied with Yun Tieqiao who studies TCM and Western medicine, and accused him of being a "maniac", a "monster" and a "traitor to TCM". The preconceived ideas hindered the exchanges between TCM and Western medicine, and intensified the debate between TCM and Western medicine since modern times.

2. Advocating the back-to-the-ancients ideology of respecting classics and regarding classics as teachers

In the sphere of ideology and culture, the Qing government advocated the back-to-the-ancients ideology of respecting classics and carrying out textual research on historical records, and launched the literary inquisition to maintain its feudal rule. In order to avoid arousing suspicion, scholars buried their heads in textual research. During this period, most TCM practitioners were immersed in the collation of medical classics and textual research on the medical books of the past dynasties. Influenced by textology, TCM practitioners of the Qing dynasty made great achievements in the research and compilation of medical classics through verifying the medical books of the past dynasties. During this period, *Gu Jin Tu Shu Ji Cheng* (*The Complete Classics Collection of Ancient China • Complete Records of Medical Volume*), a medical encyclopedia, was published. Some mistakes in the medical books of the past dynasties were revised. For example, Yao Zhian wrote *Su Wen Jing Zhu Jie Jie* (*The Annotation of Plain Conversation*) in the early Qing dynasty to revise many mistakes in *Su Wen* (*Plain Conversation*) written by Wang Bing.

In addition, the completion of *Yellow Emperor's Canon of Medicine* marks the birth of the theoretical system of TCM, while *Treatise on Febrile and Miscellaneous Diseases* establishes the syndrome differentiation and treatment system, promoting the completion of clinical medicine. The perfect combination of both classics in theory and practice makes TCM prematurely at the top of the pyramid. The precociousness of TCM makes it impossible for later TCM practitioners to establish a new system, so they can only repeat the previous successful experience to affirm its rationality and explain the new experience with old theories. Physicians of various dynasties performed well in these two aspects since the Qin and Han dynasties. The historical achievements of the theoretical system of TCM and its role in guiding later TCM practitioners in both theory and practice make later TCM practitioners follow and respect medical classics and regard the classics as teachers. As the last feudal dynasty in Chinese history, the Qing dynasty adopted the centralization regime to preserve its old order, and advocated and respected ancient classics. Therefore, the TCM practitioners in the Qing dynasty were more conservative in the study and practice of medical theories than those of any other dynasty. They showed great interest in the explanation, interpretation and explication of classics. For example, many TCM practitioners studied *Treatise on Febrile and Miscellaneous Diseases*, but they just compiled it in different ways without any attempt to change its original meaning. There were many monographs and views on *Yellow Emperor's Canon of Medicine* and *The Classic of Difficult Issues*, which praise the original meanings of the classics. Xu Dachun opposed Zhang Jingyue's abuse of ginseng and warm tonification, but highly valued *Treatise on Febrile and Miscellaneous Diseases* of Zhang Zhongjing, and insisted that any additions or deletions to this book should be avoided. He put forward the conservative idea that "words must be based on the classics and ancient treatments must be followed". Zhang Zhicong believed that books other than *Su Wen* (*Plain Conversation*) and *Ling Shu* (*Spiritual Pivot*) "were the dross". Lu Jiuzhi advocated paying supreme tribute to *Treatise on Febrile and Miscellaneous Diseases*, and criticized that *Yi Lin Gai Cuo* (*Correcting the Errors in the Forest of Medicine*) written by Wang Qingren with independent thinking was a book of saving people in a pile of skeletons and studying medicine on the execution ground. All of these manifest the conservatism of the back-to-the-ancients ideology of respecting classics and maintaining the academic viewpoint of traditional medicine of the Qing dynasty, which hinders the enrichment and development of traditional Chinese medical ethics.

3. Strong patriotism

During the transition from Ming to Qing, many TCM practitioners were unwilling to become officials of the Qing government and insisted on fighting against the Qing dynasty to restore the Ming dynasty. They carefully summarized and thought about the causes of the collapse of the Ming dynasty, and put forward many progressive ideas that enlightened the people, pursued democracy and transformed the society, which were radical, open, and inspiring. So some TCM practitioners cared about social reform, sympathized with people's sufferings, served the working masses, and became well-received TCM practitioners, including Fu Qingzhu, Lü Liuliang, Gao Gufeng, and Li Yan. They cared about medical progress, criticized unhealthy social atmosphere, and dared to stand up for justice.

After the Qing army invaded the Central Plains, Fu Qingzhu, a patriotic TCM practitioner, was determined not to be an official. When he saw the epidemic after the war, in order to save the country with medicine and safeguard livelihoods, he devoted himself to studying medicine and treating people with medical books collected by him. He secretly carried out the anti-Qing activity while saving lives with a "medicine cage" on his back. He traveled almost half of China. He was a well-skilled TCM practitioner and known as an "immortal TCM practitioner", making achievements in obstetrics and gynecology. With the noble medical ethics, he built a harmonious relationship with civilians. He was deeply loved by civilians. On the day of his funeral, thousands of people joined the funeral procession.

In the late Qing dynasty, Gong Zizhen, Wei Yuan, and others once again launched the enlightenment movement in the face of domestic turmoil and foreign aggression. Kang Youwei, Liang Qichao, Yan Fu and others vigorously publicized the idea of reformist experiments and advocated political reform to strengthen the country. They actively introduced western politics and culture, to liberate the thoughts of intellectuals. Under the influence of this ideological trend, the medical community began to break the situation of self-imposed seclusion and complacency. Many people studied abroad and received modern medical education. Some TCM TCM practitioners advocated learning from Western medicine, and put forward the idea of integrating TCM with Western medicine. This accelerated the modernization of TCM and the progress of medical ethics.

8.2 Evaluation of Medical Practitioners and Their Medical Ethics

In ancient China, medical skills were regarded as benevolent skills to help the world and save the people. Medical practice was practicing benevolence. The idea of "either to be a good prime minister or to be an excellent TCM practitioner" has been widely recognized by the society since the Song dynasty. Due to the high openness of the medical industry in the Qing dynasty, many Confucian scholars, who failed in the imperial examination could not realize the ambition that "first-class TCM practitioners can solve social maladies", sought to become good TCM practitioners to benefit the local. During the Qing dynasty, some TCM practitioners come from medical families, some are wandering practitioners traveling across the streets, some are monks and Taoists with religious backgrounds, and some are witch TCM practitioners using superstitious treatments. The medical skills of these TCM practitioners vary in quality. Some TCM practitioners can bring a dying patient back to life with their miraculous cures, but some quack TCM practitioners are able to deteriorate patients' health and hasten their death. Their medical practices have been recorded in words and used as historical materials, which also reflected the evaluation of medical ethics of TCM practitioners by their contemporaries.

8.2.1 Carriers of Medical Ethics Evaluation

In the Qing dynasty, many TCM practitioners had a strong sense of self-awareness and social responsibility. They dared to criticize the problems and malpractices in their time and produced considerable insights through a constant study and induction of their and the whole society's medical ethics consciousness and medical ethics practice in their academic research and medical practices. The abundant historical materials of medical ethics evaluation they left have been of great value to future generations in various forms. Several carriers of medical ethics evaluation are briefly introduced below.

1. Biographies of TCM practitioners

Biography is a typical and comprehensive form to evaluate a person.

Biographies of TCM practitioners are of great significance in helping to better understand the value orientation of social medical ethics at that time. As an important carrier of medical ethics evaluation, biographies of TCM practitioners have become very popular in the Qing dynasty. There are both brief biographies of TCM practitioners in book series and encyclopedias, and full-length biographies focused on a comprehensive study of TCM practitioners. *Yishu Mingliu Liezhuan* (*Biography of Medical Celebrities*) from *Gujin Tushu Jicheng: Yixue Quanlu* (*Complete Collection of Illustrations and Writings of All Times: Medical Science*) published during the reign of Emperor Yongzheng of the Qing dynasty, included more than 1,000 famous TCM practitioners and briefly evaluated their medical skills and medical ethics. *Siku Quanshu Zongmu Tiyao: Zibu Yijia Lei* (*Annotated Catalog of the Complete Library of the Four Treasuries: Masters and Philosophers—Medicine and Pharmacology*) also included more than 1,000 TCM practitioners from ancient to modern times, recorded and made objective comments on their academic achievements and medical ethics thoughts. During the reign of Emperor Kangxi of the Qing dynasty, *Gujin Mingyi Jicui* (*Collection of Ancient and Modern Famous TCM Practitioners*) recorded more than 100 famous TCM practitioners and evaluated the merits and deficiencies of each TCM practitioner's medical thoughts. During the reign of Emperor Qianlong of the Qing dynasty, Xu Dachun's *Yixue Yuanliu Lun* (*Discussion on the Origin of Medicine*) provided the evaluation and judgment of the famous TCM practitioners since Bianque, especially those in recent times, such as Zhang Jiebin and Xue Ji. There are also such works as *Gujin Yishi* (*History of Ancient and Modern Medicine*), *Yixue Yuanliu Lun* (*The Collected Biographies of Medical Practitioners*), *Gujin Mingyi Liezhuan* (*Biographies of Ancient and Modern Famous TCM Practitioners*), etc. *Ye Xiangyan Zhuan* (*Biography of Ye Xiangyan*) by Shen Deqian and *Xu Lingtai Xiansheng Zhuan* (*Biography of the Honorable Xu Lingtai*) by Yuan Mu during the reign of Emperor Qianlong conducted a comprehensive study on a certain TCM practitioner.

2. Local chronicles (chorography)

Due to the prevalence of Kaoju (evidential scholarship) in the Qing dynasty, the compilation of local chronicles and the record of celebrities at that time became a major event for the local governments and the gentry society. The TCM practitioners included in the local chronicles are mainly locally famous TCM practitioners, with their family history, social relations, personal positions, achievements and reputation, medical skills, medical ethics, etc. The TCM practitioners recorded in the local chronicles were mainly praised and recognized, and rarely criticized. Thus, it was also an honor for TCM practitioners at that time to be recorded in local chronicles. It played a positive role in guiding folk TCM practitioners to improve their medical skills and medical ethics. For example, according to *Jing'an County Chronicles*, Yu Jiayan, a TCM practitioner, said, "The treatments were unexpectedly effective, and the clinic was always crowded with patients." According to the records and statistics of the local chronicles of Shanghai, there were more than 1,000 TCM practitioners in this area during the Qing dynasty. It can be seen that local chronicles have become an important carrier for medical ethics evaluation in the Qing dynasty.

3. Medical cases

Medical cases, or medical records, are the continuous records of syndrome differentiation, determination of treating method, and prescription medication in TCM practitioners' treatment of diseases. There were works on medical cases in the Ming dynasty, but the number was small. In the Qing dynasty, TCM medical cases were more popular, developed and matured. In this period, not only the number of medical cases was far greater than that in the Ming dynasty, but the overall quality was significantly improved. There are two kinds of medical cases that have come down from the Qing dynasty: individual medical cases and mixed medical cases of many TCM practitioners. The former is usually compiled by the TCM practitioners themselves or their disciples, while the latter is mostly compiled from clinical practice materials collected by others. The collection and publication of medical cases represent the recognition of TCM practitioners' medical skills and medical ethics, and also leave valuable research materials for future generations.

In the Qing dynasty, famous personal medical cases included Ma Chu's *Yin Ji Cao*, Gao Gufeng's *Siming Medical Cases*, Lü Liuliang's *Dongzhuang Medical Cases*, Ye Tianshi's *Guidelines for Clinical Medical Cases*, Xu Dachun's *Hexi Medical Cases*, Cheng Xingxuan's *Xingxuan Medical Cases*, and Yu Tinghong's *Zhen Yu Ji*. For example, Ye Tianshi's *Guidelines for Clinical Medical Cases* is the most famous personal medical case in the Qing dynasty, which recorded 2,571 medical cases of Ye's treatment of various diseases and provided incisive arguments and many original ideas. Yu Tinghong's *Zhen Yu Ji* collected more than 120 cases, which not only offered principles and rules for people to follow, but also inspired people to be flexible and dexterous. It was well received by medical practitioners.

The most influential medical cases in the Qing dynasty include Wei Zhilin's *Supplement to Classified Case Records of Celebrated Physicians* and Yu Zhen's *Notes on Ancient and Recent Medical Cases. Supplement to Classified Case Records of Celebrated Physicians* is the most extensive medical cases book in China. The medical cases it selected were mainly those that came into being after the Ming dynasty, with a special focus on the medical cases of warm diseases. Each kind of disease is exemplified by several medical cases, which help people to understand the changes and treatment of diseases from various aspects, and can also be used to learn the academic experience of different medical schools. Many medical cases are accompanied by notes, which extend, rebut and revise the cases. They are important references for understanding the medical ethics of the Qing dynasty. More than 1,000 medical cases of famous TCM practitioners in the past dynasties have been selected in *Notes on Ancient and Recent Medical Cases*, and great efforts were made in the completion of the book in both the selecting and noting parts. Most of the cases selected were noted with commentary, inventive and innovative ideas. They were detailed and clear in terms of syndrome differentiation, excellent in terms of treatment, and influentially exemplary. The notes added contained judgments about the academic thoughts of various schools and efforts in emulation of the good.

The detailed facts recorded in the medical cases in the Qing dynasty reflected the true picture of the medical skills and medical ethics of TCM practitioners. Most of the medical cases were compiled by TCM practitioners too. And the characteristics of medical cases also reflected the author's medical ethics. The magnitude of the medical cases in the Qing dynasty left abundant historical materials for the research into the medical ethics evaluation of TCM practitioners in the Qing dynasty.

4. Medical essays

A medical essay is a kind of medical note that is not restricted to style. It includes research experience, study notes, clinical syndrome treatment, anecdotes, elucidation of textual evidence, etc. The variety of styles of medical essays enabled the TCM practitioners to express their ideas and understandings. That's why they were very popular in the Qing dynasty. Famous medical essays in the Qing dynasty include *Youyuzhai Yihua* (*Youyuzhai Medical Essays*) by Huang Kaijun, *Liuzhou*

Yihua (*Liuzhou Medical Essays*) by Wei Zhilin, *Chongqing Tang Suibi* (*Chongqing Hall Essays*) by Wang Xuequan, *Qian Zhai Yihua* (*Qianzhai Medical Essays*) by Wang Shixiong, *Leng Lu Yihua* (*Lenglu Medical Essays*) by Lu Yihuai, etc.

For example, Huang Kaijun pointed out 24 ethical standards to which TCM practitioners should adhere in *Youyuzhai Yihua*, "Good prescriptions are validated by their effects on patients. It is necessary to prepare good prescriptions. For emergency patient, set forth immediately once asked for. Do not be hasty or unmindful when taking the patient's pulse. Do not reduce the dosage because the medicine is expensive. Do not delay your trip even if the remuneration is petty. Do not medicate your patients so that you can cover up the mistakes you have made in syndrome differentiation. Do not be unwilling to treat a patient who is far away because you do not want to endure the coldness of winter or the mugginess of summer. Do not excuse yourself for not treating the patient because you want to go to a banquet and have fun. For those who are poor, give them medicine and treat them for free. Do not let patient's recovery be delayed because you are rigid in medicating your patient. Do not use strong medicines to seek quick effects. Do not make capital of the occasion when the patient is critically ill. Do not horrify the patient and his or her family. Do not sell bogus medicines to the patient and, by doing so, preclude the patient from recovery. Do no remiss the patients who are in critical conditions. Do not dislike filthy patients. Do not delay your patients' recovery because there is discord between you and your fellow TCM practitioners. Do not use medicine causing miscarriage. Do not slander the Shiyi (opportunist TCM practitioners, who pursue personal gains and temporary effects rather than medical skills and the well-being of patients). Do not fail to differentiate the syndrome nor medicate your patient with strong medicines. Do not charge your patient for traveling expenses if your patient's place is within your walking distance. Do not distribute the medicine to your patient only when you get money."

For another example, Lu Yiqian in *Leng Lu Yihua* mentions that "medical practitioners must be knowledgeable and well-informed", and if "you use the medicine with all your heart, you can avoid harming your patients". In addition to studying, Lu diligently recorded the medical prescriptions, saying that "I am not able to save the people from their sufferings. I should widely spread the good prescriptions in the hope of fulfilling my responsibilities for benefiting and helping the people". These are sufficient reflections of his noble medical ethics.

In the Qing dynasty, works on medical cases often not only evaluated others' medical ethics, but also described TCM practitioners' personal views on medical ethics. Therefore, medical cases also became an important approach to evaluate the medical ethics of TCM practitioners in the Qing dynasty.

5. Prefaces

There are two kinds of prefaces in medical books: prefaces by the authors and those by others. In the prefaces by the authors, the author mostly describes his own medical skills and medical ethics. They are the embodiment of the self-consciousness of the TCM practitioner. For example, Xu Dachun said in the preface of *Shanghanlun Leifang* (*Classified Prescriptions from Treatise on Febrile Disease Caused by Cold*), "After having finished the compilation of these prescriptions, I had reexamined them for seven years and revised the draft for five times, so I have no regrets at all." This manifests his truth-seeking spirit in his earnest search for textual evidence. Prefaces written by others in medical works during the Qing dynasty were more common, and their contents were more objective and credible. For example, in the Qing dynasty, Ji Shufu wrote a preface for Zhang Nan's *Yimen Banghe*, "Master Zhang had spent years carefully reading, expounding, correcting many books. His analysis was logical and thorough, and his writings were clear and inspirational. If TCM practitioners are not upright, lives will not be saved and if rules are not to be obeyed, the medical art will be groundless. What a rare champion of medical art he was in the medical field! Provided that the works of Master Zhang are not to be widely spread, those so-called TCM practitioners who are bigoted and inflexible would consider themselves as learned. How can you expect those people to wake up and practice introspection when they are openly and bitterly criticized."

6. Novels

The novel was an important literary genre in the Ming and Qing dynasties. It emerged with the rise of the civil class. Novels in the Ming and Qing dynasties either reflected the reality of society or criticized historical facts. They had a profound impact on later generations. Compared with the novels of the Ming dynasty, the novels of the Qing dynasty have made more brilliant achievements. The novels written in the classical Chinese language and those in the plain Chinese language influenced each other and, evolving together, reached their heydays. What a considerable part of the novels in the Qing dynasty recorded was the stories of TCM practitioners. Although they were not as realistic as the medical cases or medical records in medical works, to a certain extent they reflected the public's opinions on TCM practitioners' medical ethics. For example, the novel *Hu Zhongtian* tells the situation of a TCM practitioner in the late Ming dynasty. Gong Xin, the protagonist of the novel, started his new career as a medical practitioner after having failed the imperial examination. This reflects the phenomenon of the Confucian scholar becoming TCM practitioners at that time. In Guangxu period of the Qing dynasty, Yu Wenyao wrote in the preface of his *Yijie Xianxingji*, "This book aims to describe the true features of the medical field. It is an indispensable book for it distinguishes clearly the medical skills of TCM practitioners." In addition, well-known novels such as *Yuewei Thatched Cottage Notes* (*Fantastic Tales* By Ji Xiaolan) and *Liaozhai Zhiyi* (*Strange Tales from a Chinese Studio*) also present us with the images of many folk TCM practitioners.

7. Appointment to bureaucrat offices and conferment of titles

Chinese rulers in all dynasties often attempted to influence highly respected TCM practitioners and express their official recognition of TCM practitioners' medical ethics by conferring official posts on them. For example, Xu Dachun had been summoned to the imperial palace to give treatment two times. For the first time, he was commended for his honesty and outspokenness and was appointed to the official position, but he did not take up the appointment. For the second time, he died of old age 3 days after having arrived in Beijing, and Qianlong gave him a hundred taels of gold and let him be buried in his hometown. In Qianlong period, Wu Qian, a TCM practitioner, accepted the position of judge in the Right Courtyard of the Imperial Academy of Medicine and was entrusted by Emperor Qianlong to edit the *Yixue Jinjian*. At that time, there were two cases of conferment of titles: First, it was conferred by the authority to highly respected TCM practitioners. For example, Emperor Qianlong gave Huang Yuanyu, a TCM practitioner, a plaque with his personal inscription "Miao Wu Qi Huang", and issued an edict ordering him to be an imperial physician. In the second case, the honorary title was given by the people. For example, Fu Shan was commended by the people as a "godlike TCM practitioner" and "medical sage" because he had dedicated himself to treating the poor with extraordinary medical skills. Due to his consummate medical skills, Ye Tianshi was hailed as "a Heavenly medical practitioner who has descended on the earth" by the people. Qi Zan of Jiangyin, a famous TCM practitioner, was honored as "the Grand Master". Sheng Wujiu of Kunshan, a virtuous old man who helped people with medical skills, was called "the Centenarian".

8.2.2 Criteria for Medical Ethics Evaluation

During the Qing dynasty, there were TCM practitioners of different origins and with varied medical skills active in society. According to virtuousness, they were called famous TCM practitioners, good TCM practitioners, opportunist TCM practitioners and quack TCM practitioners. The images of TCM practitioners vary according to different criteria, which also offer a basis for the conductibility of medical ethics evaluation.

1. Famous TCM practitioners

In the Qing dynasty, TCM practitioners believed that a famous TCM practitioner should be knowledgeable, skilled and well-known. Tan Yiyuan, a TCM practitioner in the late Qing dynasty and the early Republic of China, believed that "A so-called famous TCM practitioner must be a man of the highest integrity and willing to exert painstaking efforts to benefit the world. His prescriptions and methods must be excellent. His works must be extensive, sufficiently influential for the future generations to emulate, and indelible like the sun and moon passing through heaven and rivers flowing on earth." To become a famous TCM practitioner, there are quite strict requirements of medical ethics and skills. The TCM practitioner Xu Dachun once sighed, "It is difficult to be a TCM practitioner, especially a famous TCM practitioner." It is because famous TCM practitioners often have a very high reputation and social status and thus hard to make an appointment with them, so that the family of the patient will not invite them to treat the patient at once if it is a minor disease; and only when the illness becomes fatal, the TCM practitioners at hand are powerless, and the whole family thinks that the patient is in danger will the famous TCM practitioners be asked for. However, if a famous TCM practitioner is only asked for when the patient is terminally ill, how can he bring the dying back to life? But if a famous TCM practitioner is unable to perform something extraordinary in this case, he will not stand out from those common TCM practitioners. If he is to shrink back and avoid his responsibilities, he will be accused of being unworthy of his reputation.

If the famous TCM practitioner treats it, when there is still a glimmer of hope for the patient to survive this terminal illness, if the TCM practitioner uses weak medicine to shirk from his responsibilities, he will be full of remorse for not having offered the patient a chance to survive. If he uses strong medicine as a last-ditch attempt and the patient's condition worsens, he will be accused and to blame for all the errors made by previous TCM practitioners." Therefore, whatever he does, he will be blamed. He is truly on the horns of a dilemma. Therefore, it is more difficult for famous TCM practitioners to treat diseases than common TCM practitioners. In order to avoid the potential risk of "potent medicine to cure chronic diseases", famous TCM practitioners in the Qing dynasty often chose "gentle medicine to protect their name". The prescriptions were "mostly similar, all of which were extremely gentle and weak, with each flavor of 3 to 5 fen into one dose, with a total of a little over 3 qian." Only a few medicines were given according to the usual routine, and even for a person who was almost dying of asthenia cold, they still prescribed several clear and refreshing flavors of medicine. Although the disease cannot be cured, and the life cannot be saved, it would never be bad for the patient. Although there was no merit, nor fault either. However, the patient was vaguely ignorant. If they were cured, they would attribute it to famous TCM practitioners. If not, he would be resigned to fate.

2. Good TCM practitioners

In the Qing dynasty, TCM practitioners believed that good TCM practitioners were the ones with noble medical ethics and certain skills. Huang Kaijun said in *You Yu Zhai Yi Hua*, "Medical practitioners must be benevolent, reasonably smart and honest, otherwise, they cannot be trusted. So in ancient times, people preferred the TCM practitioners who cared for patients more than their name. They were benevolent enough to express love and wise enough to give comfort and relieve worries. They could tell the real condition of patients, determine the trend of the disease progress and the severity of the original disease so as to decide the appropriate dose of medicine. They were too meticulous to miss any details. Only in this way can they be called good TCM practitioners." Hua Xiuyun, a TCM practitioner, referred to the three deeds to immortality of Confucianism, namely to set one's virtue, to set one's meritorious, and to expound one's ideas in writing, and pointed out that the three deeds to immortality of good TCM practitioners in dealing with affairs are "Neglect of name and interests to set one's virtue, treatment and cure of diseases to set one's meritorious, and elaboration on deep thoughts and becoming an author to expound one's ideas in writing." In response to the TCM practitioners' "gentle medicine to protect their name", Wu Tianshi, a TCM practitioner, believed that "the use of medicine is like the use of soldiers, what matters is whether the medicine is appropriate instead of whether it is poisonous or not". The use of potent medicine can better show the superior judgement of a good TCM practitioner. Under the value system of TCM practitioners in the Qing dynasty, a good TCM practitioner was a combination of noble medical ethics and superb medical skills, which was the highest realm that medical practitioners should pursue.

3. Opportunist TCM practitioners

In the Qing dynasty, TCM practitioners believed that the opportunist TCM practitioners were those who pursued fame and fortune rather than learning. Wu Jutong, a TCM practitioner, pointed out, "The opportunist TCM practitioners were arrogant and mean. He put a high price on themselves and asked for more money, even some refused to come without 300 jin a day." The TCM practitioner Yu Tingju sighed, "They did what they wished without restraint, but they rarely even never read. Even though Confucian scholars placed great emphasis on reading books, it was quite common for some to praise themselves to be an expert after reading only a few books. Alas! They are even ignorant of Yin and Yang, and treat patients with the least respect on lives. How ironic it is!" Xu Dachun believed that opportunist TCM practitioners were those who catch up with fashion, cater to the trend of the times, and do not learn skills.

Li Zhongyue, a TCM practitioner, criticized opportunist TCM practitioners, "They did not move with the times but stick in the mud with rare changes." Zhao Xuemin also regarded the official TCM practitioners who "travel by palanquin, live with servants and guards, wear high hats, crave fame, play up to persons in power, and enjoy high salaries" as opportunist TCM practitioners. During the Qing dynasty, opportunist TCM practitioners were able to fish in the medical circle, which even fully revealed the lack of medical management of the Qing government from the central government to the local government.

4. Quack

TCM practitioners in the Qing dynasty believed that quacks were TCM practitioners who were incompetent, low-level, fraudulent, and extremely irresponsible for the life of patients. When talking about quacks, Shen Jinao said, "The quacks practiced with their mediocre qualification, stubborn opinions and greedy hearts. They were even unable to understand what they read, so they just mistook and spread the false information. Every time a quack tried to cure a disease, he would fail and cause a death. Even if he succeeded by luck once in a while, he didn't know why. However, he just claimed credit for himself, and thought only he could treat the disease, which is really a shame." In the late Qing dynasty, TCM practitioner Mao Duishan attacked the three bad habits of quacks, "Writing prescriptions with a wild scribble, applying rare medicine, and claiming to know the pulse without asking about the condition. He didn't delve into medical ethics but claimed himself to be in charge of people's life, so he didn't take it seriously, which also revealed his medical ethics."

In the Qing dynasty, quack TCM practitioners widely existed without restraints. Since quacks went their own way, and medical road became gloomy, and the name of TCM practitioners became light. Especially in the late Qing dynasty, the mistreatment and killing of individuals by TCM were regarded as the inferiority of TCM groups. People's disappointment at some TCM practitioners developed into the denial to the achievements of TCM in the Ming and Qing dynasties, and then a question to the whole TCM, which brought great negative impacts on the development of TCM.

8.3   Representative Medical Practitioners and Their Medical Ethics

During the Qing dynasty, there were many famous TCM practitioners. While helping the world, they also focused on summarizing treatment experience and expounding medical ethics, leaving valuable heritage for later generations. At the same time, with the development of commodity economy, traditional medicine shops represented by Tong Ren Tang, Hu Qing Yu Tang, Xing He Tang and Lei Yun Shang have gradually emerged across the whole country. In the process of operation, these medicine shops mostly put integrity first, observed ethics and inherited their respective medical ethics culture, which is the genetic code of their operation to date.

8.3.1 Representatives of Medical Ethics

In the Qing dynasty, a large number of TCM practitioners with noble medical ethics and excellent medical skills emerged, and medical ethics were also elaborated in their works. The following is a brief introduction to some representative figures.

1. Yu Jiayan

Yu Jiayan, a famous TCM practitioner in the late Ming and early Qing dynasties, with courtesy name Jiayan, was born in Xinjian County, Nanchang Prefecture, Jiangxi Province (now Xinjian County, Nanchang City). Because Xinjian was originally called Xichang, he called himself Xichang Elderly in his twilight years. Yu was brilliant since childhood. In Tianqi period, he passed the examination and became a tribute student. Although he was ambitious, his official career was not smooth. He once wrote to the imperial court in the name of all students, stating the political opinions on state governance and asking for "renovation of the rule of law", but he did not attract the attention of the rulers of the Ming dynasty because of his humble position. Later, when the Qing army entered the pass, Yu turned to Zen and later went out of Zen to study medicine. At the age of 50, he became a monk and devoted himself to studying Buddhism and medicine.

Yu Jiayan, who treated patients regardless of rich or poor, was of noble character and excellent skills, and was deeply recognized by his peers. He was proficient in curing intractable diseases and busy with out-call. He was enthusiastic that he never turned others' requests down. In his later years, he was not satisfied with clinical practice, and said, "I held the prescription to cure people, and my merit is temporary, but if I write books to teach people, the merit will be ever-lasting." Therefore, he began to write books and set up a theory and recruit disciples widely. He has successively written the self-ordered medical case Yu Yi Cao, and successively completed the composition of *Shang Lun Pian* and *Principle and Prohibition for Medical Profession*.

The *Principle and Prohibition for Medical Profession* is Yu Jiayan's representative work, which is also the epitome of his medical ethics. This book is of unique style and points out the medical ethics that TCM practitioners should have when they are in clinical practice. In this book, Yu put forward the thought of "adhering to sincerity", which established his position in the history of medicine. *The*

Annotated General Catalog of the Complete Library of the Four Treasures commented on the book that: "It was specially written for quack medical practitioner to avoid misleading people. It distinguishes things from subtle differences and deeply illustrates that a millimeter miss is as good as a thousand miles so that the clinical practitioners dare not make mistakes."

2. Fu Qingzhu

Fu Qingzhu, a TCM practitioner in the intersection of Ming and Qing dynasties, was originally named Fu Shan, and later styled his name from Qingzhu (the rising tone) to Qingzhu (the entering tone). He was a native of Yangqu, Shanxi (now Taiyuan City, Shanxi Province). After the demise of the Ming dynasty, in order to resist the rule of the Qing dynasty, Fu Qingzhu sold his asset, put on priest frock, called himself Taoist priest and lived in seclusion in Juewei Mountain with his mother. Fu Qingzhu, nearly 40 years old, witnessed years of wars and epidemics, determined to learn medicine to treat the patients. He devoted himself to studying medical records, enthusiastically diagnosed and treated diseases for the people, and constantly accumulated clinical experience, eventually becoming a famous TCM practitioners. He also used the name of practicing medicine to contact others in Shaanxi, Shanxi and other places in the struggle against the Qing dynasty.

Fu Qingzhu's main medical works include *Fu Qingzhu's Obstetrics and Gynecology, Secret Prescriptions of Qingzhu*, and *The Andrology*, among which *Fu Qingzhu's Obstetrics and Gynecology* is his representative work, which is an ancient book of gynecology in TCM with high clinical practical value. In addition to his medical achievements, Fu also has great attainments in poetry, compositions, calligraphy and painting. For poetry, he thought it was "the voice of life". As for writing compositions, he put forward that "it is better to be frank than gorgeous". As for calligraphy and painting, he advocated that "people should learn how to conduct themselves because the style is the man himself". This is actually a reflection of Fu Qingzhu's lofty moral sentiment, and common people have commented on him that "Everyone knows that the character of Fu is exquisite, but they do not know none of his calligraphy, poetry, painting and medical skills are as good as himself." This shows his moral character.

Fu Qingzhu treated patients equally. Those who came to ask for help made his house crowded. But he never felt tired and treated them equally regardless of rich or poor. He often treated the poor free of charge, and said, "If someone wants to buy it, I will offer it without considering the price." He went to out-call for ordinary people regardless of the distance. Sometimes he went hundreds of miles away to out-call at night. Yang Sijian, a scholar, was seriously ill and asked Fu Qingzhu to treat him. It was a scorching summer day and he lived hundreds of miles away from Fu Qingzhu's house. Fu Qingzhu went to the rescue immediately after hearing about it. It took five days and nights of bad weather before he arrived at the destination.

Together with Gu Yanwu, Huang Zongxi, Wang Fuzhi, Li Zhuan and Yan Yuan, Fu Qingzhu was called the "Six Masters of the Early Qing dynasty" by Liang Qichao.

3. Ye Tianshi

Ye Tianshi was a warm disease expert of Chinese traditional medicine in the Qing dynasty. His given name is Gui, the courtesy name is Tianshi, the pseudonym is Xiangyan and the alias is Nanyang Gentleman, later he was called Shangjin Elderly in his old age. He was born in Wuxian County, Jiangsu Province (now Suzhou City, Jiangsu Province). Ye Tianshi has read *Yellow Emperor's Canon of Medicine*, *The Classic of Difficult Issues* and other classic medical works since childhood, and he was modest and virtuous. He has learned from 17 TCM practitioners successively, and later generations praised his "learning widely from others". In the process of studying and practicing medicine, Ye Tianshi paid attention to absorbing the strengths of different TCM practitioners and abandoned their shortcomings without sectarian bias. In the Qing dynasty, there was a strong trend of returning to ancient times and respecting scriptures, while Ye Tianshi had a spirit of reform. At that time, many TCM practitioners believed that *Treatise on Febrile and Miscellaneous Diseases* could cure thousands of diseases in the world. However, Ye believed that the methods involved in the book could not adapt to the treatment of febrile diseases such as plague. He put forward many new ideas in the field of febrile diseases with the spirit of "not learning from the ancients and not following the normal examples", which provided valuable experience for later generations to treat febrile infectious diseases. Although some of his views were criticized by other TCM practitioners, his spirit of seeking truth and innovation is commendable. His representative works include On *Febrile Diseases* and *Guide to Clinical Medical Case*, which were collected and sorted out by his disciples and descendants.

As a TCM practitioner with innovative spirit, Ye Tianshi had distinctive personality. Historical records show that he was "playful, lazy. Sometimes he was unwilling to out-call even the patients were in extreme danger, so he was criticized by others. However, his treatment methods were of wonderous effect, so slander cannot hide his fame". This shows the unruly side of his personality.

Ye Tianshi left a last word before passing away, "One can't be a TCM practitioner easily. He must be talented, intelligent, and have read enough books to guide the practice of medicine with superb medical skills. Otherwise, he can kill people with medicine as a knife. My decedents should be cautious about being a TCM practitioner after I die!" This reflects his highest level in medical ethics and even in philosophy of life.

4. Xu Dachun

Xu Dachun, who was formerly known as Daye and styled his name Lingtai, was called Hexi Elderly as his pseudonym. He was born in Wujiang, Jiangsu Province. Xu has worked since he was young and has read countless books. Although he had blurred vision, he still could not stop reading. Xu Dachun studied astronomy, geography, philosophy, calendar, historical records, music, poetry, calligraphy and painting, and had the highest medical attainments. He had been summoned twice to cure diseases under imperial edicts. He has written *The Interpretation of the Classic of Difficult Issues, The Hundred Species of Shennong's Herbal Classics, Prescriptions of Typhia, The Medical Case of Hexi, Annotation of Medicine, The Theory of Medical Origin, The Criterion of Lantai, The Discussion on Diseases*, etc.

In Xu Dachun's opinion, medical ethics was more important than medical skills. He put forward in *The Theory of the Origin and Development of Medicine*, saying that: Being a TCM practitioner can help build upright character. A TCM practitioner may be insufficient in his skills, but he will never intend to harm others. If you can learn with an open mind, you will learn more and make progress. As you learn more, you will cure the patients every time you treat them. Since you become famous, there will be more people seeking for interview and more benefits. If you are dedicated to seeking benefits, you will lose both fame and wealth. Which one is more important?: He believed that the primary requirement for medical practitioners was being of integrity. At the same time, he also emphasized that practicing medicine was a life-and-death matter, opposed the low requirement of taking medicine as the livelihood, and believed that learners should be prudent to learn medical skills. Those who were not smart and nimble, profound and knowledgeable, modest and flexible, diligent and good at memorizing, and precise and accurate cannot learn.

Xu Dachun studied with a sincere attitude and practiced medicine with a prudent spirit, leaving a model for future generations. Yuan Mei commented that he was experienced in preparing the prescription and choosing medicine, Before his death, he wrote an elegiac couplet, "The mountain is full of fragrant herbs, and I will lie at rest in the refreshing breeze." This can be described as his lifetime.

5. Zhao Xuemin

Zhao Xuemin, a famous medical scholar in the Qing dynasty, whose courtesy name is Shuxuan and pseudonym is Yiji, was born in Qiantang (now Hangzhou, Zhejiang Province). His father once served as Sima (minister of warfare in ancient China) in Yongchun and later the magistrate of Longxi County. In Qianlong period, there was a plague in Xiasha, and thousands of people survived because of his father practicing medicine and filling the prescription. Zhao Xuemin and his younger brother, Zhao Xuekai, both took orders from their father to study Confucianism and medicine. When Zhao Xuemin was young, he had no interest in scholarly honor or official rank. He stopped studying literature and began to study medicine and was particularly interested in medicines. He collected herbs widely and cultivated, observed and tested some of them. He was well-read and devoted to doing research on all the books of ephemeris, medicine and pharmacy collected by his family. Every time he gained knowledge, he would compile them into volumes, and thousands of manuscripts have been accumulated. There was a Nutrient Garden in his house, which was a place for testing and planting medicine. It was easy for him to observe the shape and nature of the herbs. There was a Li Ji Hall in his house, which was a place for diagnosis and treatment of diseases. He extensively collected the knowledge and experience of folk medicine, compiled 12 kinds of medical books, called *Twelve Kinds of Li Ji*.

Zhao Xuemin was rigorous about medical practicing and scholarship. His collection of folk prescriptions and proven prescriptions have been carefully selected. Once, Zhao Huamin came to Fenghua and knew that the Monochasma sauatieri Franch had the effect of heat-clearing and detoxicating. He bought a bunch of Monochasma sauatieri Franch for a hundred cents and used it for clinical trials. During an epidemic, he decocted a stem with fruits and achieved good results. Later, he tried it again and again before he included it. In order to compile *The Collection* of *Compendium of Materia Medica*, Zhao has read more than 600 ancient books, including more than 280 medical books and more than 340 classics. In order to check the shape, performance and efficacy of some medicine, he not only tried them in the Nutrient Garden, but also visited the folk. In order to identify Spatholobus suberectus Dunn, he once entrusted relatives and friends to bring it back from Yunnan, Sichuan and other places. After he completed the compilation of *The Collection of Compendium of Materia Medica* in 1765, he made it more complete after more than 30 years of revision. Zhao Xuemin said in *The Collection of Compendium of Materia Medica: Notes*, "Although the collection is mainly for collecting, it was selected carefully. Some of them came from local record and the others came from skilled TCM practitioners. I must examine its validity before collecting them and I'll attach their names to show validity. If there is any doubt, they will be omitted immediately. For example, there are enough prescriptions for Yin Han, Ding Shuang, eggs, excreta of bees, nepheline, realgar oil, etc., but the effect has been verified, and those that are similar to above-mentioned medicines should be deleted. It is better to leave a deficiency uncovered than to have it covered without verifying. Herbs are of the widest range, different people hold different opinions on them, I am always skeptical. *Mirror to Herbs* is the most detailed collection, the collected herbs had been tested in the garden, so they were recorded. Otherwise, it is better to omit them rather than deceive others."

It can be seen that Zhao Xuemin has always attached great importance to testing medical theory by practice. His systematic experience in folk medical treatment has provided an important source of information for the further development of TCM. At the same time, his spirit of "must examine its validity" can be regarded as a model of medical ethics, which is in sharp contrast to the academic fraud such as fabricating data and subjectively choosing experimental results.

6. Chen Xiuyuan

Chen Xiuyuan, a famous TCM practitioner in the Qing dynasty, is a representative of the school of venerating ancient classics. His given name is Nianzu, courtesy name is Xiuyuan and pseudonym is Shenxiu, and he is a native of Changle, Fujian. Chen studied traditional books and records when he was young. He once learned medicine from Cai Mingzhuang, a famous TCM practitioner in Quanzhou. In

1792, he passed the provincial civil service examination but failed in the metropolitan examination, and later lived in the capital. In 1801, he was appointed as the candidate of the county magistrate in Baoyang (now Baoding City, Hebei Province). It was midsummer, and the plague was rampant. Chen compiled the *Song of the Current Prescriptions* with simple rhymes to teach TCM practitioners to treat according to the method, saving lots of people. Since then, he has served as magistrate of the prefecture in Zhengding, and in addition to his busy official duties, he still wrote medical books and treated people. In 1819, he returned to his hometown and gave lectures at the Jingshang Thatched Cottage of Songshan Mountain in Changle, cultivating a large number of medical talents.

Chen Xiuyuan attached equal importance to medicine and literature. His works are of both high theoretical value and literariness. On the basis of studying ancient medical books, Chen has compiled a large number of medical introductory textbooks, such as *Synopsis Explain of Typhoid Medicine*, *Three Character Classic of Medicine*, *The Readable Medicine*, and *Medicine for the Public*, which have popularized the knowledge of TCM and enlightened the descendants.

Chen Xiuyuan venerated the ancients all his life. He was critical of those who deviated from Zhang Zhongjing's theory. However, he focused on the things only and was honest with his colleagues. On his deathbed, he told his descendants to publish his medical books without reservation, which showed his noble medical ethics. Later generations compiled his medical books into *The Complete Collection of Medical Books of Nanyatang*, which was widely spread. Some of its contents were also translated into foreign languages and became famous overseas. Lin Zexu commented on him, "No one studying medicine in recent years can be comparable to him."

7. Wang Qingren

Wang Qingren, an anatomist and medical scientist with innovative spirit in the Qing dynasty, also known as Quanren, was a native of Yutian, Zhili (now Yutian County, Hebei Province). Wang practiced martial arts since he was young. He took the position of Qianzong and was honest and upright. He began to learn medicine when he was about 20 years old, and later became famous in Beijing. Based on his rich clinical experience, Wang had unique views on the causes and pathology of diseases, and believed that the structure of human organs was very important for medical treatment. He went to the mass graves and death penalty grounds of the dead of epidemic diseases for many times to observe the internal organs of the human body. After more than 40 years of hard exploration and unremitting efforts, he finally wrote two volumes of *Corrections on the Errors of Medical Works*. No one can be comparable to his concentration. The book describes some human tissue structures he observed, and attaches 25 pictures of human organs. The book corrects some of the previous misconceptions about the human body. Although there are still many fallacies in the book compared with modern medicine, most of them were affected by the social background and observation and research conditions at that time. This book is still of great significance for promoting the development of TCM from empirical medicine to empirical medicine.

Wang Qingren said when explaining the purpose of writing *Corrections on the Errors of Medical Works*, "The reason I depict the pictures is not for the purpose of expressing my own opinions. I don't mind the future generations criticizing me when commenting on the strengths and weaknesses of the ancients. I only hope that TCM practitioners can be enlightened and follow the clinical evidence, so as to reduce the death." He was skeptical of antiquity and did not fear filth and was indifferent to people's praise or blame. For medical workers, his spirit is particularly valuable. It will not be outdated in any era and should be followed by future generations.

8. Wang Shixiong

Wang Shixiong, a Chinese medicine febrile disease expert in the Qing dynasty, was born in Qiantang, Zhejiang Province (now Hangzhou City, Zhejiang Province). Wang's ancestors were famous TCM practitioners for three generations. When Wang Shixiong was 14 years old, his father passed away. He told him on his bedtime, "You are supposed to do good to the society in your lifetime. If you bear the words in mind, I will die without regret." After his father died, Wang Shixiong followed his parental instructions and studied medicine. However, due to poverty of his family, he went to the Salt Affairs Bureau of Xiaoshun Street in Jinhua to work as an accountant in the same year. In 1830, he left Jinhua to practice medicine in Hangzhou. In 1837, cholera was rampant in Jiangsu and Zhejiang provinces. Wang Shixiong was afraid of the epidemic and did his best to cure the disease, and collected his treatment experience to write a book—*On Cholera*. In 1862, when Wang lived in Shanghai, cholera was rampant then. Because the commander didn't know the measures, and there were many dead people, he revised the original book and renamed it *Revising the Theory of*

Cholera in Residency.

In his life, Wang Shixiong has experienced many epidemics such as febrile disease and cholera. He has accumulated a lot of valuable experience in the treatment of these diseases, especially his unique views on the syndrome differentiation and treatment of cholera. He attached great importance to sanitation, put forward many valuable views on disease prevention, and was praised as a representative physician in the heyday of the School of Febrile Disease. In addition to *Revising the Theory of Cholera in Residency*, his main works include *Compendium on Epidemic Febrile Disease, Recipe in Residency, Qianzhai Medical Notes, Wang's Medical Cases*, etc.

Wang Shixiong lived in the era of Western Learning Spreading to the East. He did not have sectarianism on western medicine that was introduced into China at that time, and dared to criticize the idea of respecting classics and ancient Chinese medicine and rejecting foreign medicine. In his life, he did not care about power and wealth, and always took curing diseases as his own duty. In his life, the vast majority of people who he diagnosed and treated were toiling massed. He was not afraid of the plague and tried his best to cure them. Wang once said, "I'm passionate for nothing in the world except for curing the patients without selfishness, and I don't mind any resentment." "Without selfishness" showed his noble medical ethics of treating patients wholeheartedly. Zhou Guangyuan, who was in charge of Jinhua Salt Affairs Bureau, praised Wang, "Mengying is very knowledgeable and warm-hearted. He never gives up when encountering dangerous diseases. He is the most hard-working people." Yuan Fengtong, a friend of Wang Shixiong, wrote an inscription for Wang Shixiong's book *The Records of Observing Inkstone* and noted, "Shixiong showed benevolence to the toiling masses. If there were people who asked for medical advice from afar, and he would go there by boat regardless of distance and weather." Wang Shixiong's enthusiasm for the sick was evident.

8.3.2　Medical Ethics Culture of the Four Medicine Brands

During the Ming and Qing dynasties, with the development of commodity economy, a large number of traditional medicine shops began to flourish. Some of them have disappeared in the long process of history while others became time-honored brands well known at home and abroad. Among the time-honored brands, the most famous are Chen Li Ji, Tong Ren Tang, Lei Yun Shang, Hu Qing Yu

Tang, etc. In their development process, these time-honored medicine stores mostly adhere to the principle of honest management, leaving many stories of medical ethics.

1. Chen Li Ji

Founded in 1600, Guangzhou Chen Li Ji has a history of more than 400 years, and is one of the earliest time-honored brands in China's TCM industry.

In 1600, Chen Tiquan, a businessman from Nanhai (now Nanhai District, Foshan City, Guangdong Province), returned to Guangzhou after receiving payment. After the ship arrived in Guangzhou, he hurried ashore. The money was left on the ship and was picked up by a fellow passenger named Li Shengzuo. Li Shengzuo was also a native of Nanhai County. He was proficient in medicine and had a Chinese herbal medicine store in Guangzhou. Li Shengzuo found the money and waited at the dock all day. He eventually returned the money to the owner. Chen Tiquan was moved by Li Shengzuo's noble character and wanted to reward him. He was politely declined, so he sincerely proposed to give half of the money to invest in Li's Chinese herbal medicine store. It was hard for Li to turn down the earnest offer. So they signed the agreement on a red paper with the words, "Each pays his own equity and both can share the interests, and works together to do good to the society." The store was named "Chen Li Ji", which means "Chen and Li work together to do good to the society". Since then, the store "Chen Li Ji" has been established at the foot of the memorial archway at the end of the Great South Gate of Guangzhou.

It can be said that honesty is the soul of the foundation, inheritance and development of Chen Li Ji. In Chen Li Ji's Traditional Chinese Medicine Museum, there is a pair of hundred-year-old wooden couplets written with the words "Making medicine with scrupulous precision". These words are full of philosophy and ambition as well as the core of Chen Li Ji's spirit of doing good to the society.

Chen Li Ji, adhering to the purpose of doing good to the society, takes "the process can't be deleted regardless of the complex craft, and the material can't be reduced regardless of the various herbs" as the purpose of management. The elaborate pharmaceutical process and superb herbs can make the quality of medicine keep improving. The famous medicine produced by Chen Li Ji are all products of excellence under the guidance of this spirit.

The first store of Chen Li Ji was located in the center of Guangzhou, and thousands of pedestrians passed by it every day. When there were many hungry people and refugees, pedestrians often fainted and became unconscious. The employees of Chen Li Ji would help them so there were Zhuifengsuhe Pill (for cold), Xingjun Power (for heat-clearing and detoxicating), Wanying Balm, Lijue Pill and other medicines for emergencies. The climate was humid in Guangzhou especially in summer. Chen Li Ji supplied tea for free for the pedestrians, and the good deed has lasted for hundreds of years.

The Emperor Tongzhi of the Qing dynasty took Chen Li Ji's Zhuifengsuhe Pill on the recommendation of the imperial physician after he got a cold. The medicine cured him. The emperor granted Chen Li Ji the title of "Xing He Tang" to show his recognition. Chen Li Ji became famous all over the country. In Guangxu period, the teacher of the emperor Weng Tonghe inscribed "Chen Li Ji". The gilded characters have been preserved for years, witnessing the cultural heritage of a time-honored brand.

As the representative of Lingnan (south of the Five Ridges) TCM culture, Chen Li Ji has a long history of development and profound cultural accumulation. Its honest attitude, spirit of doing good to the society and excellent workmanship have won the public praise.

2. Tong Ren Tang

Beijing Tong Ren Tang was founded in 1669. Its founder was Le Xianyang, whose ancestral home was in Ningbo, Zhejiang. When Zhu Di, an emperor of the Ming dynasty, relocated the capital during Yongle period, the twenty sixth generation of Le's family Le Liangcai moved from Ningbo to Beijing. After settling down, the family worked as itinerant medical practitioners. When the clan passed on to Le Xianyang, he became an official in the Imperial Academy of Medicine of the Qing dynasty, ended his ancestral life as an itinerant medical practitioner, and founded Tong Ren Tang medicine shop.

Le Xianyang, the founder of Tong Ren Tang, was proficient in medicine. He once proposed that "medicine is the most important for regimen and doing good to the society", laying a good foundation for the establishment of Tong Ren Tang. Later, his son, Le Fengming, compiled *The Formula for the Ingredient of Le's Ancestral Pill, Powder, Unguent and Pellet*. The book collected 362 kinds of secret prescriptions handed down by Le's family, imperial physician, and the court. It had strict pharmaceutical standards of these prescriptions, and put forward the ancient maxim "the process can't be deleted regardless of the complex craft and the material can't be reduced regardless of the expensive herbs". The Chinese herbal medicine, pills, powders, unguents and pellets and other Chinese patent medicines operated by the store were famous for their authentic materials, exquisite processing. Its products were famous at home and abroad for their unique formula, superior materials, exquisite workmanship and remarkable curative effect, and were sold all over the world. Therefore, Tong Ren Tang has become a symbol of quality and reputation.

The spirit of Tong Ren Tang is reflected in many details of the operation. According to historical records, the first store of Tong Ren Tang was just a bungalow with three front doors. It had painted beams and columns, and black tiles and grey bricks. It was a traditional Chinese style building. However, its storefront was lower than the block. When customers entered the door, they had to go downstairs, which was called "Low-lying Gate". Inadvertently, people in the shop found that this "low-lying gate" was just suitable for many patients who came to the pharmacy to buy medicine. They were in poor health, and it was easier to go downstairs than go upstairs. After buying the medicine of Tong Ren Tang, going out from the store was a good omen for getting better and better. The counter for filling the prescriptions in the pharmacy had two layers: the dispenser filled the prescriptions in the inner layer and the customers waited in the outer layer. In the middle of the two layers of counters, an experienced pharmacist checked and verified the prescriptions one by one. Only after the prescriptions were confirmed to be correct, can the medicines be wrapped and handed over to the customers. This method can effectively avoid accidents caused by filling the wrong prescriptions.

In the history of more than 300 years, Tong Ren Tang has combined traditional medical ethics culture with production and operation, formed its own distinctive corporate culture, and built itself into one of the time-honored brands of TCM at home and abroad.

The culture of Tong Ren Tang has nourished the enterprise spirit of "cultivating benevolence and benefiting the world", the self-discipline consciousness of "improving self-training without feeling regretful", the business philosophy of "putting justice first and combining justice with benefit", and the operation principle of "being benevolent with one idea and one will", which have played a vital role in the development of Tong Ren Tang.

3. Lei Yun Shang

Like Tong Ren Tang, Lei Yun Shang is a time-honored TCM store with a high reputation in the field of TCM. It has a history of more than 280 years from the Song Fen Tang Pharmacy established in 1734 to the current Lei Yun Shang Pharmaceutical Group Co., Ltd.

Lei Dasheng, with the courtesy name Yunshang and the pseudonym Nanshan is the founder of Lei Yun Shang. He was born in Kangxi period. He was intelligent, diligent and especially liked reading medical books. Once he was the apprentice of Wang Zijie, a famous TCM practitioner in Suzhou. In the long process of out-call and selling medicines, he has accumulated a lot of folk prescriptions and collected many Chinese herbal medicines especially pills, powders, unguents and pellets. In 1734, Lei Dasheng opened a pharmacy called "Song Fen Tang" at the entrance of King Zhou Temple in front of the Tianku, Zhuanzhu Lane, Changmen, the ancient city of Suzhou. Lei Dasheng was a kind person. He often provided free medicine for patients. There was a stoker in the pharmacy to make pills. He can practice medicine and sell medicine at the same time. The pills, powders, unguents and pellets he cultivated were made of exquisite materials and effective. They were highly praised by the people then and were regarded as "life-saving medicines". Because of his excellent skills and moral integrity, Lei shot to fame. Over time, people linked Lei Yun Shang with the name of the store Song Fen Tang, and called it "Song Fen Tang of Lei Yun Shang".

In 1860, the descendants of Lei's Family took refuge in Shanghai. The next year, they opened Song Fen Tang of Lei Yun Shang in Xingsheng Street (now Yongsheng Road, the new north gate) of the French Concession in Shanghai. After the war was subsided, some of the clansmen returned to Suzhou and reset the store at the original site. Since then, Song Fen Tang of Lei Yun Shang was divided into two stores, the one in Suzhou and the other in Shanghai. The one in Shanghai was a subbranch.

"Being faithful and strict with the quality" is the ancestral precept and the core of medical ethics culture of Lei Yun Shang. For more than two hundred years, the descendants of Lei Yun Shang, adhering to the ancestral motto and with the mission of "gathering hundreds of herbs and benefiting the people", have selected authentic medicinal materials, piously made unguents and pellets, operated in good faith and kept improving, and created a large number of famous prescriptions and medicines with precise and appropriate prescriptions and remarkable effects, making important contributions to the development of the Chinese medicine.

4. Hu Qing Yu Tang

There is a saying, "Tong Ren Tang in the north and Qing Yu Tang in the south." Hu Qing Yu Tang, known as the "King of Medicine in Jiangnan (the regions south of the Yangtze River)", was founded by Hu Xueyan in 1874 and is located in Qinghen Lane, a historical and cultural block in Hangzhou.

As for the founding of Hu Qing Yu Tang by Hu Xueyuan, there was a story of "founding the medicine shop in a pet". Once, one of Hu Xueyan's family was ill. He appointed someone to the store to get some medicine. When he got the medicine, he found that two kind of medicines were shoddy, so he asked the store to replace them. However, the boss of the store retorted, "If you want to replace them, please set up a store yourself." Hu Xueyan was furious when he heard this, so Hu Qing Yu Tang was established.

Hu Xueyan's founding of Hu Qing Yu Tang was essentially his benevolent act of doing good to the society. As a rich Zhejiang businessman, Hu Xueyan was also deeply influenced by Hangzhou's long TCM culture. In addition, due to wars, diseases and other reasons, Hu Xueyan decided to save the dying and heal the wounded. He invited famous TCM practitioners in Jiangsu and Zhejiang provinces to develop Zhuge Xingjun Powder, Babao Hongling Pill and other medicines, and presented them to Zeng Guofan, Zuo Zongtang and other ministries of the Hunan Army and the people in the affected areas.

Under the leadership of Hu Xueyan, Hu Qing Yu Tang brought out 14 categories of patent medicines. It gave away free "standing medicines", such as anti-plague pills and blood stasis-removal medicine, and made a big-layout advertisement on *Shun Pao*, making Hu Qing Yu Tang famous.

What made Hu Qing Yu Tang inherit for a hundred years was its business philosophy of doing good to the society and treating people with sincerity. The name of Hu Qing Yu Tang came from the saying in the *Book of Changes* that "one good turn deserves another", which also laid the foundation for the management of the medicine shop. The plaque hanging in the hall can reflect the medical ethics of Hu Qing Yu Tang. The four characters "that is benevolent skill" written by Hu Xueyan was reserved on the door of Hu Qing Yu Tang, which came from *Mencius: King Hui of Liang*, "The TCM practitioners must be of benevolent skill." This reflects the purpose of the founding of the store. He regarded the pharmaceutical industry as a cause to help all people, and also reflected honesty, trustworthiness and benevolence of Hu Qing Yu Tang in curing the sick and saving the people. Another famous plaque "No Deceiving" was the shop motto written by Hu Xueyan. All the plaques in Hu Qing Yu Tang were undisguised, only this one was for the staff. It reminded everyone in Hu Qing Yu Tang all the time, "All trades are not allowed to cheat others. The pharmaceutical industry is vital to life, so cheating is forbidden. If you are ready to do good to the society, you are not allowed to use inferior products to make exorbitant profits. Wish all of you can be honest and keep improving. If you don't deceive others, one good turn deserves another."

The motto of "being pragmatic in procurement, being meticulous in processing" of Hu Qing Yu Tang fully reflects its moral character of being honest. In order to buy quality medicine, Hu Xueyan stipulated that the medicinal materials should be purchased from the place of origin. In the process of production, the staff were required to strictly abide by the process flow, and cheating in work, cutting down materials and shoddy products were forbidden.

The concept of no deceiving covers all aspects of the business of Hu Qing Yu Tang. There is a plaque of "the fixed price", which means valuing honesty in business. This is Hu Qing Yu Tang's commitment to customers and the witness of its honesty.

From "That is benevolent skill" to "The fixed price", Hu Qing Yu Tang has been adhering to the ancestral motto of "no cheating".

8.4　Medical Management and Medical Education

The Qing dynasty was both the end of ancient Chinese history and the beginning of modern Chinese history. In the transitional period, the medical management and medical education in the Qing dynasty also presented a diversified and unified, changeable and stable state.

8.4.1　Medical Management System

In the early Qing dynasty, after the Manchu rulers took over the Central Plains, their systems and policies basically continued the old practices of the Ming dynasty, showing the typical characteristics of "the Qing dynasty inherited the system from the Ming dynasty". After the Opium War, China was forced to open up and was gradually involved in the wave of Western-centered modernization. Facing the impact of the West, the Qing government also began to launch a series of new policies, try to reform the system, set up a new health management organization, and the medical administration began to enter the track of modernization.

1. Central medical management institutions

As the highest medical institution in the country during the Qing dynasty, the Imperial Academy of Medicine was endowed with the power to manage the medical administration of the country. And its main responsibility was to provide daily health care services for the emperor and his relatives.

There was an envoy of the Imperial Academy of Medicine. He was a fifth-rank official and the senior official of the Imperial Academy of Medicine. There were two judges, the left judge and the right judge. Both of them were deputy officials of sixth rank. The above officials were also called "Tang Guan". The subordinate medical officers were 15 imperial physicians, who were of the seventh rank (the eighth rank before the seventh year of Emperor Yongzheng's reign) and the sixth rank with the crowns and belts. Besides, 30 minor officials (15 actually-awarded eighth-rank officials and 15 pre-awarded ninth-rank officials). In addition, there were 40 medics who had no rank and were given the title of ninth grade. They can be regarded as quasi medical officers. Sometimes they were also called medical officers together with imperial physicians and minor officials. TCM practitioners were students studying in the Imperial Academy of Medicine and practicing medical chores. There were 30 TCM practitioners who were not medical officers. In the eighth year of Yongzheng period (1730), another 30 Shiliang TCM practitioners, also called Enliangsheng, were added. In the 23rd year of Daoguang period (1843), 2 imperial physicians, 4 minor officials and 20 Shiliang TCM practitioners were dismissed. In addition, four scribes, called Jingcheng, were appointed to manage the administrative official documents and miscellaneous affairs.

In the early Qing dynasty, the Imperial Academy of Medicine was divided into 11 clinical departments: Dafang Mai (It is specialized in treating adult diseases, which is equivalent to the current internal medicine), Xiaofang Mai (Specialized in treating children's diseases), typhoid, gynecology, sore and ulcer, acupuncture, ophthalmology, dentistry, pharyngeal and laryngeal, orthopedics and pox and rash. In 1797, the pox and rash department was merged into the Xiaofang Mai, and the pharyngeal and laryngeal department and the dentistry department were merged, so there were 9 departments. Later, the orthopedic department was assigned to Shangsi Hospital, and the TCM practitioners of orthopedics department were not managed by the Imperial Academy of Medicine. In 1822, the acupuncture department was repelled by the Imperial Academy of Medicine because of the statement that "acupuncture and moxibustion are not suitable for the emperor". Since then, acupuncture can only be used in the folk, but not for the emperor.

In addition to treating the royal staff, eunuchs, palace maids, officials and bodyguards who have lived in the imperial court for a long time, the imperial physicians would also treat the nobility, minority nobles, royal relatives, officials and their families. Moreover, if there was an epidemic in the capital Beijing, the emperor would also send the imperial physician to treat the ordinary people.

The place where the imperial physicians were on duty in shifts in the palace was the Imperial Pharmacy. The Imperial Pharmacy was the medicine administration organ in the Qing dynasty. According to the *Records of the Imperial Academy of Medicine*, the Imperial Pharmacy managed the purchase, storage and preparation of medicines. It was divided into two branches, the east and the west. Senior medical officials such as envoys, judges, imperialphysician and minor officials in the Western Pharmacy worked in shifts. In the Eastern Pharmacy, the imperial physician, minor officials and physician were on duty in shifts. The Imperial Pharmacy was set up in 1653 and belonged to the Imperial Academy of Medicine. Medicinal materials produced in various provinces were brought to the Imperial Academy of Medicine every year. After the medical officers identified the quality of the medicinal materials, they were stored in the raw medicine warehouse. In the 10th year of Kangxi period (1671), the Imperial Pharmacy did not belong to the Imperial Academy of Medicine. There were 2 chief eunuch physicians, 2 warehouse leaders, 1 head eunuch, and 1 eunuch physician, 19 eunuchs and 34 servants. In addition to the above responsibilities, the Imperial Pharmacy also distributed medicines when the plague occurred.

Before the implementation of the new policies in the late Qing dynasty, the Imperial Academy of Medicine was an independent central medical administration. After the reforms, in the 31st year of Guangxu's period (1905), the Patrol Ministry was set up, with a patrol division and a health section in the department. The responsibility of the health section was to assess the medical school, manage road cleaning, epidemic prevention, plan and review all health regulations. The following year, the official system was set up and the Patrol Department was changed to the Ministry of Civil Affairs with five divisions, and the Health Section was upgraded into the Department of Health. The Department of Health has three sections: health and fitness, inspection and quarantine and divination. During this period, the old and new systems coexisted, and the Department of Health and Imperial Academy of Medicine coexisted to jointly implement medical administration. In the 34th year of Guangxu period (1908), the Ministry of Civil Affairs of the Qing dynasty issued *The Rules for Banning Medical Practitioner*. At the same time, the Imperial Academy of Medicine was blamed for the deaths of Guangxu and Cixi in a few days, and all the following officials were dismissed. Since then, as a symbol of the medical administration in the old era, Imperial Academy of Medicine has become the past records forever, and the Department of Health has become the only central medical administration.

2. Local medical management institutions

The local medical management institutions in the Qing dynasty inherited from the Ming dynasty, which was mainly the Medical Bureau. Generally speaking, the government had one section member (the ninth-rank official), the prefecture had one official physician, and the county had one physician. The three officials were all physicians. There was a People Benefiting Medicine Bureau attached to the Medical Bureau, and most of the time, they coexisted. In the 13th year of Kangxi period (1674), the appointment method of local medical officials was clearly stipulated and explained, "It was approved in the 13th year of Kangxi period that officials such as the external Yin and Yang study should be appointed from the candidates of administrative department. The department should carefully investigate and register them, transfer them to the administrative department and appoint them... Physicians, selected by provincial and local officials, should be inferior to principles of medical science, and the way was the same as the selection of the Yin and Yang study."

To the first year of Yongzheng period (1723), the Qing government made arrangements for medical affairs once again, "The grand coordinators at the provincial level are ordered to inspect the TCM practitioners and conduct examinations. The questions come from *Notes to the Inner Canon*, *Compendium of Materia Medica*, and *Treatise on Febrile Diseases*. The superior will be awarded as the professor of medical officer. There is one professor for each province and they can get salary for three years. If they are diligent and prudent, they will be appointed to the Imperial Academy of Medicine, and are awarded as imperial physicians. And the professors will be selected from the apprentices in the province. If there are trainees in the health centers that belong to prefectures and counties, they can be appointed as Three Book professors according to the law of the Ming dynasty. Those who are proficient in medical science can be reported to the grand coordinators and take examinations in the Imperial Academy of Medicine. The superior will be awarded lower ranking titles or as medical officers. Those who are unable to go to Beijing because of the age will be the probationary professors of the province." It can be seen that, in addition to the provincial medical institutions regularly recommending TCM practitioners to the hospital, the outstanding TCM practitioners among the public from different states and counties can be reported to the provincial units and provided opportunities to participate in the selection examination of the Imperial Academy of Medicine. The imperial court hoped to establish a standardized link with the Imperial Academy of Medicine through the Medical Bureau. However, the official aimed to select medical talents to supplement the system of the Imperial Academy of Medicine, and the local medical departments have not benefited from such decrees. In fact, the local medical management system in the Qing dynasty was not perfect, and it was only symbolic. When the reform was implemented in the late Qing dynasty, the local medical administration was reorganized and the examination system for local medical practitioners was formed.

3. Employment restrictions and penalties

The Qing government had certain conditions for the selection of imperial physicians, TCM practitioners and local medical officers of the Imperial Academy of Medicine. For example, the Qing government stipulated that "Anyone who enters the Imperial Academy of Medicine and works as a TCM practitioner should be investigated from the aspects of moral ethics and medical skills. He will be appointed by the officers of the Imperial Academy of Medicine. He will be ordered to enter the academy and study, and the envoy and judges can decide whether he can work here." The apprentices would be examined by the officials of the Imperial Academy of

Medicine four times each season. The questions came from *Yellow Emperor's Canon of Medicine, The Classic of Difficult Issues, The Pulse Classic, The Shennong's Herbal Classic* and other books. After grading, they would be registered by the Ministry of Rites. The officials of the Ministry of Rites would come to the academy to hold examination every three years. The winners would be TCM practitioners, and those who failed would continue studying. In the fifth year of Tongzhi's period (1866), after the establishment of the medical school, the examination was reduced to two times each two seasons, that is, the examinations were conducted in mid spring and mid autumn. In the Year of the Tiger and the Year of the Rooster, the judges of the Imperial Academy of Medicine, together with the officials of the Ministry of Rites, would take an examination of all officials and students below the minor officials except the imperial physicians. There were also strict regulations on the specification of the papers, the content of questions, the discipline of the examination halls, the time of the examination, etc. As for the stipulation of recommendation of TCM practitioners in local places, the Imperial Academy of Medicine stipulated that the recommended person should generally be recommended by fellow villagers of sixth rank or higher, and the Manchu people should be recommended by his chief, and the officials of the Imperial Academy of Medicine should act as a guarantor. The chief officer should interview to confirm if he has a good command of medical books and is proficient in Mandarin before he can enter the academy. In the first year of Yongzheng period, according to the imperial edict, "A good TCM practitioner must be mature and experienced." It can be seen that it was not easy for people to become imperial physicians of various rankings in the Imperial Academy of Medicine.

However, at the local level, the official medical administration of the Qing dynasty was in a state of decline, especially the long-term absence of grass-roots medical management. It made the access mechanism for TCM practitioners' practice missing and lacking strict requirements for access. Anyone can became a TCM practitioner easily, or take part-time jobs to treat patients around. The government basically abandoned the effective management of the medical market, and only used the medical industry as the government's emergency response means in the process of large-scale and sudden disasters such as plague, flood and drought, and only in the disaster relief period would the government use its power to organize relevant personnel to provide medical assistance for the people. As for daily medical care services, people relied more on groups of different levels and categories that played the role of TCM practitioners in daily life. This directly led to the proliferation of quack TCM practitioners in the Qing dynasty, seriously undermining the prestige of TCM.

In order to curb the proliferation of quack TCM practitioners, the Qing government made some regulations at the legal level. For example, *The Criminal Law of the Qing Dynasty* stipulated that, "A mediocre TCM practitioner who uses acupuncture or medication by mistake and makes people die, other TCM practitioners will be ordered to identify and test the medicine. If there is no cause for harm, the quack TCM practitioner will be judged as negligent homicide. He must redeem the family of the dead according to the law, and he is not allowed to practice medicine. If there is no cause for violating the prescription, treating the patients with deception and taking advantage of danger to take property, the quack medical practitioner will be convicted larceny. If he uses the fake medicine that makes patients die, he will be sentenced to death."

According to *The Criminal Law of the Qing Dynasty*, TCM practitioners will be severely punished for wrongly treating patients. Ten cases of quack TCM practitioners have been collected in *The Collection of Criminal Cases of the Qing Dynasty*. For example, in the 56th year of Qianlong period (1791), Li Xiuyu from Sichuan wrongly used Radix Aconiti powder to make Wu Guixiang and others die. Li was sentenced to make several times of compensation, be flogged for one hundred times and flailed for three months. In the tenth year of Jiaqing period (1805), Ding Erwa from Yunnan who wrongly used medicine and poisoned Zhang Chengjian and others to death. As a result, Ding Erwa was fined three cents of silver for compensation, to be flogged for one hundred times and flailed for three months. In the seventeenth year of Jiaqing period (1812), Xue Chuannian from Anhui Province went to Beijing to present the case of Ye Chongguang, a TCM practitioner in charge, making his son Xue Jiayu die by acupuncture. As a result, Ye Chongguang was convicted of manslaughter. In the 23rd year of Jiaqing period (1818), Zhejiang Du Zhang was sentenced to be flogged for one hundred times, and he was not allowed to get the remuneration. However, due to the lack of professional medical knowledge of local officials, and the lack of medical standards as the basis for the wrong treatment of quack TCM practitioners, the government often took a conciliatory attitude in dealing with medical lawsuits. Only 10 cases of killing and injuring of quack TCM practitioners in *The Collection of Criminal Cases* was the evidence. As the people of that time said, "Medicine is belittled in China and it isn't treated seriously. If the quack TCM practitioners are not forbidden, and are only flogged and allowed to get the remuneration, they will be indifferent and unscrupulous. According to the low, the murders should be sentenced to death, and there are also specific rules on how to punish a quack TCM practitioner who kills people. But now, the regulations are ignored by people and don't show the warning effect."

In general, although the punishment of quack TCM practitioners in the Qing dynasty had a certain deterrent effect on medical practitioners, it was not enough. The defects of the legal system itself and the lack of judgment basis have greatly limited the role of criminal law, and patients can only rely more on the medical ethics of TCM practitioners.

8.4.2 Medical Education

The medical education in the Qing dynasty generally inherited the medical education system of the Song and Ming dynasties, but it also developed, especially under the impact of western medicine, which brought some changes to Chinese medical education. Medical education in the Qing dynasty mainly took the form of education from teachers, school education, academy education, and self-teaching.

1. Education from teachers

TCM is a subject with practicality. In the process of its inheritance and development, it has formed a unique form of education—education from masters (teachers). Medical education in ancient China has always been based on the inheritance from teachers, and continued its theory and experience in the way of teacher passing on disciples and father passing on son, as was the case in the Qing dynasty. For example, Ye Tianshi, an outstanding medical expert in the Qing dynasty, was born in a medical family. His grandfather Ye Shi and father Ye Chaocai were both proficient in medical skills. He began to learn medicine with his father at the age of 12. He was modest and eager to learn, and he studied with 17 teachers within 10 years. Another example is Chen Xiuyuan, a famous TCM practitioner in Fujian, who learned medical science under the influence of his grandfather in his early years and learned from Cai Mingzhuang, a famous TCM practitioner in Quanzhou in his later years. Under the guidance of their teachers, these masters have read the classics of Chinese medicine, understood the wonders of medicine, and had their own characteristics in medical skills.

Of course, there were also shortcomings in education from teachers. First of all, the education mode of teachers leading apprentices was far from meeting the actual needs of society in terms of the scale and effectiveness of talent training. Secondly, education from teachers took recitation, memory, etc. as the main way of imparting knowledge, and it's of the typical characteristics of accumulation and inheritance, being inaccessible and conservative, lacking of pioneering and competitiveness. Thirdly, there was a narrow range of knowledge between teachers and apprentices, emphasizing that only for men, and secret recipes should not be passed on to others. They should pay attention to understanding tacitly and teaching by personal example as well as verbal instruction, which should not be widely publicized. This has also led to the gradual loss of many important medical prescriptions under this model. At the same time, the teacher's personal words, deeds and thoughts greatly affected the students' way of thinking. The teacher's limitations in knowledge and thought had a negative impact on the students' vision. On the whole, as a subject with strong experience, education from teachers has played an important role in inheriting TCM and cultivating TCM.

2. School education

There was no special medical education institution in the Qing dynasty, and the central medical education was in the charge of the Imperial Academy of Medicine. The Teaching and Learning Department in the Imperial Academy of Medicine performed educational functions. The Teaching and Learning Department was divided into two parts: the internal one and the external one. The internal one taught eunuchs in the palace and the external one taught medical officials and their families. Talents for teaching were selected from the imperial physicians and minor officials, and those who were of fine qualities and fine scholar were preferred. In addition to training the medical officials and their families, the external division also taught ordinary people and staff in the department. The department mainly taught medical classics, various subjects of TCM and their specialized medical books. These students also undertook part of the work of writing and repairing the bait. At the end of the three-year study period, students who passed the exam can be filed in the Imperial Academy of Medicine to fill the vacancy of personnel in the academy when necessary. In short, before the Opium War, Imperial Academy of Medicine was not only a medical service institution, but also responsible for medical education and training medical talents. Although this kind of training was only to select excellent medical talents for the royal family, it also undertook the important task of the central government running TCM education to a certain extent.

After the Opium War, the Qing government signed a series of unequal treaties with the West. These treaties forced China to open trade ports, and allowed foreign missionaries to open hospitals, establish churches and preach freely at trade ports. As a result, church hospitals were increasing in modern China. The development and establishment of missionary hospitals needs a large number of TCM practitioners, but it is far from enough to send TCM practitioners from abroad alone. So the church began to invest in the selection of foreign students and set up medical schools in China, which also brought vitality to China's medical education.

In 1866, the Chinese Medical Missionary Association established Boji Medical School in Guangzhou Boji Medical Bureau, which was the first missionary medical school established by a foreign church in China. Peking Union Medical College, West China Medical Center, Xiangya School of Medicine, Medical College of Aurora University, Cheeloo College of Medicine, etc., which have an important influence in the field of medical education in China, were all established with the support of the church. These schools imitate the educational system and teaching materials of Britain, the United States, Germany, Japan and other countries. While teaching western medicine knowledge and skills, they also enrich China's medical education model.

In 1881, Li Hongzhang invited Ma Genji, a missionary TCM practitioner, to set up the Beiyang Medical School, the first official medical school in China. Medical science was also included in *The Constitution of Founding Schools* issued in 1904. The official medical education in China has gradually changed from the traditional mode of taking the Imperial Academy of Medicine as the core to the track of modern school medical education.

3. Academy education

The academy education was originally a way of Confucian classics education, which was between school education and teacher education and played an important role in the history of ancient Chinese education. After the Ming dynasty, some TCM practitioners applied this form to medical education. The rulers of the early Qing dynasty, in view of the lessons learned by the members of Donglin Party at the end of the Ming dynasty, adopted a policy of restraining the academy from giving lectures in order to prevent the academy from gathering students to ridicule the government, and stipulated that it was not allowed to found other academies. After the rule was consolidated, the Qing government changed its negative policy towards the academy and adopted a policy of actively establishing and strengthening control of academy.

At the end of the Ming dynasty and the beginning of the Qing dynasty, Lu Zhiyi, a famous TCM practitioner, set up a academy-style medical forum in Zhejiang. Later, Zhang Zhicong and Gao Shihang, famous TCM practitioners, developed it into a lecturing-style education of TCM—"Lvshan Hall" education. This kind of education attached great importance to the teaching and research of the basic theories of classical Chinese medicine, and created a precedent for TCM education of the classical medical school in the Qing dynasty. However, as for traditional Chinese education, the number of traditional Chinese education academies was far less than those serving the imperial examinations. Academy education did not occupy the dominant position in the medical education system of the Qing dynasty. Nevertheless, academy education still had an important impact on medical education in the Qing dynasty. First, the mainstream academies have trained many famous TCM practitioners. For example, Chen Xiuyuan, a TCM scholar, once studied in Fuzhou Aozhao Academy. Ding Fubao, Yang Ruhou and Cao Yingfu graduated from Jiangyin Nanpu Academy successively and contributed a lot to the education of Chinese medicine. The experience of these TCM practitioners in the academy in studying scripture and poetry has undoubtedly laid a deep cultural foundation for their study of medicine. Second, the academies that taught Chinese medicine and spread Chinese medicine culture played an irreplaceable role in the popularization of Chinese medicine education and academic exchanges in the Qing dynasty.

4. Self-study

Self-study was also a special form of medical education in ancient China to learn medical knowledge, master medical skills and join the ranks of TCM practitioners. For example, the famous TCM practitioner Xu Dachun became famous in this way. After self-study, many TCM practitioners also wrote many books to popularize medical knowledge for later generations. For example, Li Yingguan, a Confucian TCM practitioner, selected medical classics, formulated rules, and compiled The

Thirty-six Words Verse for Medical Introduction, which was concise and catchy. It not only assisted teaching, but also became a means of popularizing medical knowledge. There are also books of this kind, such as *The Readable Materia Medica* and *Tang Tou Verse* compiled by Wang Ang, *The Three-Character Medical Verse* and *The Readable Medicine* compiled by Chen Xiuyuan. In addition, there are monographs dedicated to collecting and studying medical cases, summarizing and passing down the rich practical experience of famous TCM practitioners, such as Wei Zhizhen's *Classified Medical Records of Distinguished Physicians*, You Zaijing's *Medical Cases of Jingxiang Tower*, etc. The issuance of these popular medical books has reduced the difficulty of studying medicine, made it easier for medical enthusiasts to learn medicine by themselves, and promoted the popularization of medical education. However, on the other hand, the reduction of the difficulty in employment has also contributed to the proliferation of quacks to a large extent.

Chapter Summary

The Qing dynasty was the last feudal dynasty in Chinese history. Influenced by the invasion of Western powers, it gradually became a semi-colonial and semi-feudal society. Chinese medicine in this period entered the historical stage of summary and criticism under the impact of its own development laws and Western medicine, and the Chinese medical ethics culture in the same period also showed distinctive characteristics of the times.

During the Qing dynasty, the discussion on medical ethics was gradually improved. TCM practitioners had the spirit of criticizing the current situation and focusing on the truth. Under the aggression of western powers, many TCM practitioners also showed strong patriotism. However, conservative sectarianism and back-to-the-ancients ideology of respecting the classics shackled by feudal ideology were also the distinctive characteristics of the medical ethics culture in this period.

There were many famous TCM practitioners in the Qing dynasty. They practiced medicine to help the patients. They also focused on summing up treatment experience and elaborating medical ethics. They left behind a large number of classic works, enabling people today to understand the essence of medical ethics culture in the Qing dynasty. At the same time, with the development of the commodity economy in the

Ming and Qing dynasties, medicine brands such as Tong Ren Tang, Hu Qing Yu Tang, Xing He Tang, Lei Yun Shang, etc. emerged. These medicine brands strictly abide by the principle of honesty and adhere to moral ethics, and also carried and inherited the medical ethics culture of the Qing dynasty.

In the system of medical administration, the medical administration of the Qing dynasty had the characteristics of inherting the system from the Ming dynasty. After the Opium War, China was forced into the wave of modernization. The Qing government also began to try to reform the medical administration system, set up new health management institutions, and made the medical administration enter the exploration of modernization.

Medical education in the Qing dynasty mainly took the form of education from teachers, school education, academy education, self-study. The TCM practitioners cultivated by these education methods varied in medical skills. People at that time divided them into famous, good, common TCM practitioners and quacks. Different images of TCM practitioners also directly showed different evaluations on medical ethics.

In general, the medical ethics culture in the Qing dynasty not only inherited the tradition, but also reflected the characteristics of the new era. The end of the feudal dynasty was not the summary of the traditional medical ethics culture, but the starting point of its continuation and innovation.

Application in Contemporary Times

1. The thought of "adhering to sincerity" and the orientation of "valuing justice over benefit" are still the values of TCM practitioners in the new era

This chapter describes the main contents of medical ethics culture in the Qing dynasties. Chinese medicine in this period entered the historical stage of summary and criticism under the impact of its own development laws and Western medicine, and the Chinese medical ethics culture in the same period also showed distinctive characteristics of the times. There were many famous TCM practitioners in the Qing dynasty. These TCM practitioners practiced medicine to help and save the sick. They also focused on summing up treatment experience and elaborating medical ethics, leaving behind a large number of classic works. *Principle and Prohibition for Medical Profession* by Yu Jiayan is a prominent representative of medical ethics in the Qing dynasty. He put forward the thought of "devoting to sincerity", emphasizing that TCM practitioners should have sympathy and compassion for patients and think from the standpoint of patients. This idea has a positive guiding significance for building a harmonious medical practitioner-patient relationship. At the same time, in view of the increasing phenomenon of "disregarding moral principles in pursuit of profit" in medical activities, the responsible TCM practitioners in the Qing dynasty also dared to point out problems and persuade wrongdoers to correct them, praise virtue and punish, expose and criticize many adverse factors that affect the development of medicine, and played a positive role in correcting the unhealthy medical style.

The medical students and medical workers in the new era should learn and inherit the medical ethics thought of "devoting to sincerity", respect life and patients, have a sense of benevolence, learn to think on the position of others, adhere to the value orientation of "valuing justice over profit", abandon the wrong idea of taking the sacred medical cause as a profit-making tool, and interpret the original intention of doctors with the spirit of "practicing medicine is showing benevolence".

2. Caring for the toiling masses and having the sense of patriotism demonstrate the social responsibility of TCM practitioners

This chapter reviews the characteristics of medical ethics culture in the Qing dynasty. The Qing dynasty was the last feudal dynasty in Chinese history, and in the late Qing dynasty, influenced by the invasion of Western powers, the country gradually became a semi-colonial and semi-feudal society. Influenced by the times, many TCM practitioners in this period showed strong patriotism. They generally cared about medical progress of the country, the future and destiny of the nation, show sympathy for the people suffering from the turbulence, and insisted on serving the toiling masses. This spirit fully demonstrated the responsibility of TCM practitioners.

General Secretary Xi Jinping has repeatedly encouraged college students in the new era to devote themselves to what the Party and the people need most. Medical students in the new era should keep in mind the instructions of General Secretary Xi Jinping, inherit the sense of patriotism of their predecessors, actively integrate their personal ideals into the cause of the Party and the country, and contribute their youth and power to the great rejuvenation of the Chinese nation and the strategic planning of a healthy China.

3. The business philosophy of honesty first of the time-honored brand inherits and enriches the spiritual core of national medical culture

This chapter introduces in detail the famous TCM practitioners in the Qing dynasty and their thinking on medical ethics. Different from other historical periods, in the Qing dynasty, with the development of the commodity economy, medicine brands such as Tong Ren Tang, Hu Qing Yu Tang, Xing He Tang, Lei Yun Shang emerged. These medicine brands strictly abide by the principle of honesty and adhere to moral ethics, inherited and enriched the spiritual core of national medicine culture. Chen Li Ji's business philosophy of "making medicine with scrupulous precision", the corporate spirit of "cultivating benevolence and benefiting the world" of Tong Ren Tang, Lei Yun Shang's ancestral motto of "being faithful and strict with the quality", and Hu Qing Yu Tang's eight-character motto and "benefiting the world" of Tong Ren Tang, Lei Yun Shang's ancestral motto of "being faithful and strict with the quality", and Hu Qing Yu Tang's motto of "being pragmatic in procurement, being meticulous in processing" have been passed on from generation to generation, and also enriched and carried forward the essence of TCM culture.

The business philosophy prioritizing honesty is the exact reason why the time-honored medicine brands can last for a hundred years. At the same time, these interesting and inspiring medical ethics stories can also inspire medical workers and medical students in the new era to abide by the principle of honesty and adhere to moral ethics, and inherit and promote the excellent medical ethics.

References

[1] BAI SHOUYI. General History of China[M]. Shanghai: Shanghai People's Publishing House, 2015.

[2] BIAN QUE. Nan Jing (The Classic of Difficult Issues)[M]. Beijing: China Medical Science and Technology Press, 2018.

[3] CAO ZHIMING. Collection of Gong Zizhen[M]. Zhengzhou: Henan University Press, 2016.

[4] CHEN PINGYUAN. Collected Works of Heroine Qiu Jin[M]. Guiyang: Guizhou Education Press, 2014.

[5] CHEN SHIGONG. Authentic Surgery[M]. Beijing: China Medical Science and Technology Press, 2018.

[7] CHEN XIAOBAO, YAO MINJIE, ETAL. History of Medical Ethics and Moral Principles in Ancient China[M]. Xi'an: Sanqin Press, 2002.

[7] CHEN XIUYUAN. Collected Works of Chen Xiuyuan's Medical Books[M]. Beijing: Traditional Chinese Medicine Classics Press, 2017.

[8] DUAN YISHAN. Ancient Medical Prose[M]. Beijing: China Press of Traditional Chinese Medicine, 2007.

[9] FAN YUQIANG, CHEN JINGLIN. Cultural Relics of Chinese Medicine[M]. Tianjin: Tianjin Academy of Social Sciences Press, 2015.

[10] FU SHAN,YIN XIE. Pandect of Fu Shan[M]. Taiyuan: Shanxi People's Publishing House, 2016.

[11] HU BING. Medical Ethics of Famous TCM Experts from Pre-Qin Period to Sui and Tang Dynasties[M]. Beijing: Intellectual Property Publishing House, 2014.

[12] HUANG TIANHUA. History of China's Financial System[M]. Shanghai: Shanghai People's Publishing House, 2017.

[13] JU BAOZHAO. Compilation of Historical Data of Medical Figures in Qing Dynasty[M]. Shenyang: Liaoning Science and Technology Press, 2013.

[14] LI HONGTAO. A Collection of Vintage Medical Books[M]. Beijing: Traditional Chinese Medicine Classics Press, 2016.

[15] LI YANSHOU. History of the Northern Dynasties[M]. Beijing: Zhonghua Book Company, 2013.

[16] MIAO XIYONG. Shennong's Herbal Classics[M]. Beijing: Traditional Chinese Medicine Classics Press, 2017.

[17] QIU PEIRAN. Grand Dictionary of Chinese Medicine[M]. Shanghai: Shanghai Science and Technology Press, 2002.

[18] WANG MINGQIANG. History of Medical Education Thought in Ancient China [M]. Beijing: China Press of Traditional Chinese Medicine, 2018.

305